MRCS Part A

550 SBAs and EMQs

SECOND EDITION

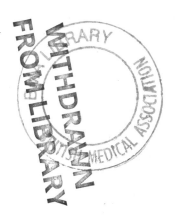

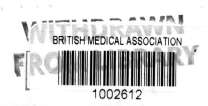

MRCS Part A

550 SBAs and EMQs

SECOND EDITION

Pradip K Datta MS FRCS(Ed) FRCS(Eng) FRCS(Ire) FRCS(Glasg)
Honorary Consultant General Surgeon
Caithness General Hospital
Wick, UK

Sherif Elsobky MB ChB MS MRCS(Ed)
Specialty Registrar in Radiology
St George's Hospital
London, UK

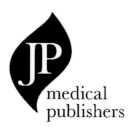

JP
medical
publishers

London • New Delhi • Panama City

ISBN: 978-1-909836-67-9

British Library Cataloguing in Publication Data
A catalogue record for this book is available from the British Library

Library of Congress Cataloging in Publication Data
A catalogue record for this book is available from the Library of Congress

Commissioning Editor: Steffan Clements
Editorial Assistants: Adam Rajah, Katie Pattullo
Design: Designers Collective Ltd

Preface

Surgery is a popular postgraduate specialty. This is almost certainly because of the number of subspecialties it has to offer, all of them hugely interesting in their own right. To commence basic surgical training, every aspiring surgeon has to pass the intercollegiate Member of the Royal College of Surgeons (MRCS) examination, which is taken in two parts: Part A and Part B. In 2017, the structure of the Part A exam changed: the number of questions increased from 270 to 300, and the time available for sitting the exam increased from 4 hours to 5 hours.

MRCS Part A: 550 SBAs and EMQs has been written to assist trainees in their preparation for the Part A examination. The book provides a wealth of practice questions to test candidates' knowledge of applied basic sciences and principles of surgery, thereby ensuring they are thoroughly prepared for the exam. The book covers each module in the syllabus, and the questions are written in the same format as those in the examination. Along with the correct answer, the reader is also provided with an explanation: as well as being a self-assessment tool, this book also acts as a personal tutorial.

For this second edition, we have improved and replaced over 200 questions. We have also added chapters on orthopaedic and trauma surgery to ensure that the exam syllabus is fully covered, and replaced many of the images with better examples. As with the first edition, the contributors of this book range from trainees on the brink of becoming consultants, to educators and examiners with many decades of experience in helping trainees pass the intercollegiate surgery exams.

We are confident that the revisions made in the second edition of this book make it an even more useful revision tool than the first, and will help trainees on the road towards a rewarding and worthwhile career.

Pradip K Datta
Sherif Elsobky
December 2017

Contents

Contents

Section B   PRINCIPLES OF SURGERY IN GENERAL

Principles of surgery in general

Contents

Contributors

Marilyn A Armstrong BSc PhD
Former Senior Lecturer in Immunology
School of Medicine and Dentistry
Queen's University
Belfast, UK

Christopher JK Bulstrode CBE MCh FRCS(Orth)
Professor and Honorary Consultant
Orthopaedic Surgeon
University of Oxford
Oxford, UK

Catherine Collinson BSc(Hons)
Specialty Trainee in Anaesthesia
Royal Infirmary of Edinburgh
Edinburgh, UK

Andrew Duckworth MSc BSc(Hons) MBChB
MRCSEd
Trainee and Clinical Research Fellow
Edinburgh Orthopaedic Trauma Unit
South-East Scotland, UK

Yan Li Goh MBChB MRCS PG Dip Clin Edu
Specialty Trainee in General Surgery
West Midlands Deanery
UK

Yan Mei Goh MBChB MRCS PG Dip Clin Edu
Specialty Trainee in General Surgery
Thames Valley Deanery
UK

Rong R Khaw MBChB(Hons) MRes Med Sci(Dist)
MRCSEd
Senior Clinical Fellow
Wythenshawe Hospital
Manchester, UK

Pawanindra Lal MS DNB MNAMS MNASc
FRCS(Ed) FRCS(Glasg) FRCS(Eng)
Professor of Surgery
Maulana Azad Medical College
New Delhi, India

Ian Leeuwenberg FRCA
Consultant Anaesthetist
Victorial Hospital
Fife, UK

Alistair May FCARCSI
Specialty Trainee in Anaesthesia
West of Scotland Deanery
UK

Iain Nixon FRCS(Ed) (ENT and Head & Neck)
Clinical Fellow
Memorial Sloan Kettering Cancer Centre
New York, USA

Anirudh Sharma MS(Orth) DNB(Orth) MRCSEd
Senior Resident
Vardhman Mahavir Medical College and
Safdarjung Hospital
New Delhi, India

William FM Wallace BSc MD FRCP FRCA FCAI
FRCSEd
Professor Emeritus of Applied Physiology
Queen's University
Belfast, UK

Introduction to the MRCS Part A

The Intercollegiate MRCS Part A is a 5-hour multiple choice question (MCQ) based exam, which is sat over a 1-day period. The exam takes place at each of the colleges throughout the UK at the same time, with identical questions asked.

The exam consists of two papers that cover the MRCS syllabus, including questions that cover the core applied knowledge of surgical sciences, as well as the recommended core knowledge of the nine surgical specialties. Questions are in either a single best answer (SBA) format or in an extended matching question (EMQ) format, with equal marks available for each question. Details of the two papers are:

1. **Applied Basic Sciences**
   a. 3 hours in length
   b. 180 SBA questions with five possible answers per question
   c. Questions are clinically based but test core theoretical knowledge of surgical sciences

2. **Principles of Surgery in General**
   a. 2 hours in length
   b. 120 questions
   c. Themed EMQs consisting of 2–5 questions per theme, with a selection of potential answer options (average 8)
   d. Questions are more clinically based

On the day of the exam, remember to bring proof of identity, e.g. passport or driving license, so you can register. Leave all personal belongings, including bags and mobiles phones (turned off), outside in the designated area. All stationery will be provided but bring in some hydration if you think you will need it.

On your table will be the exam paper, an answer sheet, a pencil and a rubber. Remember to check all these items are correct and working, and then complete your candidate details at the top of the answer sheet. You will be required to complete your answers on an electronic marking sheet, using a clear horizontal pencil line in the appropriate box on the answer sheet; for example, if you think the answer to question 15 is D, a mark should be placed in box of column D in the row labelled 15. Only one mark is allowed per question/row. The paper is not negatively marked. During the exam, you are not permitted to leave in the first 60 minutes or in the last 15 minutes.

For a candidate to progress to the MRCS Part B Objective Structured Clinical Examination (OSCE), a pass in Part A is necessary. For a pass, you need to pass both papers individually, as well as achieving the minimum overall mark set for the exam (combined mark for Papers 1 and 2).

How to answer SBAs and EMQs

Firstly, always carefully check the instructions – they may be different from what you expect! The questions are based on short clinical vignettes. Read them with care, as each item of information is critical and should influence your choice. Particularly when making your final choice, perhaps between two options, do not make assumptions which are not supported by the information given. Although your general approach should be similar for the two types of question, they will now be dealt with separately because the detailed approach is somewhat different.

Single best answer

Here the situation is simple – for each vignette, you must decide which one of five answers is 'best', e.g. the most likely diagnosis, or the most effective management. It follows that the other answers are inferior. Some may be less complete, or incorrect in some aspect, but each option to be rejected is flawed, irrelevant, or just wrong. Be on the lookout for options which:

- Conflict with the information given in the vignette, including gender and age
- Require assumptions for which there is no foundation in the vignette

Once you have read the initial vignette and question, before you go to the options, think in your mind what the correct answer should be. Once you have that in your mind, look at the list of options to see if your answer is in the list. If it is, then most likely this is the correct option, but check the others carefully to make sure one is not better than your initial instinctive choice.

When you read a vignette and question and you feel that you are not comfortable with the topic and do not know a lot about it, then do not waste time in thinking about it. It will get you down mentally and you will lose valuable time. Just go ahead and answer the questions you know. Come back to the unanswered questions later.

The correct options are randomly distributed, so don't be surprised if you have a preponderance of Cs or Ds over a group of questions, and don't bother to work out whether you have the same numbers of As and Es.

Extended matching questions

With these there is a list of options which are to be used for each of a number of vignettes, but again the requirement is to pick the single best option from the list for each particular vignette. Remember, an option can be picked to match more than one vignette and some options may not be used.

With EMQs it is a good method to read the clinical scenarios first and not the list on top. Once you read a scenario, you should have an idea about the possible option, e.g. the diagnosis. Then look at the list of diagnoses. Look for the diagnosis that you made. If that is present in the list, then that is probably the correct answer. Do not start by reading all the scenarios one after another. Finish each scenario and make the diagnosis.

Tactical points

First, be alert. As with any exam your mental state as you start the exam is much more important than any final revision in the last few minutes before you start. Your preparation for this alert state starts several days before.

Candidates are asked to use a pencil and the aim is to make a mark, usually horizontal, so that the answer is unequivocal when the sheet is being read by the optical marker. The test you should apply is this – would there be the slightest doubt to someone reading your completed paper about whether one and only one option is marked? Bear in mind that the machine will be faced with erased options which can still be seen faintly and it is programmed to ignore these. For this reason avoid pencils which have been sharpened to a very fine point, which may not give a readable response especially if little pressure is exerted. The box should be very clearly marked and this is best done with a worn rounded pencil, so don't hesitate to do an initial wearing down of a fine point. It's not necessary to fill 99.9% of the box area, but very slight marks may not register with the machine, resulting in no mark. Of course, there will be no mark if two or more boxes could reasonably be interpreted as filled.

You may like to mark the options on the question sheet initially and then copy them to the optically read sheet. No extra time, of course, is allowed for this, so be very sure you have time to do this!

Some people, if the time is not up, will re-read and modify their answers. Unless you have obviously marked a different box from the one intended, changes of mind at this stage very rarely improve results.

And, finally, of course, make sure you answer all the questions, or you are throwing away potential marks.

Acknowledgements

The figures listed below have previously been published in the following books and are reproduced with permission.

Datta PK, Bulstrode CJK, Kaur, V. How to Pass the MRCS OSCE Volume 1. Oxford: Oxford University Press; 2011. Figures 34.1, 46.1, 47.2a, 47.3, 47.13, 47.14, 48.3, 49.5, 49.11, 58.1.

Datta PK, Bulstrode CJK, Praveen BV. MCQs and EMQs in Surgery. London: Hodder Arnold; 2010. Figures 49.10, 54.1, 58.1, 58.2

Goodfellow JA. Pocket Tutor Neurological Examination. London: JP Medical; 2012. Figure 3.1.

Misra RR, Uthappa MC, Datta PK. Radiology for Surgeons. Cambridge: Greenwich Medical Media; 2001. Figures 46.7, 47.1, 49.8, 49.10, 54.1, 58.1.

Tunstall R and Shah N. Pocket Tutor Surface Anatomy. London: JP Medical; 2012. Figure 3.2.

We thank Christopher JK Bulstrode and William FM Wallace for editing the first edition, and Vasha Kaur, Zahid Raza, Alex Laird, Diptendra Sarkar, Grant Stewart and Ben Stutchfield for their contributions to the first edition.

Section A

Applied basic sciences

Chapter 1

Skull and brain

Questions

For each question, select the single best answer from the five options listed.

1. A 25-year-old footballer was injured while heading a ball. He was unconscious for less than a minute and then continued to play. At the end of the game he felt drowsy and was brought to the emergency department unable to be aroused, with a Glasgow Coma Score of 13. A CT scan shows an extradural haemorrhage.

    Rupture of which blood vessel has caused the extradural haematoma?

    A   Internal carotid artery
    B   Middle cerebral artery
    C   Middle meningeal artery
    D   Superficial temporal artery
    E   Superior sagittal sinus

2. A 35-year-old woman with an untreated infected lesion on her face complains of severe ocular pain, fever and chemosis, and has a pulsating proptosis.

    Which one of the following structures is involved?

    A   Cavernous sinus
    B   Optic nerve
    C   Pituitary gland
    D   Superior sagittal sinus
    E   Trigeminal nerve

3. A 70-year-old man, a smoker, presents with intermittent amaurosis fugax (temporary visual loss) in the form of a shutter dropping in front of his eye. He has a systolic carotid bruit on the same side.

    The main artery that is affected enters the orbit through which one of the following foramina?

    A   Foramen rotundum
    B   Foramen spinosum
    C   Inferior orbital fissure
    D   Optic canal
    E   Superior orbital fissure

4. A 45-year-old woman is diagnosed with a space-occupying lesion at the cerebellopontine angle.

   The lesion is arising from which one of the following structures?

   A   Basilar artery aneurysm
   B   Cerebellum
   C   Glossopharyngeal nerve
   D   Hypoglossal nerve
   E   Vestibulocochlear nerve

5. A 55-year-old man presents with sudden onset of severe thunderclap headache, which he likens to a 'hammer blow' to the back of the head. A gadolinium-enhanced MRI shows a haemorrhagic lesion in the anterior cranial fossa.

   Which one of the following vessels is involved?

   A   Anterior communicating artery
   B   Basilar artery
   C   Internal carotid artery
   D   Middle cerebral artery
   E   Posterior communicating artery

6. A 48-year-old man, after investigations for persistent early morning headaches, is found to have raised intracranial pressure from a pituitary adenoma. Recently he finds that he is bumping into the sides of doorways and people.

   Pressure by the tumour into which of the following structures is causing his specific visual problem?

   A   Cavernous sinus
   B   Ophthalmic nerve
   C   Optic chiasma
   D   Optic nerve
   E   Visual cortex

7. A 30-year-old man, a recent immigrant from Africa, presents with an advanced right-sided nasopharyngeal carcinoma. A CT scan shows widespread extension into the right posterior fossa at the base of the skull. On protruding the tongue, it deviates towards the side of the lesion.

   Which one of the following nerves is affected by the growth?

   A   Glossopharyngeal nerve
   B   Hypoglossal nerve
   C   Spinal part of accessory nerve
   D   Superior cervical sympathetic nerve
   E   Vagus nerve

8. A 30-year-old man presents with anosmia, after sustaining a fracture of his anterior cranial fossa in a road traffic accident 5 weeks ago. At that time he had cerebrospinal rhinorrhoea.

   Fracture of which one of the following bones is causing his anosmia?

   A   Cribriform plate of the ethmoid bone
   B   Frontal process of the zygomatic bone
   C   Nasal bones
   D   Orbital plate of the frontal bone
   E   Squamous part of the temporal bone

Answers

1. C Middle meningeal artery

The middle meningeal artery is a branch of the maxillary artery which, along with the superficial temporal artery, is one of the terminal branches of the external carotid artery. It enters the middle cranial fossa through the foramen spinosum and divides into an anterior and posterior branch. It is the cause of bleeding in extradural haemorrhage because it lies deep to the squamous part of the temporal bone which is a very thin part of the cranium, and therefore easily fractured. This patient has typically suffered from lucid interval, a common feature of extradural haemorrhage. The ideal surgical procedure is to carry out a craniotomy in the neurosurgical unit. In a critical emergency, however, a burr hole can be made at the pterion to access the middle meningeal artery and stop the bleeding.

2. A Cavernous sinus

The cavernous sinus is vulnerable to thrombosis in any serious infections of the face in the 'danger area' – upper lip, nose and medial part of cheek. This is a very serious condition and may lead to proptosis and ophthalmoplegia. The structures of the cavernous sinus are: internal carotid artery, ophthalmic division (1st division) and maxillary divisions (2nd division) of the 5th cranial nerve and the 3rd, 4th and 6th cranial nerves. The other surgical condition that can occur within the cavernous sinus is an aneurysm of the internal carotid artery, resulting in a caroticocavernous fistula presenting clinically as a pulsating proptosis.

3. D Optic canal

The central artery of the retina is affected. It is a branch of the ophthalmic artery which enters the orbit through the optic canal inferolateral to the optic nerve within a common dural sheath. It supplies the extraocular muscles, the lachrymal gland and the eye. The eye is supplied by the central artery, an end artery (which supplies the optic nerve and retina) and the anterior and posterior ciliary arteries. The venous drainage from the orbit is by the superior ophthalmic vein which passes through the superior orbital fissure and the inferior ophthalmic vein that passes through the inferior orbital fissure.

4. E Vestibulocochlear nerve

The lesion is arising from the vestibulocochlear nerve at its entrance to the auditory meatus. The auditory meatus is situated in the posterior cranial fossa in the petrous part of the temporal bone. In that area a cerebellopontine angle tumour arises from the nerve sheath of the 8th cranial nerve (schwannoma, acoustic neuroma); it may press on the adjacent 7th cranial nerve, causing facial numbness or weakness.

5. A Anterior communicating artery

This patient has a classical presentation of a ruptured berry aneurysm resulting in subarachnoid haemorrhage. The commonest site for a berry aneurysm is the anterior communicating artery. Congenital berry aneurysms (so-called because of their resemblance to the fruit) occur in the circle of Willis, particularly at the junction of the vessels where the tunica media is lacking; turbulent blood at the bifurcation also contributes to the development of these aneurysms. Patients present with features of subarachnoid haemorrhage: complaining of a severe and sudden headache, where they feel a hammer-blow on the back of the head. Patients fast become unconscious. Unless suspected by clinical awareness, promptly investigated by MRI and immediately treated as an emergency, it carries a poor prognosis.

6. C Optic chiasma

This patient's pituitary adenoma is compressing on the optic chiasma causing bitemporal hemianopia (blindness in the temporal half of both visual fields). The optic chiasma lies on the optic groove. The tumour expands upwards from the pituitary fossa, compressing the inferior midline of the chiasma. This causes the nasal fibres from both retinas to be interrupted, thus narrowing the outer part (temporal) of each visual field. The optic nerve fibres on the nasal side of each retina cross over to the opposite side of the brain via the optic nerve at the optic chiasma (decussation of medial fibres) to enter the contralateral optic tract. This explains why a tumour of the pituitary, by compressing the central part of the chiasma, causes bitemporal visual loss (**Figure 1.1**).

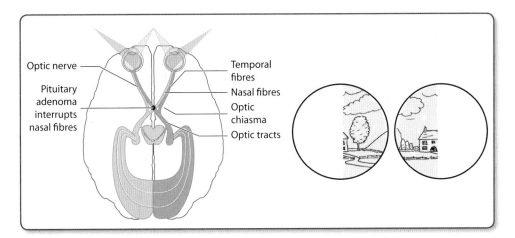

Figure 1.1 Diagrammatic representation of the optic chiasma showing how a pituitary adenoma causes bitemporal hemianopia.

7. B Hypoglossal nerve

The hypoglossal nerve exits the posterior cranial fossa through the hypoglossal canal. This is a separate foramen seen at the edge of the foramen magnum. Direct extension of the growth into the base of the skull infiltrates the hypoglossal nerve which may also be invaded by secondary lymph nodes. The nerve supplies all the intrinsic and extrinsic muscles of the tongue except the palatoglossus because the latter is essentially a muscle of the palate and hence supplied by the pharyngeal plexus. Iatrogenic damage can occur during excision of the submandibular salivary gland and this would cause the tongue to deviate to the paralysed side with atrophy of the tongue.

8. A Cribriform plate of ethmoid bone

After recovery from a head injury, the patient suffers from anosmia. This means that the olfactory (1st cranial) nerve has been damaged as a result of fracture of the cribriform plate of the ethmoid bone. The olfactory bulb may be separated from the olfactory nerves or the nerves may be torn as a result of the fracture. Such an injury will cause cerebrospinal rhinorrhoea at the time of initial injury. The midline of the cribriform plate projects up as a sharp triangle of bone called the crista galli for attachment of the falx cerebri. Up to 20 olfactory nerve filaments on each side of the nose perforate the dura and arachnoid mater over the cribriform plate to pass upwards through the subarachnoid space and enter the olfactory bulb.

Chapter 2

Head and neck

Questions

For each question, select the single best answer from the five options listed.

1. A 45-year-old man underwent simple excision of the submandibular salivary gland for sialadenitis. On the first postoperative day, the patient is drooling saliva from the angle of the mouth on the side of the operation.

    Which of the following anatomical structures is most likely to be damaged?

    A   Buccal branch of the facial nerve
    B   Hypoglossal (12th cranial) nerve
    C   Lingual nerve
    D   Marginal mandibular branch of the facial (7th cranial) nerve
    E   Maxillary (2nd branch of 5th cranial) nerve

2. A 35-year-old woman is undergoing a hemithyroidectomy. During the procedure, the surgeon has to ligate the inferior thyroid artery.

    Which one of the following structures is in danger of being damaged while doing so?

    A   Ansa hypoglossi
    B   Cervical branch of facial nerve
    C   External laryngeal nerve
    D   Pharyngeal branch of the glossopharyngeal nerve
    E   Recurrent laryngeal nerve

3. A 50-year-old man presents with recent onset of pain in his face over the upper and lower jaws. This is brought on by washing, shaving, eating or cold wind blowing on his face.

    Which one of the following nerves is the cause of this symptom complex?

    A   Ansa cervicalis
    B   Cervical plexus
    C   Facial (7th cranial) nerve
    D   Spinal branch of accessory (11th cranial) nerve
    E   Trigeminal (5th cranial) nerve

4. A 58-year-old man, a smoker, presents with severe cramp-like pains in his right upper limb, associated with fainting attacks and visual disturbances. These are particularly strong when he uses the limb vigorously, such as when painting the ceiling. Vascular investigations have shown an atheromatous obstruction to the first part of the subclavian artery, resulting in a diagnosis of subclavian steal syndrome.

    From which of the following branches of the subclavian artery is blood being redirected as a result of retrograde flow?

    A   Costocervical trunk
    B   Dorsal scapular artery
    C   Internal thoracic artery
    D   Thyrocervical trunk
    E   Vertebral artery

5. A 70-year-old woman complains of sudden bouts of severe coughing in the middle of the night while asleep when undigested food tends to regurgitate into the back of her throat. This is associated with halitosis and recurrent chest infections. A diagnosis of pharyngeal pouch was made.

    At what anatomical point does a pharyngeal pouch occur?

    A   Between middle and inferior constrictor muscles of the pharynx
    B   Between right and left palatopharyngeus
    C   Between superior and middle constrictor muscles of the pharynx
    D   Between thyropharyngeus and cricopharyngeus (two parts of the inferior constrictor) muscles
    E   Between two heads of the sternocleidomastoid

6. An open carotid endarterectomy is being carried out for internal carotid artery stenosis causing transient ischaemic attacks (TIAs).

    Which one of the following structures is most vulnerable to iatrogenic damage during the operation?

    A   Ansa cervicalis
    B   Glossopharyngeal nerve
    C   Hypoglossal nerve
    D   Sympathetic trunk
    E   Vagus nerve

7. A 28-year-old man undergoes an endoscopic transthoracic sympathectomy for palmar hyperhidrosis. Postoperatively, he has developed ptosis of his eye.

    This is due to iatrogenic damage to which one of the following nerves?

    A   8th cervical nerve
    B   1st thoracic nerve
    C   Lower cord of brachial plexus
    D   2nd thoracic ganglion
    E   7th cervical nerve

8. A 35-year-old man has been investigated for hypercalcaemia from primary hyperparathyroidism. A technetium-labelled sestamibi scan shows a parathyroid adenoma in the superior mediastinum.

    The adenoma has developed from which of the following sites of origin of the parathyroid?

    A   1st pharyngeal pouch
    B   4th pharyngeal pouch
    C   2nd pharyngeal pouch
    D   3rd pharyngeal pouch
    E   Ultimobranchial body

Answers

1. D Marginal mandibular branch of the facial (7th cranial) nerve

The patient is drooling saliva because the depressor anguli oris has been paralysed from damage to the marginal mandibular branch of the facial nerve. As the most superficial nerve this can be damaged if the skin incision is made incorrectly. To avoid damaging the nerve, a horizontal skin crease incision is made two fingers breadth below the ramus of the mandible, and the incision deepened down to the body of the gland. The superior flap consisting of the skin, platysma and fascia investing the gland is then lifted up to the ramus of the mandible. Damage to the nerve which lies between the platysma and the fascia is thus avoided (**Figure 2.1**). The other two nerves that lie within the gland and are in danger of iatrogenic damage are the lingual and hypoglossal nerves.

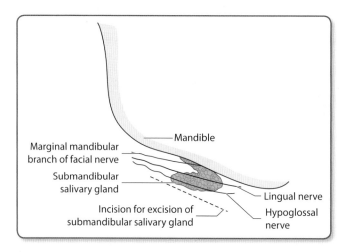

Figure 2.1 Nerves that are vulnerable during excision of the submandibular salivary gland: the marginal mandibular branch of the facial nerve, hypoglossal nerve and lingual nerve.

2. E Recurrent laryngeal nerve

The inferior thyroid artery is the last vascular pedicle sought during thyroid surgery. It is ligated in continuity. The thyroid lobe is rotated medially out of its bed and the carotid sheath retracted laterally to display the inferior thyroid artery and the recurrent laryngeal nerve (RLN) which lies in the tracheo-oesophageal groove. Ligation of the inferior thyroid artery must always be carried out under full visualisation of the RLN.

On the right side, the RLN hooks round the subclavian artery and on the left it hooks round the ligamentum arteriosum under the arch of the aorta. This asymmetry in the course of the two RLNs is due to the difference in the fate of the arch arteries of the neck in foetal life. The RLNs enter the pharynx by passing under the lower border of the inferior constrictor behind the cricothyroid joint.

3. E Trigeminal (5th cranial) nerve

The three divisions (or branches) of the trigeminal nerve, ophthalmic, maxillary and mandibular supply the skin of the face in three zones. The sensations from the front, near the orbit, are carried by the ophthalmic, division; sensations from the lower lid, mid-face, nose and upper lip and gum by the maxillary division and the mandibular division carries sensations from the temporal region, both surfaces of the lower lip and gum and mucous membrane of the floor of the mouth and the lingual gum. Hence in trigeminal neuralgia (*tic doloureux*) the face is the most affected. The pattern of a facial capillary haemangioma (port-wine stain) and the distribution of vesicles when herpes zoster affects the trigeminal ganglion fit the pattern of sensory supply of the facial skin.

4. E Vertebral artery

Subclavian steal syndrome results from retrograde flow of blood from the vertebral artery of the vertebrobasilar system. In this condition, there is atheromatous obstruction of the first part of the subclavian artery. Therefore, when extra blood is required due to excessive use of the upper limb, particularly in activities involving manual labour, blood is provided by the vertebral artery by reversal of its flow into the subclavian artery. This causes ischaemic cerebral symptoms from vertebrobasilar insufficiency.

5. D Thyropharyngeus and cricopharyngeus (two parts of the inferior constrictor) muscles

A pharyngeal pouch occurs through the Killian's dehiscence (first described by Gustav Killian). This is potentially a triangular-shaped weakness between the cricopharyngeus (transverse fibres) and thyropharyngeus (oblique fibres) parts of the inferior constrictor muscle of the pharynx. The inferior constrictor encloses the middle and superior constrictor muscles with its fibres, curving backwards and upwards around them. The cricopharyngeus is continuous with the circular muscle coat of the oesophagus and acts as a sphincter. It is always closed, relaxing only during deglutition. After excision of a pharyngeal pouch, cricopharyngeal myotomy is an essential part of the operation to prevent recurrence.

6. E Vagus nerve

In open carotid endarterectomy exposure is usually through a longitudinal incision parallel to the anterior border of the sternocleidomastoid. Within the carotid sheath lies the common carotid artery on the medial part, with the internal jugular vein lateral to it and the vagus nerve deeply placed in the groove between the two vessels. It is during the exposure of the three carotid arteries that the vagus nerve is most vulnerable to injury. The sympathetic trunk lies outside the carotid sheath and behind the artery. The vagus nerve descends straight down the neck. On the right side at the root of the neck it gives off the RLN which hooks round the subclavian artery; on the left side the vagus nerve gives off the RLN in the superior mediastinum to hook round the ligamentum arteriosum under the arch of the aorta.

7. B 1st thoracic nerve

During this operation, the 1st thoracic nerve has been inadvertently damaged resulting in division of the sympathetic fibres which ultimately supply the smooth muscle part of the levator palpebrae superioris (Muller's muscle). Paralysis of this part of the muscle causes partial ptosis. This is one of the features of Horner's syndrome, the others being constriction of the pupil and absence of sweating in the forehead. The syndrome, described in 1869 by Johann Friedrich Horner, can also occur from compression of the T1 nerve root by a space-occupying lesion such as a carcinoma of the apex of the lung (Pancoast tumour), carcinoma of the thyroid or oesophagus, metastatic lymph nodes or pressure from thoracic inlet/outlet syndrome.

8. D 3rd pharyngeal pouch

The inferior parathyroid gland would be the site of the adenoma. This is because, it is less constant in its position and hence more likely to be in the mediastinum. The inferior glands develop from the 3rd pharyngeal pouch. The thymus also develops from the 3rd pharyngeal pouch. This close association between the two results in the inferior parathyroids descending with the thymus. Therefore, they may be found in the thorax, superior or posterior mediastinum and in front of the trachea or oesophagus.

The superior parathyroids develop from the 4th branchial pouch and are much more constant in position. Therefore, the superior parathyroids are sometimes referred to as parathyroid IV and the inferior parathyroids as parathyroid III. The glands are very close to the anastomosis between the superior and inferior thyroid arteries on the posterior border of the thyroid gland.

Chapter 3

Upper limb and breast

Questions

For each question, select the single best answer from the five options listed.

1. A 29-year-old man presents complaining of pain in his left neck and shoulder region following a forced abduction injury to his arm, resulting from a fall from his motorbike at high speed. Subsequent imaging demonstrates an upper brachial plexus lesion.

    Which of the following nerves is a branch of the lateral cord of the brachial plexus?

    A Axillary
    B Musculocutaneous
    C Radial
    D Thoracodorsal
    E Upper subscapular

2. A 35-year-old woman presents with winging of the right scapular due to paralysis of the serratus anterior muscle.

    A lesion to which nerve would result in this presentation?

    A Dorsal scapular
    B Long thoracic nerve of Bell
    C Nerve to subclavius
    D Suprascapular
    E Thoracodorsal

3. A 23-year-old man presents following a fall onto his left shoulder whilst playing rugby. He complains of pain throughout the shoulder and on examination has weakness when testing internal rotation of the arm compared to the contralateral side. Radiographs are negative.

    Injury to which tendon would explain his symptoms?

    A Deltoid
    B Infraspinatus
    C Subscapularis
    D Supraspinatus
    E Teres minor

4. A 38-year-old woman presents following a twisting injury during a fall from her horse at low speed. She complains of pain in the region of the fracture and on examination has a wrist drop in the ipsilateral hand. Radiographs reveal a fracture of the humeral diaphysis.

   An injury to which nerve would explain her presentation?

   A   Axillary
   B   Median
   C   Musculocutaneous
   D   Radial
   E   Ulnar

5. An 18-year-old man presents following a deep penetrating stab injury to the anterior aspect of his left forearm.

   Which of the following muscles of the forearm is supplied by the ulnar nerve?

   A   Flexor carpi radialis
   B   Flexor carpi ulnaris
   C   Flexor digitorum superficialis
   D   Palmaris longus
   E   Pronator teres

6. An 18-year-old man presents with a posterior dislocation of the left elbow. He complains of decreased sensation and weakness throughout the left hand. On examination, there is a weakness to abduction and adduction of the fingers.

   Which of the following nerves has been injured as a result of the dislocation?

   A   Anterior interosseous
   B   Posterior interosseous
   C   Median
   D   Radial
   E   Ulnar

7. A 48-year-old woman presents with a 1-year history of numbness and tingling affecting the radial three and half digits of her left hand. She has signs of atrophy to the thenar eminence of the hand and has a positive Tinel's and Phalen's tests.

   Compression of which structure is causing the patient's symptoms?

   A   Flexor carpi radialis tendon
   B   Flexor digitorum profundus tendons
   C   Flexor digitorum superficialis tendons
   D   Flexor pollicis longus tendon
   E   Median nerve

8. A 49-year-old woman has a unilateral mastectomy for carcinoma of the breast.

   Which of the following is the primary contributor to the arterial supply of the female breast?

   A Dorsal scapular artery
   B Internal thoracic artery
   C Suprascapular artery
   D Thoracodorsal artery
   E Transverse cervical artery

Answers

1. B Musculocutaneous

The brachial plexus is formed from the ventral rami of the lower four cervical nerve roots (C5–C8) and the first thoracic nerve root (T1). It provides muscular and cutaneous innervation to the pectoral girdle as well as to the rest of the upper limb. The plexus is divided into zones with roots (C5–T1), trunks (superior C5–C6, middle C7, inferior C8–T1), divisions (anterior or posterior divisions of the three trunks) and cords (lateral, posterior, medial). The cords are named according to their location in relation to the second part of the axillary artery. Branches arise from these zones as shown in **Figure 3.1**. The branches of the posterior cord include the upper subscapular nerve that supplies subscapularis, the lower subscapular nerve that supplies subscapularis and teres major, the thoracodorsal nerve that supplies latissimus dorsi, the axillary nerve that supplies teres minor and deltoid, and the radial nerve that supplies the extensors of the elbow, wrist and hand. The musculocutaneous nerve is a branch of the lateral cord, which also gives rise to the lateral pectoral nerve, along with the medial cord and the median nerve.

There are three types of injury that can occur to the brachial plexus: upper, lower or whole. Excessive lateral flexion of the neck (downward traction of arm) away from the pectoral girdle can lead to an upper plexus injury (C5/C6). The clinical presentation is known as an Erb–Duchenne paralysis with the arm in a 'waiter's tip' position due to dysfunction of the suprascapular nerve, musculocutaneous nerve and axillary nerve leading to paralysis of the rotator cuff muscles and unopposed elbow extension and forearm pronation. A forced traction injury on an abducted arm (upward traction) can lead to a lower plexus injury (C8/T1) and the clinical presentation is known as Klumpke's palsy. A characteristic sign is that of an ipsilateral clawed hand due to loss of the ulnar nerve leading to paralysis of the intrinsic

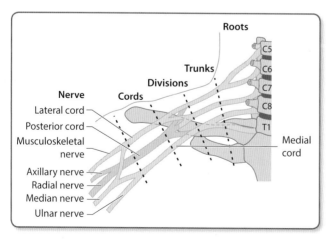

Figure 3.1 The brachial plexus. The roots are located between scalenus anterior and medius, the trunks in the posterior triangle of the neck, the divisions posterior to the clavicle and the cords in the axilla.

muscles of the hand. T1 involvement can lead to Horner's syndrome (sympathetic chain involvement) with ptosis, miosis and anhydrosis. Such a presentation can be associated with a cervical rib or Pancoast's tumour.

The reflexes of the upper limb are:

- Biceps (C5–C6, musculocutaneous, biceps)
- Triceps (C7–C8, radial, triceps)
- Supinator (C7–C8, radial, brachioradialis)

2. B Long thoracic nerve

The serratus anterior muscle originates on the surface of the first 8–9 ribs on the lateral aspect of the chest wall and inserts on the anterior medial border of the scapula. The muscle protracts and stabilises the scapula, and also assists with arm abduction past 120° by rotating the scapula and forcing the glenoid cavity to point superiorly. A winged scapula (scapula alata) is caused by paralysis of the serratus anterior muscle, commonly secondary to a lesion of the long thoracic nerve of Bell (C5–C7, see **Figure 3.1**). Injury can be traumatic (blunt trauma, subscapular bursitis, or iatrogenic, e.g. mastectomy with axillary clearance), nontraumatic (viral illness, radiculopathy, coarctation of the aorta) or idiopathic. A palsy of the accessory nerve (affecting the trapezius muscle) and dorsal scapular nerve (rhomboid) can lead to a clinical winged scapula also.

3. C Subscapularis

The rotator cuff is a mesh of four tendon insertions that insert into the greater and lesser tuberosity of the humerus, covering the shoulder capsule and reinforcing the stability of the glenohumeral joint. The four muscles of the rotator cuff are:

- Subscapularis
- Infraspinatus
- Supraspinatus
- Teres minor

Features of the four muscles are shown in **Table 3.1**.

Table 3.1 Origin, insertion, innervation and action of the four rotator cuff muscles				
Muscle	Origin	Insertion	Innervation	Movement
Subscapularis	Scapular subscapular fossa	Lesser tuberosity	Upper and lower subscapular nerve (C5–C6)	Internal rotation
Infraspinatus	Scapula infraspinous fossa	Greater tuberosity (middle facet)	Suprascapular nerve (C5–C6)	External rotation
Supraspinatus	Scapula supraspinous fossa	Greater tuberosity (superior facet)	Suprascapular nerve (C5–C6)	Abduction
Teres minor	Lateral border of scapula	Greater tuberosity (inferior facet)	Axillary nerve (C5)	External rotation

4. D Radial

The radial nerve arises from the posterior cord of the brachial plexus (C5–T1), passes through the lower triangular space of the axilla, passes posteriorly between the long and medial head of triceps, enters the arm posterior to the axillary artery and branches to give the posterior cutaneous nerve of the arm. It travels on the posterior medial aspect of the humerus giving a branch to the medial head of biceps and then passes into spiral groove of the humerus, circumnavigating the humerus with the deep brachial artery and providing innervation to the lateral head of triceps. It emerges posteriorly on the lateral aspect of the distal humerus and pierces the lateral intermuscular septum, running between brachialis and brachioradialis in the anterior compartment of the arm. During this course, motor innervation to elbow extensors (anconeus, triceps), brachioradialis and extensor carpi radialis longus are provided, as well as sensory cutaneous branches to the posterior forearm and the lateral arm. It then passes anterior to the lateral epicondyle of the humerus, traversing the antecubital fossa posterior to brachioradialis, entering the forearm. The nerve divides into a deep and superficial branch, with the deep branch continuing as the posterior interosseous nerve after penetration of the supinator muscle and innervates the muscles in the posterior compartment of the forearm. The superficial branch of the radial nerve descends the forearm posterior to brachioradialis, emerges just above the wrist and then provides sensory cutaneous innervation to the lateral dorsum of the hand including the first dorsal web space.

Injury to the radial nerve predominantly occurs at two levels with a distinct clinical picture:

- At the axilla, resulting in loss of elbow extension, wrist extension and metacarpophalangeal joint (MCPJ) extension
- At the spiral groove of the humerus, resulting in loss of wrist extension and MCPJ extension, but with preservation of elbow extension

5. B Flexor carpi ulnaris

The muscles of the flexor compartment of the forearm are divided into a superficial and deep layer, as outlined in **Table 3.2**.

The muscles of the flexor compartment of the forearm are supplied by the median nerve except for:

- Flexor carpi ulnaris (ulnar nerve)
- Flexor digitorum profundus medial two digits (ulnar nerve)

6. E Ulnar

The ulnar nerve arises from the medial cord of the brachial plexus (C8–T1), entering the arm medial to the axillary artery. It travels down the posterior medial aspect of the humerus (medial to brachial artery), pierces the medial intermuscular septum, and descends distally anterior to the triceps, giving off no branches in the arm. It passes posterior to the medial epicondyle of the humerus, entering the anterior compartment of the forearm between the two heads of flexor carpi ulnaris. The nerve

Table 3.2 Origin and insertion of the muscles of the flexor compartment of the forearm

	Muscle	Origin	Insertion
Superficial	Pronator teres	Medial epicondyle of humerus	Lateral body of radius
	Flexor carpi radialis	Medial epicondyle of humerus	Bases of 2nd and 3rd metacarpals
	Palmaris longus	Medial epicondyle of humerus	Palmar aponeurosis
	Flexor carpi ulnaris	Medial epicondyle of humerus	Pisiform
	Flexor digitorum superficialis	Medial epicondyle of humerus	Base middle phalanges four fingers
Deep	Flexor digitorum profundus	Upper third of volar ulna	Base distal phalanges four fingers
	Flexor pollicis longus	Middle third of volar radius	Base distal phalanx thumb
	Pronator quadratus	Anteromedial surface ulna	Anterolateral surface radius

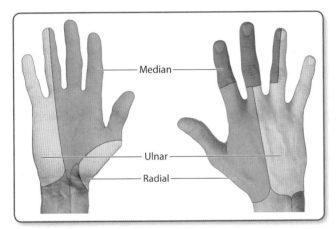

Figure 3.2 Cutaneous nerve supply to the hand.

descends through the forearm alongside the ulna and ulnar artery deep to flexor carpi ulnaris, which it innervates along with the medial two digits of the flexor digitorum profundus. Approximately 5 cm above the wrist, the nerve gives off the palmar and dorsal branches of the ulnar nerve, which provide cutaneous innervation to the hand (**Figure 3.2**). At the wrist, the ulnar nerve and artery pass through Guyon's canal, superficial to the flexor retinaculum. In the hand the superficial and deep branches of the ulnar innervate the intrinsic muscles of the hand (hypothenar muscles, 3rd and 4th lumbricals, adductor pollicis, interossei). The interossei muscles are responsible for abduction (dorsal) and adduction (palmar) of the fingers. Dysfunction of the ulnar nerve in the hand can also be tested using Froment's sign (test pinch grip and patient compensates by flexing the interphalangeal joint of thumb using flexor pollicis longus, which is innervated by the median nerve).

When severe lesions of the ulnar nerve occur at the wrist a classic clawing appearance to the hand is observed. However, if the lesion is more proximal at the elbow, the claw like appearance of the hand is reduced due to the loss of innervation to flexor digitorum profundus medial two digits. This is known as the ulnar paradox.

7. E Median nerve

The carpal tunnel is found on the volar or palmar aspect of the wrist and connects the anterior forearm to the volar aspect of the hand. It is formed through the flexor retinaculum and its attachments radially to the scaphoid tubercle and the trapezium, and on the ulnar side to the pisiform and hook of hamate. The contents of the carpal tunnel include the median nerve, four tendons of flexor digitorum profundus, four tendons of flexor digitorum superficialis and the tendon of flexor pollicis longus. The tendon of flexor carpi radialis is adjacent to, but not within the carpal tunnel.

The median nerve arises from the medial and lateral cords of the brachial plexus (C6–T1), entering the arm anterior to the distal third of the axillary artery. It travels down the arm lateral to the brachial artery, moving to the medial side at the mid-humeral level. The median nerve exits the antecubital fossa and passes into the forearm between the heads of pronator teres, giving off the anterior interosseous nerve. It then travels down the forearm between flexor digitorum superficialis and flexor digitorum profundus, before emerging near the wrist medial to flexor carpi radialis and entering the carpal tunnel. In the forearm the nerve innervates some of the muscles in the flexor compartment of the forearm along with one of its branches (anterior interosseous nerve). It then enters the hand via the carpal tunnel (inferior to the flexor retinaculum) and innervates some of the small muscles of the hand (thenar eminence, 1st and 2nd lumbricals). The palmar cutaneous branch of the median nerve is given off prior to the carpal tunnel and explains the preservation of sensory innervation to the central and radial aspect of the palm in patients with carpal tunnel syndrome (**Figure 3.3**).

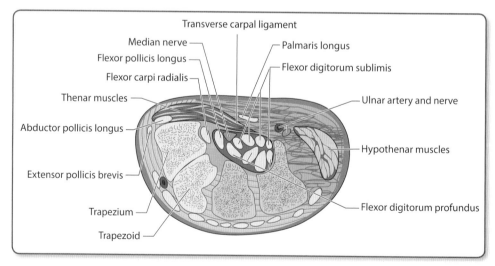

Figure 3.3 The carpal tunnel.

8. B Internal thoracic artery

The arterial supply of the female breast is through the:

- Internal mammary/thoracic artery
- Intercostal arteries
- Axillary artery (lateral thoracic and acromiothoracic)

The dorsal scapular artery arises from the subclavian artery and supplies the levator scapulae, rhomboids, and trapezius. The thoracodorsal artery is a branch of the subscapular artery and supplies the latissimus dorsi. The transverse cervical artery is an upper branch of the thyrocervical trunk and has contributions to trapezius and sternocleidomastoid. The suprascapular artery is a lower branch of the thyrocervical trunk and has contributions to supraspinatus, sternocleidomastoid and subclavius.

Chapter 4

Thoracic cavity

Questions

For each question, select the single best answer from the five options listed.

1. A 35-year-old man needed a routine annual medical examination for his employment. His ECG result showed prolongation of the PR interval to more than 0.22 s (normal = 0.12–0.20 s).

   In which one of the following sites in the heart is the abnormal conducting system situated?

   A   The left atrium
   B   The right atrium
   C   The right ventricle
   D   The left ventricle
   E   The aortic sinus

2. A 35-year-old woman presents with shortness of breath and is diagnosed with mitral stenosis. On auscultation, she has an opening snap with mid-diastolic murmur with presystolic accentuation.

   At which one of the following anatomical sites will these auscultatory findings be best heard?

   A   Sternal end of the 2nd left intercostal space
   B   5th left intercostal space in the midclavicular line
   C   Sternal end of 2nd right intercostal space
   D   Left lower sternal border at the 5th intercostal space
   E   Opposite the 4th left costal cartilage behind the sternum

3. A 50-year-old man complains of symptoms of heartburn and gastro-oesophageal reflux disease (GORD). He is due to have an oesophagogastroduodenoscopy (OGD).

   At what level from the incisors will the normal gastro-oesophageal junction be found?

   A   36 cm
   B   38 cm
   C   40 cm
   D   37 cm
   E   42 cm

4. A 45-year-old man is due to undergo a laparoscopic Nissen fundoplication as an anti-reflux operation for his gastro-oesophageal reflux disease (GORD).

   Which one of the following structures is in danger of being damaged?

   A   Hemiazygos vein
   B   Phrenic nerve
   C   Sympathetic trunk
   D   Thoracic duct
   E   Vagus nerves

5. A girl is born with severe respiratory distress as a result of a congenital diaphragmatic hernia. This was diagnosed antenatally.

   Through which one of the following foramina in the diaphragm has the hernia occurred?

   A   Aortic hiatus
   B   Bochdalek's foramen
   C   Inferior vena cava hiatus
   D   Morgagni's foramen
   E   Oesophageal hiatus

6. A 60-year-old man, a smoker, presents with a 3-day history of worsening headaches and shortness of breath with swelling of his face, upper chest and neck.

   Which one of the following structures is compressed causing his symptoms?

   A   Azygos vein
   B   Bifurcation of the trachea
   C   Both lung hila
   D   Superior vena cava
   E   Thoracic duct

7. A 62-year-old man complaining of dysphagia has been diagnosed with carcinoma of the middle third of the oesophagus.

   Which group of lymph nodes will this cancer spread to in the first instance?

   A   Brachiocephalic nodes
   B   Diaphragmatic nodes
   C   Internal thoracic nodes
   D   Paratracheal nodes
   E   Posterior mediastinal nodes

8. A 60-year-old man presents with a large carcinoma of the upper left lung. A chest X-ray confirms the diagnosis and also shows marked elevation of the left hemidiaphragm.

   Which one of the following nerves is affected by the carcinoma causing elevation of the left dome?

   A   Greater splanchnic nerve
   B   Phrenic nerve
   C   Recurrent laryngeal nerve
   D   Thoracic sympathetic trunk
   E   Vagus nerve

Answers

1. B Right atrium

This patient has a first degree atrioventricular (AV) block. This denotes that the site of abnormality is the AV node. This is situated in the right atrium on the interatrial septum above the attachment of the septal cusp of the tricuspid valve. It receives impulses from the sinoatrial node, the pacemaker of the heart which is situated in the right atrium just below the superior vena cava. From the AV node runs the AV bundle of His, which divides into right and left branches that travel down the respective sides of the interventricular septum (**Figure 4.1**). The bundle is the means of conducting the contractile impulse from atria to ventricles. The right branch becomes subendocardial on the right side of the septum. The left branch breaks up into a sheaf of subendocardial fibres. Abnormalities of heart rhythms are due to malfunctioning of the conducting system.

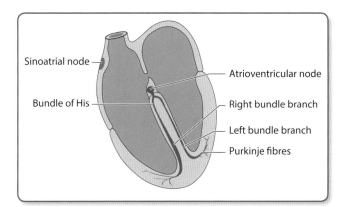

Figure 4.1 Conduction system of the heart.

2. B 5th left intercostal space in the midclavicular line

This patient has mitral stenosis. Hence the mitral valve needs to be auscultated to maximum benefit. The mitral valve sounds are best heard over the apex of the heart at the 5th left intercostal space in the midclavicular line (**Figure 4.2**). The sites of auscultation for the heart valves do not correspond to the surface anatomy of the valves because the intensity of the sounds is influenced by the direction of blood flow. The sites for hearing the other sounds are: the pulmonary–sternal end of the 2nd left intercostal space; the aortic–sternal end of the 2nd right intercostal space and the tricuspid–left lower sternal border at the 5th intercostal space.

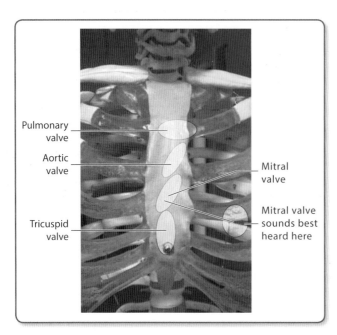

Figure 4.2 Surface markings of the heart valves. Mitral valve sounds are best heard over the apex of the heart at the 5th left intercostal space in the midclavicular line.

Pulmonary valve

Aortic valve

Tricuspid valve

Mitral valve

Mitral valve sounds best heard here

3. C 40 cm

The normal gastro-oesophageal junction is 40 cm from the incisors. It is situated to the left of the midline behind the 7th costal cartilage at the level of the T11 vertebra. This is an important anatomical landmark on OGD. In gastro-oesophageal reflux disease, the junction will be encountered earlier indicating that the oesophagus has been shortened due to oesophagitis from reflux. Biopsies will be taken from the abnormal, inflamed mucosa to look for the presence and extent of dysplasia. The oesophagus has certain normal anatomical sites of constriction where foreign bodies may get lodged. From the incisors, these sites are: commencement at the cricopharyngeal sphincter 15 cm; where it is crossed by the aortic arch 22 cm; where it is crossed by the left main bronchus 27 cm; at its entrance into the abdomen through the diaphragmatic hiatus at the level of the 10th thoracic vertebra 38 cm.

4. E Vagus nerves

The anti-reflux operation of Nissen fundoplication can be done through the chest or abdomen by open surgery or laparoscopically. Whatever the approach for the procedure, both the vagus nerves are vulnerable to inadvertent damage because of their proximity to the oesophagus. Below the pulmonary hila, the vagus nerves descend in contact with the oesophagus – the right behind and the left in front. The anterior vagal trunk is the left vagus which may be in two or three branches – hepatic, gastric and pyloric branches, their configuration being likened to a crow's foot. The posterior vagal trunk is the right vagus. It is usually a single thick cord and lies behind and to the right, and is not in contact with the posterior surface of the oesophagus. It gives off coeliac branches, and branches to the body and fundus.

5. B Bochdalek's foramen

This is a congenital diaphragmatic hernia which occurs through the foramen of Bochdalek. This results from a failure of development of the pleuroperitoneal membrane. The defect is posterior and occurs much more commonly on the left side due to the presence of the liver on the right. The diaphragm develops from four sources. The major part of the central tendon is developed from the septum transversum. This septum is invaded by the 3rd, 4th and 5th cervical myotomes which carry their own nerve supply which constitute the phrenic nerve. The thoracic and abdominal parts of the coelom are closed by mesodermal folds called pleuroperitoneal membranes thus separating the abdomen from the thorax. The oesophageal mesentery also makes a contribution to the diaphragm's development. Failure in union between the xiphoid and costal parts results in the foramen of Morgagni, a smaller hernial site.

6. D Superior vena cava

This is the classical acute presentation of superior vena cava syndrome (SVC syndrome) caused by compression of the superior vena cava by enlarged mediastinal secondary lymph nodes from a presumed carcinoma of the lung. A lymphoma from mediastinal lymph nodes can also present in a similar manner. The SVC starts at the lower border of the 1st costal cartilage by the union of the right and left brachiocephalic veins. It passes vertically downwards behind the right border of the sternum; at the level of the 2nd costal cartilage it pierces the pericardium to enter the upper border of the right atrium at the lower border of the 3rd costal cartilage. Behind the sternal angle the azygos vein enters the SVC. The patient requires an urgent chest X-ray followed by a CT scan of the chest and CT guided biopsy of the enlarged lymph nodes.

7. E Posterior mediastinal nodes

These lymph nodes are situated behind the pericardium on the oesophagus and descending aorta. Lymph from the middle one third drain first into the posterior mediastinal nodes. However, there are lymphatic channels within the oesophageal walls which enables lymph to pass along the viscus thus allowing cancer to spread through the submucosal lymphatic channels. Therefore, cancer spread into the lymph nodes is not segmental. A cancer of the middle one-third of the oesophagus may have lymph nodal secondaries which may be extensive from the neck to the abdomen.

8. B Phrenic nerve

Elevation of the left hemidiaphragm denotes paralysis of the left dome. The motor supply of the diaphragm is from the phrenic nerve which has been paralysed by infiltration with the lung cancer (**Figure 4.3**). The nerve arises in the neck from the 3rd, 4th and 5th cervical rami, the main contribution coming from the 4th. Approximately, two-thirds of the nerve fibres are motor to the diaphragm; the remainder of the nerve is sensory to the diaphragm, mediastinal

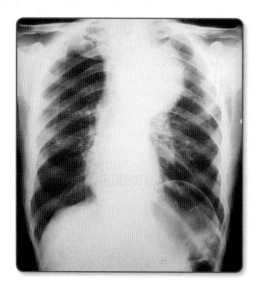

Figure 4.3 Chest X-ray showing large carcinoma of left lung with raised left hemi-diaphragm from infiltration of left phrenic nerve.

and diaphragmatic pleura, serous and fibrous pericardium and diaphragmatic peritoneum. Pain from irritation of the diaphragmatic peritoneum, as in perforation of a hollow viscus, collection of blood or pus in the subphrenic space is referred to the shoulder tip (C4).

Chapter 5

Abdomen

Questions

For each question, select the single best answer from the five options listed.

1. A 55-year-old man, a chronic alcoholic, presents to the outpatient clinic complaining of upper abdominal discomfort and swelling. He recovered from an attack of recurrent acute pancreatitis 6 weeks ago. On examination, he has a smooth fixed lump in his epigastrium, confirmed on ultrasonography to be a fluid-filled cyst of 6 cm diameter.

   In which one of the following intraperitoneal spaces is this fluid collection most likely to be situated?

   A   Left subhepatic space (lesser sac)
   B   Left subphrenic space
   C   Right paracolic gutter
   D   Right subhepatic space (hepatorenal pouch of Morison)
   E   Right subphrenic space

2. A 60-year-old man presents following two bouts of upper gastrointestinal haemorrhage, from which he recovered with conservative management. Oesophagogastroduodenoscopy (OGD) shows a puckered ulcer in the first part of the duodenum penetrating posteriorly with a large blood clot in the middle of the floor of the ulcer.

   Which one of the following arteries is the most probable cause of the bleeding?

   A   Common hepatic artery
   B   Gastroduodenal artery
   C   Right gastric artery
   D   Right gastroepiploic artery
   E   Superior pancreaticoduodenal artery

3. A 50-year-old man presents with severe acute upper gastrointestinal haemorrhage. After resuscitation, an OGD shows a large penetrating gastric ulcer on the posterior wall in the middle of the body of the stomach with pulsatile arterial blood.

   Which one of the following vessels is the cause of the bleeding?

   A   Coeliac artery
   B   Left gastric artery
   C   Left gastroepiploic artery
   D   Splenic artery
   E   Superior mesenteric artery

4. A 70-year-old woman presents with painless obstructive jaundice and a distended gallbladder. Ultrasound has shown a solid 3 cm mass arising from the head of the pancreas.

   Which part of the extrahepatic biliary tree is being compressed by the mass causing the obstructive jaundice?

   A   Common hepatic duct
   B   Infraduodenal common bile duct
   C   Left extrahepatic duct
   D   Right extrahepatic duct
   E   Supraduodenal common bile duct

5. A 45-year-old man presents with a lump protruding from his abdomen into his groin and the upper part of the scrotum.

   Through which one of the following spaces would the lump have extruded out of the peritoneal cavity?

   A   Deep inguinal ring
   B   Femoral ring
   C   Inguinal triangle
   D   Interparietal space
   E   Superficial inguinal ring

6. A 30-year-old man is undergoing a laparotomy for a crush injury to his upper abdomen. He is bleeding actively from a torn liver. The surgeon is in the process of controlling the haemorrhage by placing their index finger into the foramen of Winslow.

   Which one of the following structures is the surgeon trying to compress to control the bleeding?

   A   Coronary ligament of the liver
   B   Falciform ligament
   C   Gastrosplenic ligament
   D   Greater omentum
   E   Lesser omentum

7. A 25-year-old man, a cyclist, presents after being hit on the left side of his lower chest when involved in a collision with a car. He complains of pain in his left lower chest, left upper abdomen and left shoulder tip. He has a full range of movements of his left upper limb. A FAST (focused abdominal sonography in trauma) scan shows free fluid under the left hemidiaphragm.

   Which one of the following is the most likely cause of his left shoulder tip pain?

   A   Diaphragmatic rupture
   B   Left acromion fracture
   C   Left kidney rupture
   D   Left lower rib fractures
   E   Splenic rupture

8. A 70-year-old man is undergoing an elective open repair of an infrarenal abdominal aortic aneurysm.

Which one of the following structures is most likely to be adherent to the aneurysm neck?

A Left renal vein
B Neck of pancreas
C Third part of duodenum
D Portal vein
E Pylorus of stomach

Answers

1. A Left subhepatic space (lesser sac)

This collection is a pancreatic pseudocyst which is most commonly located in the left subhepatic space or lesser sac. Pancreatic pseudocyst has no epithelial lining and lined by granulation tissue. They contain collections that occur as a consequence of moderate to severe acute pancreatitis, which results in disruption of parenchyma and ductal system causing extravasation of pancreatic enzymes and autodigestion of surrounding tissue. This results in a collection rich in pancreatic enzymes, blood and necrotic tissue. These collections are usually peripancreatic and typically found in the lesser sac.

The left subhepatic space (lesser sac or omental bursa) is an irregular potential space found posterior to the stomach and lesser omentum, and anterior to the pancreas, left kidney, left adrenal gland and diaphragm. It is bounded antero-superiorly by the liver including the caudate lobe and inferiorly by the transverse mesocolon. It communicates with the greater sac though the epiploic foramen of Winslow.

2. B Gastroduodenal artery

A duodenal ulcer penetrates posteriorly into the gastroduodenal artery which is a short but large branch of the common hepatic artery. It lies between the first part of the duodenum and the pancreas and supplies the pylorus and upper half of the duodenum. It terminates at the lower border of T1 when it branches into the right gastroepiploic artery and the superior pancreaticoduodenal artery, which supplies the upper half of the duodenum and pancreas.

The foregut and its derivatives are supplied by the coeliac trunk, which gives rise to the following branches – left gastric artery, common hepatic artery and the splenic artery. The right gastric artery arises from the common hepatic artery and passes along the lower half of the lesser curve. The left gastric artery courses along the upper half of the lesser curve. Both these arteries anastomose along the lesser curve within layers of the lesser omentum.

3. D Splenic artery

This patient is bleeding from the splenic artery which forms one of the constituents of the stomach bed. Posteriorly, the bed of the stomach is related to a number of clinically important structures, which form the posterior wall of the omental bursa. These structures include left crus and dome of the diaphragm, left kidney and adrenal gland, pancreas, spleen, splenic artery, the transverse mesocolon and colon. From the position of the artery and endoscopic findings, the cause of the bleeding in this patient is penetration of the ulcer into the splenic artery. It is important that the splenic artery as the source of bleeding is appreciated early by the position of the ulcer and the rate and amount of bleeding. This ulcer is at high risk of re-bleeding and may necessitate emergency surgery as the definitive treatment.

4. B Infraduodenal common bile duct

The infraduodenal common bile duct lies in close relationship to the pancreatic head and hence is compressed early in a carcinoma arising from the head of the pancreas. The right and left hepatic ducts correspondingly drain the right and left lobes of liver. Shortly after leaving the porta hepatis, the right and left hepatic ducts converge to form the common hepatic duct (CHD), which carries on caudally for approximately 2 cm. The CHD then unites with the cystic duct to form the common bile duct (CBD). The CBD is approximately 8 cm long and can be divided into four parts – supraduodenal, retroduodenal, infraduodenal and intraduodenal parts.

The supraduodenal part lies in the free margin of the lesser omentum with the portal vein posteriorly and the hepatic artery on its left. The retroduodenal part lies posterior to the first part of the duodenum and anterior to the portal vein.

5. A Deep inguinal ring

This patient's lump occupies the upper part of the scrotum and hence is an indirect inguinal hernia. Therefore, the groin lump in this patient has extruded out of the deep inguinal ring. Inguinal hernias are protrusions of abdominal cavity contents into the inguinal canal and may be classified as either direct or indirect. An indirect inguinal hernia may be seen in adults or children. They emerge through the deep inguinal ring, lateral to the inferior epigastric artery. Indirect inguinal hernias are covered by the spermatic fascia and traverse the inguinal canal, to varying degrees. Large indirect inguinal hernias may traverse the entire length of the inguinal canal and emerge from the superficial inguinal ring into the scrotum – inguinoscrotal hernias (**Figure 5.1**). Direct inguinal hernias emerge through a weakness of the posterior wall, medial to the inferior epigastric artery, in the inguinal triangle.

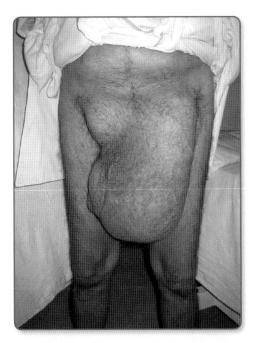

Figure 5.1 Inguinoscrotal hernia. Courtesy of Professor Pawanindra Lal.

6. E Lesser omentum

In liver trauma, at laparotomy, bleeding from the liver is controlled by squeezing the lesser omentum between the thumb and index finger by placing the index finger into the epiploic foramen of Winslow. The lesser omentum contains between its two layers the portal vein posteriorly, and in front of it the hepatic artery and bile duct, the latter to the right of the artery. This is an important anatomical landmark which is the connection between the lesser and greater sacs. The boundaries of the epiploic foramen are:

Upper – caudate process of the liver

Lower – first part of duodenum

Posterior – inferior vena cava

Anterior – right free margin of the lesser omentum containing the bile duct, hepatic artery and portal vein (as described above).

7. E Splenic rupture causing pain through the phrenic nerve

This patient's shoulder tip pain is caused by referred pain through the phrenic nerve as a result of diaphragmatic irritation from free blood under the diaphragm. In any patient with left-sided upper abdominal and lower chest trauma, there should be a high index of suspicion for splenic injury. This index of suspicion should be heightened further in a patient with these symptoms and acute left shoulder tip pain. This sign, a left sided Kehr's sign, is classically described in patients with a ruptured spleen. This occurs due to the presence of blood in the subdiaphragmatic space causing irritation of the diaphragm. The phrenic nerve provides the motor supply and most of the sensory supply of the diaphragm except peripherally where the sensory supply is from the subcostal and intercostal nerves. The phrenic nerve is formed from the 3rd, 4th and 5th cervical nerves.

8. C Third part of duodenum

While dissecting the neck of the aneurysm to put on a clamp, the third part of the duodenum is the most vulnerable. It is particularly in danger in an inflammatory aneurysm, where the duodenum is extremely adherent to the neck. The abdominal aorta is a retroperitoneal structure. It enters the abdomen at the level of T12 through the aortic hiatus of the diaphragm and terminates at the level of L4 when it bifurcates into the two common iliac arteries. It courses just to the left of the midline and descends anterior to the bodies of the L1 to L4 vertebrae and the anterior longitudinal ligament. Anteriorly, the abdominal aorta is closely related to a number of upper abdominal structures. At operation, these structures usually have to be retracted or dissected to allow access to the aorta.

Chapter 6

Pelvis

Questions

For each question, select the single best answer from the five options listed.

1. A 30-year-old woman is to have postoperative analgesia by means of a nerve block following an operation for a fistula-in-ano.

    Which one of the following nerves is the anaesthetist going to block by local anaesthetic?

    A   Common peroneal nerve
    B   Lumbosacral trunk
    C   Nerve to levator ani and external anal sphincter
    D   Obturator nerve
    E   Pudendal nerve

2. A 42-year-old man, a labourer, while at work, suddenly develops severe pain in his lower back radiating to the buttocks, back of thigh, lower leg and sole of foot. He cannot feel when he sits as he has diminished sensation on his buttocks.

    Which one of the following nerves is most likely affected?

    A   L5
    B   S1
    C   S2
    D   S3
    E   S4

3. A 65-year-old woman presents with severe pain on the inside of her left thigh for 1 week. The pain radiates from the inside of the thigh to the knee and is exacerbated by coughing. For 2 days she has had intermittent bilious vomiting and colicky left-sided abdominal pain. The pain is relieved by bending the hip and rotating it outwards. In that position, a soft lump is palpable.

    Which one of the following nerves is causing the pain?

    A   Femoral (L2, L3, L4)
    B   Genitofemoral (L1, L2)
    C   Ilioinguinal and iliohypogastric (L1)
    D   Lateral femoral cutaneous (L2, L3)
    E   Obturator (L2, L3, L4)

4. A 30-year-old man presents with left ureteric colic. A spiral CT scan shows a stone impacted at the pelvic brim.

    At which of the following anatomical sites would the stone be impacted?

    A   Common iliac artery bifurcation
    B   Fifth lumbar transverse process
    C   Ischial spine
    D   Pelviureteric junction
    E   Vas deferens crossing above the ureter

5. A 56-year-old woman is undergoing an anterior resection with total mesorectal excision for rectal carcinoma.

    During the operation which one of the following anatomical structures is vulnerable to iatrogenic damage?

    A   Fallopian tubes
    B   Ovaries
    C   Ureters
    D   Urinary bladder
    E   Uterus

6. A 25-year-old man presents following a straddle injury to his perineum having fallen astride on the beam in the gymnasium. Clinically there is a perineal haematoma with blood on his external urinary meatus.

    Which anatomical structure is most likely to be injured?

    A   Bladder neck
    B   Bulbar urethra
    C   Membranous urethra
    D   Prostatic urethra
    E   Urinary bladder

7. A 62-year-old man presents with early morning spurious diarrhoea. On clinical rectal examination, there is an easily palpable ulcerated indurated fixed mass on the anterior wall of the rectum. Biopsy showed a carcinoma.

    Through which one of the following fascial layers has the carcinoma spread?

    A   Anterior peritoneal covering
    B   Denonvilliers' fascia
    C   Lateral ligaments of the rectum
    D   Parietal pelvic fascia
    E   Waldeyer's fascia

8. A 35-year-old man is recovering from a severe motorcycle injury where he sustained major pelvic fractures and bladder and urethral injuries. He did not suffer any head injuries. 6 months after his accident his urethral catheter is removed. He is completely incontinent.

Which one of the following anatomical structures has been irreparably damaged, causing his incontinence?

A   External urethral sphincter
B   Internal urethral sphincter
C   Membranous urethra
D   Puboprostatic ligaments
E   Urinary bladder neck

Answers

1. E Pudendal nerve

The motor and sensory innervation of the perineum is derived from the pudendal nerve (S2, S3 and S4) which is the one blocked by local anaesthetic. The nerve is formed by the anterior divisions of the ventral rami of S2, S3 and S4. After its origin, it leaves the pelvis through the greater sciatic foramen to enter the gluteal region near the ischial spine. It accompanies the internal pudendal vessels into the pudendal (Alcock's) canal on the lateral wall of the ischiorectal fossa. In the posterior part of the canal it gives off its branches:

- inferior rectal nerve which innervates the external anal sphincter and the perianal skin
- perineal nerve which innervates the muscles of the perineum, skin of the labia majora and minora and vestibule
- dorsal nerve of clitoris or penis

The nerve is accessed by two approaches – transvaginal or perineal.

2. D S3

The S3 nerve root is responsible for the sensation of the sitting area of buttock. It is a constituent of the sacral plexus. The most important nerve arising from the sacral plexus is the sciatic nerve. It arises from L4, L5, S1, S2 and S3 roots of the sacral plexus. At its origin, it is 2 cm wide and is the thickest nerve in the body. It enters the gluteal region from the pelvis through the greater sciatic foramen. At a variable level in the back of the thigh proximal to the popliteal fossa it divides into the common peroneal (fibular, L4, L5, S1, S2 and tibial, L4, L5, S1, S2, S3) nerves. As an aid to remember the dermatome levels, we stand mainly on S1 (sole of foot), sit on S3 (buttocks) and wipe S4 (immediate perianal area).

3. E Obturator

The obturator nerve is causing this patient's pain. She has the clinical features of an incarcerated obturator hernia. The pain is referred to the knee by the geniculate branch of the obturator nerve (anterior divisions of L2, L3 and L4). The pain is much more pronounced in a strangulated hernia. Arising from the lumbar plexus, the obturator nerve lies on the psoas muscle and enters the obturator foramen. In the obturator canal it divides into anterior and posterior branches.

In an obturator hernia, a swelling is not often palpable unless the hip is abducted, flexed and externally rotated. The hernia can sometimes be felt as a tender swelling on rectal or vaginal examination. The pain is exacerbated by movements of the hip, coughing and abdominal straining. This is referred to as Howship–Romberg sign or syndrome.

4. A Common iliac artery bifurcation

The stone is impacted at the bifurcation of the common iliac artery where it leaves the psoas muscle. This is one of the points of natural narrowing where a stone may get arrested. The other points of natural narrowing are from above downwards: pelviureteric junction, where it is crossed by the vas deferens or broad ligament and at the ureterovesical junction.

Knowledge of the relationships of the ureter is very important, so as to prevent iatrogenic damage. On the left it underlies the apex of the sigmoid mesocolon. It then runs over the external iliac artery and vein and then down the side wall of the pelvis in front of the internal iliac artery and behind the ovary. On the right, it will be in close proximity to a pelvic appendix. Further distally at the level of the ischial spine it travels forwards and medially to enter the bladder base.

5. C Ureters

The ureters are vulnerable to iatrogenic damage by virtue of their close relationship to the rectosigmoid. Once the ureters descend to the pelvis, at the level of the ischial spine they travel forwards and medially above the pelvic floor to enter the bladder base at its upper lateral angle. Here the ureter lies at the base of the broad ligament where the uterine artery crosses it in the upper part. Under the broad ligament, the ureters penetrate the lateral cervical ligaments in close proximity to the lateral vaginal fornix being 2 cm from the cervix before entering the bladder. This is where the ureters are at greatest danger of damage, whilst ligating vessels and dividing ligaments.

The position of the ureters is of huge applied importance as they can be inadvertently damaged in operations of right hemicolectomy, sigmoid colectomy, anterior resection, abdominoperineal excision of rectum, hysterectomy and oophorectomy.

6. B Bulbar urethra

This patient has injured his bulbar urethra or anterior urethra in the perineum. This injury involves the junction of the membranous with the bulbar portion of the urethra. The anatomy of this region is such that extravasation of urine occurs, unless recognition of the injury and treatment is carried out promptly. Urine leaks between the perineal membrane and the membranous layer of the perineal fascia (Colles' fascia). As both these layers are firmly attached to the ischiopubic rami posteriorly, urine extravasates anteriorly into the loose connective tissue around the scrotum, penis and anterior abdominal wall. Should the posterior urethra be injured, urine leaks into the pelvic extraperitoneal tissues. A tear of the perineal membrane results in extravasation in the perineum. The male urethra is about 20 cm long and the female urethra is 4 cm long and 6 mm wide.

7. B Denonvillier's fascia (rectovesical fascia)

This rectal cancer has spread to Denonvilliers' fascia on the anterior wall of the rectum. This fascial layer is a condensation of the mesorectal fascia and forms a rectogenital septum called the rectovesical fascia of Denonvilliers. It is connected to the floor of the rectovesical pouch above and the apex of the prostate below. Spread of rectal cancer to this layer has a significant bearing on the management. Such a spread is diagnosed on MRI.

The lower one-third of the rectum is devoid of any peritoneal covering. The upper one-third is covered in the front and sides while the middle one-third is only covered in front. In men the Denonvilliers' fascia separates the lower rectum from the bladder base, seminal vesicles, the prostate, the termination of each ureter and vas deferens in front and the vagina in the female.

8. A External urethral sphincter

This person's urinary incontinence is due to damage to the external urethral sphincter. The internal urethral sphincter surrounding the proximal prostatic urethra is not responsible for urinary continence. This helps to prevent retrograde ejaculation by closing off the bladder neck during ejaculation.

The urethral sphincter mechanism extends from the perineum through the urogenital hiatus into the pelvic cavity. The mechanism consists of the striated and smooth muscle of the urethra and the pubourethral part of levator ani; this surrounds the membranous urethra in the male. The fibres also reach up to the lowest part of the bladder neck. The muscles are of the slow twitch variety. The innervation is from the perineal branch of the pudendal nerve and the pelvic splanchnic nerves. All these nerves originate in the S2, S3 and S4 spinal segments.

Chapter 7

Lower limb

Questions

For each question, select the single best answer from the five options listed.

1. A 62-year-old man presents with shock, secondary to acute pancreatitis. A decision is made to place a femoral line as part of his initial resuscitation in the emergency department.

   Which one of the following lies outside the femoral sheath?

   A   Cloquet's node
   B   Femoral artery
   C   Femoral canal
   D   Femoral nerve
   E   Femoral vein

2. A 75-year-old woman attends clinic 6 months following left total hip arthroplasty through a lateral approach. She is found to have a left-sided Trendelenburg gait with weakness of the ipsilateral abductors.

   Which one of the following nerves is most likely to be injured, and explains the examination findings?

   A   Femoral nerve
   B   Inferior gluteal nerve
   C   Obturator nerve
   D   Sciatic nerve
   E   Superior gluteal nerve

3. A 45-year-old man presents with a chronic swelling in the popliteal fossa, consistent with a Baker's cyst.

   Of the following muscles that comprise the borders of the popliteal fossa, which one has an insertion on the head of the fibula?

   A   Biceps femoris
   B   Gastrocnemius
   C   Plantaris
   D   Semimembranosus
   E   Semitendinosus

4. A 25-year-old man presents with significant pain and swelling to the anterior aspect of the leg following a direct blow during a football match. Clinical examination and compartment pressure monitoring confirm the diagnosis of acute compartment syndrome of the leg.

    Which of the following structures is found within the lateral compartment of the leg?

    A   Anterior tibial artery
    B   Deep peroneal nerve
    C   Peroneus tertius
    D   Superficial peroneal nerve
    E   Tibialis anterior

5. A 68-year-old woman presents with a bimalleolar fracture of the right ankle. Operative fixation is undertaken using a direct lateral approach to the lateral malleolus, with a direct incision used for the medial malleolus.

    Which one of the following structures is found anterior to the medial malleolus?

    A   Flexor digitorum longus tendon
    B   Posterior tibial artery
    C   Saphenous nerve
    D   Tibial nerve
    E   Tibialis posterior tendon

6. A 43-year-old woman presents with lumbar back pain and sciatica, with associated numbness over the lateral border of the right foot and ankle, along with an absent ipsilateral ankle jerk.

    Which spinal nerve distribution does this represent?

    A   L4
    B   L5
    C   S1
    D   S2
    E   S3

Answers

1. D Femoral nerve

The femoral sheath is 3–4 cm long (from the inguinal ligament) and is formed from a prolongation of the transversalis fascia (anteriorly) and iliacus fascia (posteriorly). It encompasses the femoral artery, femoral vein and femoral canal.

The femoral triangle is formed by the:

- Inguinal ligament (superiorly)
- Medial border of adductor longus (medially)
- Medial border of sartorius (laterally)
- Fascia lata (anteriorly/roof)
- Pectineus, iliopsoas, adductor longus (posteriorly/floor)

The femoral triangle is of major clinical significance, e.g. for arterial access in angioplasty, venous access in the shutdown patient. The following structures are contained within the femoral triangle (lateral to medial):

- Femoral nerve
- Femoral artery   Mnemonic: **NAVY** = **N**erve, **A**rtery, **V**ein, **Y**-fronts
- Femoral vein
- Femoral canal

The femoral artery is located at the mid-inguinal point (midpoint between the anterior superior iliac spine and the pubic symphysis). The femoral canal superiorly contains fat, lymphatic vessels and nodes (deep inguinal lymph nodes, Cloquet's node). The entrance to the femoral canal is known as the femoral ring, through which a femoral hernia can occur. The borders of the femoral ring are the inguinal ligament (anteriorly), pectineal ligament (posteriorly), lacunar ligament (medially) and femoral vein fascia (laterally).

2. E Superior gluteal nerve

When using the lateral approach to the hip the patient is in the lateral decubitus position. A lateral incision is made through skin, subcutaneous fat and the tensor fascia lata. The fibres of gluteus medius are then split (excess splitting to be avoided), along with the fibres of vastus lateralis, and an anterior flap is developed providing access to the hip capsule and then joint. The superior gluteal nerve (L4–S1) arises from anterior sacral foramina of the sacral plexus, exiting the pelvis through the greater sciatic foramen above piriformis (only structures above), travelling adjacent to the superior gluteal artery and vein. It then transverses between gluteus medius and gluteus minimus, passing approximately 4 cm above the greater trochanter. Muscular innervation is to gluteus medius, gluteus minimus and tensor fascia lata. Damage to the superior gluteal nerve can occur following excess splitting of gluteus medius and results in paralysis of the abductor muscles of the ipsilateral hip. A Trendelenburg gait is seen when the pelvis sags on the contralateral side of the lesion due to the lack of the abductor pull on the ipsilateral side.

The inferior gluteal nerve (L5–S2) arises from the sacral plexus, exiting the pelvis through the greater sciatic foramen below piriformis. From there it provides muscular innervation to the gluteus maximus. The sciatic nerve (L4–S3) exits the pelvis through the greater sciatic foramen below piriformis. It then transverses posterior to gluteus maximus and descends the thigh anterior to adductor magnus and posterior to the hamstrings. It supplies muscular innervation to biceps femoris, semitendinosus, semimembranosus, and adductor magnus. Sensory innervation is to the posterior aspect of the thigh and gluteal regions. The nerve divides, often just superior to the popliteal fossa, to give rise to the common peroneal and tibial nerves. The sciatic nerve is at risk during the posterior approach to the hip, with damage leading to paralysis and paraesthesia below the knee joint (sensory innervation spared medial aspect ankle and foot supplied by saphenous nerve). The femoral nerve (L2–S4) arises from the ventral rami of the lumbar plexus, passing through psoas major and emerging on the inferior lateral aspect where it then passes into the thigh posterior to the inguinal ligament. Approximately 5 cm inferior to the ligament, it provides terminal muscular (quadriceps femoris, sartorius, pectineus), sensory (intermediate cutaneous nerve, medial cutaneous nerve) and articular (hip and knee joint) branches.

3. A Biceps femoris

The popliteal fossa is a diamond shaped depression that forms the posterior aspect of the knee and is made through the following borders (**Table 7.1**):

- Semimembranosus and semitendinosus (superomedially)
- Biceps femoris (superolaterally)
- Medial head of gastrocnemius (inferomedially)
- Lateral head of gastrocnemius and plantaris (inferolaterally)
- Skin and superficial/deep fascia (roof)
- Posterior aspect of femur/knee joint and popliteus muscle (floor)

The first three muscles make up the posterior compartment of the thigh (hamstrings – semimembranosus, semitendinosus, biceps femoris). Semitendinosus, gracilis and

Table 7.1 The origin, insertion and innervation of the muscles that border the popliteal fossa			
Muscle	**Origin**	**Insertion**	**Innervation**
Semimembranosus	Ischial tuberosity	Medial aspect of tibia	Sciatic (tibial)
Semitendinosus	Ischial tuberosity	Upper part of tibia	Sciatic (tibial)
Biceps femoris Long head Short head	Ischial tuberosity Linea aspera femur	Head of fibula Head of fibula	Sciatic (tibial) Sciatic (common peroneal)
Gastrocnemius Medial head Lateral head	Distal femur Medial condyle Lateral condyle	Achilles tendon	Sciatic (tibial)
Plantaris	Supracondylar ridge femur (lateral)	Achilles tendon	Sciatic (tibial)

sartorius (posterior to anterior) insert via a conjoined tendon into an area on the anteromedial aspect of the proximal tibia known as the pes anserinus. This insertion can become inflamed and can be a source of chronic knee pain. It is also the source of tendon harvesting for anterior cruciate ligament reconstruction.

The contents of the popliteal fossa (the deepest to the most superficial) include:

- Popliteal artery
- Popliteal vein
- Sciatic nerve (superiorly)
- Tibial and common peroneal nerves (inferiorly)
- Lymph nodes
- Fat
- Popliteus bursa

4. D Superficial peroneal nerve

The leg is divided into four distinct fascial compartments (**Table 7.2**) through the interosseous membrane, the transverse intermuscular septum and the posterior intermuscular septum.

Injury to the tibial nerve leads to loss of ankle/foot plantar flexion with an associated loss of sensation on the plantar aspect of the foot. Injury to the common peroneal nerve can lead to foot drop with loss of ankle/foot dorsiflexion (deep peroneal nerve), loss of ankle/foot eversion (superficial peroneal). Loss of sensation is over the dorsum of the foot (deep peroneal = 1st dorsal web space, superficial peroneal nerve = dorsum of foot; **Figure 7.1**).

Table 7.2 The contents, neurovascular supply and action of the four leg compartments

Compartment	Contents	Neurovascular supply	Movement
Anterior	Tibialis anterior Extensor hallucis longus Extensor digitorum longus Peroneus tertius Deep peroneal nerve Anterior tibial vasculature	Deep peroneal nerve Anterior tibial artery	Dorsiflexors of ankle and toes
Lateral	Peroneus longus Peroneus brevis Superficial peroneal nerve	Superficial peroneal nerve Peroneal artery	Ankle/foot eversion and plantarflexion
Deep posterior	Tibialis posterior Flexor hallucis longus Flexor digitorum longus Popliteus Tibial nerve Posterior tibial vasculature	Tibial nerve Posterior tibial artery	Ankle/foot plantarflexion
Superficial posterior	Gastrocnemius Soleus Plantaris Medial sural cutaneous nerve	Tibial nerve Posterior tibial artery	Ankle/foot plantarflexion

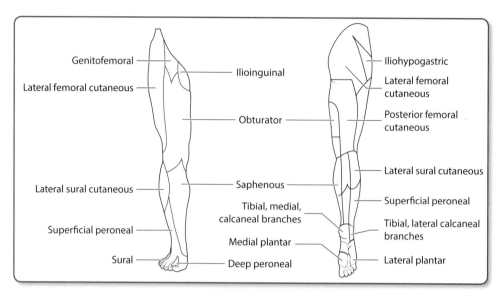

Figure 7.1 Cutaneous nerve supply of the leg and foot.

5. C Saphenous nerve

Important structures that pass anterior to the medial malleolus are the saphenous nerve and saphenous vein. This is a useful site of peripheral access in a patient with circulatory collapse, i.e. saphenous cut down. The structures that are posterior to the medial malleolus are:

- Tibialis posterior tendon   Anterior
- Flexor digitorum longus tendon
- Posterior tibial artery
- Tibial nerve
- Flexor digitorum hallucis tendon   ▼ Posterior

N.B. Mnemonic is **T**om, **D**ick **A**nd a **N**ervous **H**arry

The ankle joint is a synovial hinge type mortise joint with an articulation between the body of the talus and the distal aspects of the tibia and fibula. The ligaments of the ankle joint include:

- The medial deltoid ligament
  - Origin: medial malleolus of tibia
  - Insertion: medial aspect of the talus, sustentaculum tali of the calcaneus, calcaneonavicular ligament, navicular tuberosity
- Lateral
  - Anterior talofibular ligament
  - Posterior talofibular ligament
  - Calcaneofibular ligament

6. C S1

The sciatic nerve (L4–S3) arises from the sacral plexus. Sciatica describes a constellation of symptoms and signs associated with neural compression, due to intervertebral disc compression, of one of the five spinal nerve roots that give rise to the sciatic nerve. The most frequently affected sites are L4/L5 and L5/S1.

The dermatome distribution is shown in **Figure 7.2**. The reflexes in the lower limb are:

- Knee (L3/L4, femoral nerve, quadriceps femoris)
- Ankle (S1, sciatic nerve/tibial division, gastrocnemius)

The myotomes of the lower limb are shown in **Table 7.3**.

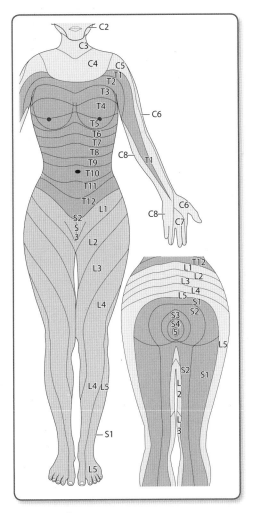

Figure 7.2 Anterior and posterior body dermatomes.

Joint movement	Muscle	Root	Nerve
Hip abduction	Gluteal muscles	L4–S1	Sciatic
Hip adduction	Adductors	L2–L3	Obturator
Hip flexion	Iliopsoas (anterior compartment muscles)	L1–L3	Femoral
Knee extension	Quadriceps femoris	L3–L4	Femoral
Hip extension	Gluteal and posterior compartment muscles	L5–S1	Sciatic
Knee flexion	Hamstrings	L5–S1	Sciatic
Ankle dorsiflexion	Anterior tibial	L4–L5	Common peroneal
Hallux extension	Extensor hallucis longus	L5–S1	Common peroneal
Ankle plantar flexion	Gastrocnemius and soleus	S1–S2	Tibial
Hallux flexion	Flexor hallucis longus	S2–S3	Tibial

Table 7.3 The myotomes of the lower limb

Chapter 8

Homeostasis, coagulation and bleeding

Questions

For each question, select the single best answer from the five options listed.

1. A 60-year-old man has been admitted to hospital unconscious after a car crash with multiple injuries and excessive bleeding in relation to his injuries. He is found to have atrial fibrillation and another occupant of the car (without serious injuries) reports that the unconscious man was taking treatment to prevent complications of his irregular heartbeat.

   Which of the following is most likely to have caused the excessive bleeding?

   A   Deficient heparin level in the blood
   B   Deficient prothrombin level in the blood
   C   Excessive calcium level in the blood
   D   Excessive haematocrit
   E   Excessive vitamin D level in the blood

2. A 60-year-old woman is having open cholecystectomy which has been prolonged by technical difficulties. It is noted that her core temperature has fallen by over a degree since the start of surgery.

   Which of the following is most likely to have caused the fall in core temperature?

   A   An operating theatre temperature in the range 25–30°C
   B   Intravenous fluids administered at around 35°C
   C   Loss of homeostasis due to the anaesthetic
   D   Reaction to propofol administered by the anaesthetist
   E   The patient's increased metabolic rate

3. A 24-year-old man undergoes an uncomplicated appendicectomy for acute appendicitis. Shortly after the end of surgery, in the recovery room, he develops violent shivering and becomes cyanotic.

   Which of the following is most likely to have caused this condition?

   A   Depression of the reflex control of blood oxygen saturation
   B   Exaggeration of the reflex control of body temperature
   C   Low temperature in the recovery room
   D   Septicaemia related to the appendicitis
   E   Undiagnosed cyanotic heart disease

4. A 45-year-old woman presents to the outpatient clinic for preoperative assessment for an elective laparoscopic cholecystectomy. She mentions that that she is concerned about the operation as she has a bleeding tendency with frequent nose bleeds, gum bleeds and commonly finds bruises that she cannot account for. She has had this problem all her life but has not got it investigated.

    Blood tests are taken and show the following:

Test	Result	Reference range
Partial thromboplastin time (PTT)	11 seconds	9.5–13.5 seconds
Activated partial thromboplastin time (APPT)	40 seconds	21–35 seconds
Platelet count	103 ×10⁹/L	15–400 ×10⁹/L
Bleeding time	Increased	
Factor VII levels	Low	

    Which of the following is the most likely diagnosis?

    A   Antiphospholipid syndrome
    B   Haemophilia A
    C   Immune thrombocytopenic purpura
    D   Protein C deficiency
    E   Von Willebrand's disease

5. A 64-year-old man presents with acute bowel obstruction and is scheduled for an emergency laparotomy. He is currently taking warfarin for a postoperative deep venous thrombosis and his INR is 4.2.

    Which of the following will be the most appropriate management of his INR?

    A   Fresh frozen plasma administration
    B   Intravenous vitamin K administration
    C   Oral vitamin K administration
    D   Proceed with surgery and omit the evening dose of warfarin
    E   Prothrombin complex concentrate administration

6. A 55-year-old woman with multiple injuries has developed disseminated intravascular coagulation leading to hypofibrinogenaemia and a risk of excessive haemorrhage.

    Which of the following is most likely to have caused this condition?

    A   Activation of the extrinsic clotting pathway by a drug (extrinsic agent) administered to her
    B   Activation of the extrinsic clotting pathway by products of tissue damage
    C   Activation of the intrinsic clotting pathway by excess calcium ions
    D   Activation of the intrinsic clotting pathway by excess factor VIII levels
    E   Excess production of prothrombin (factor II)

7. A 65-year-old man presents to the emergency department with sudden intense persistent back pain, and a blood pressure of 90/60 mmHg. On examination, a pulsatile abdominal mass is found. A ruptured abdominal aortic aneurysm is suspected. Two large bore cannula are inserted and the patient is scheduled for an immediate open abdominal aortic aneurysm repair.

Which of the following is the most appropriate fluid management?

A   Administer intravenous colloids until patient's systolic blood pressure is normalised

B   Administer intravenous compact red blood cells until patient's systolic blood pressure is high

C   Administer intravenous crystalloids allowing for a slightly lower systolic blood pressure

D   Do not administer any fluids

E   Encourage the patient to drink plenty of fluid

8. A 55-year-old woman complains of a swollen right calf five days after a right hip replacement. On examination, the right calf is enlarged and tender. A duplex ultrasound is performed and is in keeping with a diagnosis of deep vein thrombosis. The patient is very needle-phobic and finds venepuncture extremely distressful.

Which of the following would be the most appropriate management of her deep vein thrombosis?

A   Aspirin

B   Clopidogrel

C   Heparin

D   Rivaroxaban

E   Warfarin

Answers

1. B Deficient prothrombin level in the blood

A deficient prothrombin level is usually due to the effects of warfarin treatment, or to liver disease. This man is likely to be on warfarin treatment which reduces the risk of thrombi forming in his fibrillating atria and throwing off emboli either from the right atrium to the lungs, or from the left atrium to the systemic circulation, including the cerebral circulation to cause a stroke. In this case, the risk of excessive bleeding must be dealt with before surgical intervention.

Options D and E are not associated with haemorrhage; the changes in A and C are the reverse of those which cause haemorrhage.

2. C Loss of homeostasis due to the anaesthetic

Depression of brain function during anaesthesia leads to loss of various homeostatic reflexes (which maintain constancy of blood pressure, core temperature, etc.). Vasodilation produced by anaesthetic drugs leads to excessive heat loss by bringing increased flow of warm blood to the peripheries [warm operating theatres (A) help to reduce the heat loss]. With loss of temperature-regulating reflexes, the vasodilation is unopposed and increased heat production by shivering is not possible. The resting metabolic rate falls somewhat, partly due to decreased brain metabolism [reverse of (E)]. Warming intravenous fluids (B) to around core temperature helps to reduce cooling. Reactions to anaesthetic drugs are more likely to cause hyperthermia than hypothermia (D), though this is a rare problem. Even a degree fall below normal core temperature has an adverse effect on recovery, since mechanisms like haemostasis and healing are impaired.

3. A Depression of the reflex control of blood oxygen saturation

The violent, cyanotic, shivering in the recovery room, as this man recovers from the effects of his anaesthetic suggests that, during the anaesthetic, the loss of body temperature homeostasis due to suppression of brain function allowed his core temperature to fall. With recovery of reflex control of core temperature, vigorous shivering is initiated. However, recovery of homeostatic control of arterial blood oxygenation has lagged behind that of core temperature, due to residual suppression of ventilation, so oxygen intake is unable to keep up with the very large oxygen consumption associated with shivering. Thus, the shivering is normal in relation to restoring body temperature (B). There is no evidence for the other options.

4. E Von Willebrand disease

This patient has a bleeding tendency, an increased bleeding time and activated partial thromboplastin time (APPT) making von Willebrand's disease (VWD) the most likely diagnosis. VWD is a common inherited disease where there is a dysfunction of the von Willebrand factor, a protein responsible for the interaction between platelets and blood vessels. This dysfunction can translate clinically into an increased bleeding time. Another function of the von Willebrand factor is to protect factor VIII from degradation and therefore factor VIII is reduced in VWD. The reduced factor VIII levels are responsible for the increased APPT.

Antiphospholipid syndrome (A) and protein C deficiency (D) results in thromboembolic disease not bleeding tendencies. Immune thrombocytopenic purpura (C) tends to be self-limiting with a reduced platelet count. Haemophilia (B) is X-linked recessive therefore almost always seen in males.

5. E Prothrombin complex concentrate administration

This patient requires his INR reversed as soon as possible and administrating prothrombin complex concentrate (PCC) will be the best option. Prothrombin complex concentrate is derived from human plasma and contains clotting factors II, VII, IX and X. In this case, the patient is at a very high risk of haemorrhage if he undergoes a laparotomy with an INR of 4.2. The warfarin should be reversed so that the INR is 1.5 at the highest. PCC is recommended over fresh frozen plasma (A) as it has a fast onset of action, does not require cross matching of blood groups, can be prepared faster and smaller amounts required for infusion. Oral vitamin K (C) has a slow onset of action and a reduction in INR can take up to 24 hours to come into effect. It therefore has a greater role in reducing INR in elective cases. Intravenous vitamin K (B) is commonly used in combination with PCC in acute situations.

6. B Activation of the extrinsic clotting pathway by products of tissue damage

With multiple injuries, this woman is a typical candidate for the generation of products which activate the extrinsic (extravascular) clotting pathway. These products then enter the blood stream and activate the final stages of the clotting pathway (**Figure 8.1**), by passing the initial intrinsic (intravascular) pathway. Fibrin is laid down widely in the circulation, depleting circulating fibrinogen so that, paradoxically, excessive clotting leads to a risk of excessive bleeding.

7. C Administer intravenous crystalloids allowing for a slightly lower systolic blood pressure

This patient is suffering from a ruptured abdominal aortic aneurysm and it is important that the patient's systolic blood pressure remains permissively low. Keeping the systolic blood pressure slightly lower can help prevent further tearing of the aorta and reduce the blood loss into the abdomen. Giving aggressive fluid

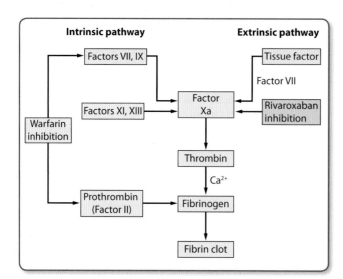

Figure 8.1 The clotting pathway.

therapy is associated with higher mortality. The high fluid input can dilute clotting factors and result in hypothermia leading to an impairment in haemostasis.

8. D Rivaroxaban

This patient needs prophylaxis and is very anxious about venepuncture, making rivaroxaban the treatment of choice. Rivaroxaban is a direct factor Xa inhibitor and is licensed for venous thromboembolism prophylaxis. Unlike warfarin, rivaroxaban is given as a standard dose and serum levels do not need to be monitored. However, there is currently no antidote for rivaroxaban and bleeding can be a challenge to control.

Aspirin and clopidogrel are not used in venous thromboembolism prophylaxis. They have a direct role on platelets and are used in the treatment of myocardial infarctions and ischaemic strokes.

Chapter 9

Temperature regulation

Questions

For each question, select the single best answer from the five options listed.

1. A 25-year-old woman presents with gangrenous changes in both legs. She reports that she has been living rough and has suffered greatly from the recent extremely cold spell (around –10°C at night).

   Which of the following is most likely to have caused this condition?

   A   Abnormal temperature-regulating centre in the basal ganglia
   B   Cerebrally-induced hypothermia
   C   Core temperature maintained by peripheral vasoconstriction
   D   Disorder of the autonomic nerves
   E   Leg skin temperature of only 20–25°C

2. Two 40-year-old men have just been admitted to the emergency department, one with immersion hypothermia and the other with haematemesis. Both have relatively cool peripheries and contracted superficial veins, from which it is difficult to obtain a blood sample.

   Which of the following is most likely to differ between the two men?

   A   Heat exchange between forearm arteries and venae commitantes
   B   Peripheral catecholamine receptors
   C   The level of activity in peripheral sympathetic nerves
   D   The part of the brain initiating vasoconstriction
   E   Total forearm and hand blood flow

3. An 18-year-old woman presents with severely excessive sweating in her hands, which interferes with her daily activities.

   Which of the following is most likely to have caused this condition?

   A   Emotional instability
   B   Over-activity of cholinergic parasympathetic nerves
   C   Over-activity of cholinergic sympathetic nerves
   D   Over-activity of temperature sensitive receptors in her hands
   E   Under-activity of noradrenergic sympathetic nerves

4. A 30-year old woman is attending the gastroenterology clinic with a complaint of severe diarrhoea and weight loss. While waiting in the clinic, she is sweating profusely. Her temperature is normal and pulse rate 110 beats per minute. The temperature in the clinic room is 22°C.

Which of the following is the most likely diagnosis?

A Anxiety neurosis
B Hyperhidrosis
C Inflammatory bowel disease
D Primary thyrotoxicosis
E Sepsis

5. A 25-year-old woman suffers intermittently from cold white hands, particularly in cold weather. During a test period of body warming in a cool environment her hand skin temperature rises, after some time, from 20°C to 35°C on both sides, her pulse rate rises from 65 to 90 beats per minute, and her blood pressure from 115/80 mmHg to 135/80 mmHg.

What is the most likely diagnosis?

A Bilateral arterial disease in the arms
B Early heart failure
C Excessive and dangerous body warming
D Intermittent vasospasm related to sympathetic nervous activity
E Thyrotoxicosis

6. A 16-year-old man is one of a group of young people who have been rescued from a hill walk after they were caught in mist, rain and wind, the environmental temperature being about 5°C. He has cold peripheries and looks exhausted, but can answer questions rationally.

Which of the following is most likely to have caused his condition?

A Early stage of infection
B Frostbite
C Hypoglycaemia
D Hypothermia
E Ventricular fibrillation

7. A 40-year-old woman has been on holiday in a warm locality, where the humidity is low. While sitting in the shade in the garden of her hotel, she began to feel seriously light-headed and nauseated and is advised by an attendant to lie down.

What is the most likely diagnosis?

A Cardiac arrhythmia
B Excessive alcohol intake
C Heat syncope
D Internal haemorrhage
E Myocardial infarction

Answers

1. C Core temperature maintained by peripheral vasoconstriction

This woman is able to respond to questions and to give a history, so her cerebral temperature has been maintained close to normal values (B). The changes in her legs are consistent with a cold injury. This is to be expected in the extremely cold circumstances in which she has been living as the temperature-regulating centres in the hypothalamus (A) have maintained core temperature by intense activity in sympathetic vasoconstrictor nerves in her peripheries. The damage is likely to be due to freezing of the superficial tissues – ice crystals produce irreversible damage. Peripheral nerves cannot conduct their impulses at such low temperatures, so intense pain is not experienced until the peripheries have warmed and the pain fibres resume function, stimulated by the products of tissue damage. 20–25°C is the normal peripheral skin temperature in a cold environment.

2. D The part of the brain initiating vasoconstriction

In the man with hypothermia it is the temperature regulating centre that initiates the peripheral vasoconstriction whereas in the man with haematemesis, it is the blood pressure regulating centre that initiates the peripheral vasoconstriction. The peripheral mechanisms are similar for both men.

Both these men's survival depends on reducing peripheral blood flow. The physiological mechanism for this is intense sympathetic activity. The sympathetic nerves release noradrenaline, which acts on the predominant α-receptors at the surface of vascular smooth muscle cells, resulting in vasoconstriction.

For the man with hypothermia, this almost arrests the blood flow through the peripheries so that core heat is retained. For the man with haematemesis peripheral vasoconstriction maximises the blood volume in the central circulation, reducing the fall in arterial pressure and maintaining the vital cerebral and coronary blood flow.

3. C Over-activity of cholinergic sympathetic nerves

This young woman has hyperhidrosis which interferes with her daily life and should be helped greatly by bilateral cervical sympathectomy. There are no parasympathetic nerves in the limbs (B). Nerves which activate sweat glands are sympathetic nerves which release acetylcholine to cholinergic receptors as an important mechanism for body cooling in a hot environment. Noradrenergic sympathetic nerves (E) are important for promoting peripheral vasoconstriction in a cold environment and also for maintaining arterial blood pressure, particularly in the upright posture. Sympathectomy also severs these constrictor nerves, so that the hand is usually noticeably warmer after sympathectomy. The effects of sympathectomy are immediate dryness and warmth of the corresponding periphery.

With time, the effects may decline. There is no evidence for emotional instability (A) or over-activity of temperature receptors (D).

4. D Primary thyrotoxicosis

A history of diarrhoea, weight loss, excessive sweating and tachycardia in a female should always alert one to the possibility of primary thyrotoxicosis or Graves' disease. This is an autoimmune disease whereby serum immunoglobulin G (IgG) antibodies are produced. These bind to and activate thyroid stimulating hormone receptors, leading to release of excess thyroid hormones – tri-iodothyronine (T_3) and thyroxine (T_4). In thyrotoxicosis, there is increase in the basal metabolic rate which makes the patient very sensitive to heat. As a result, there is increased sympathetic activity to sweat glands thus making the patient sweat profusely. Thyroid function tests should confirm the diagnosis – a rise in T_3 and T_4 and fall in thyroid stimulating hormone.

Hyperhidrosis (B) usually affects limbs, inflammatory bowel disease (C) should not produce tachycardia and the septic patient (E) would usually be very ill with pyrexia.

5. D Intermittent vasospasm related to sympathetic nervous activity

This is a relatively common problem in young women, and it may be relieved by cervical sympathectomy. A sympathetic release test can help to predict the result of sympathectomy and exclude vascular narrowing as a cause of poor blood flow. It is carried out in a cool environment which causes a reflex rise in sympathetic tone to the extremities. The patient's body is then warmed, with the arms kept exposed. In the cool environment hand skin temperature is well below core temperature. Body heating releases the sympathetic tone (a normal response) and hand skin temperature rises towards core values. Such a test confirms that the blood vessels in the arms are normal and that a sympathectomy has a good prognosis. The tachycardia and increased pulse pressure are normal responses to body warming.

6. D Hypothermia

With prolonged rain and wind there is a considerable risk of hypothermia. With serious exhaustion the ability to generate internal heat by activity and increased muscle tone is lost. Frostbite (B) requires freezing of tissues and does not occur at an environmental temperature of 5°C. Ventricular fibrillation (E) is a risk with hypothermia but is not present when the individual is conscious. The picture described does not suggest hypoglycaemia (C) as the primary problem, though exhaustion of energy stores in skeletal muscle is likely. Again the features of early infection (A) do not need to be invoked as the cause of his condition. Careful monitoring to detect cardiac arrhythmias is needed and to avoid early peripheral vasodilation which may carry cold skin blood to the core, depressing core temperature.

7. C Heat syncope

This is a classic case of heat syncope. In hot weather, the combination of reduced fluid intake and increase sweat loss, can result in a depleted blood volume. Meanwhile profound reflex vasodilation in the peripheries to maintain heat loss demands a considerable rise in cardiac output. Thus, the two components of arterial blood pressure (cardiac output and total peripheral resistance) are reduced and blood pressure tends to fall. This can reduce cerebral blood flow in the upright posture.

The combination of mild cerebral ischaemia and a developing vasovagal reflex produce presyncopal symptoms with eventual loss of consciousness and a fall, unless remedial action is taken rapidly. This remedial action consists of adopting the horizontal posture (ideally with the feet raised to augment venous return), drinking a considerable quantity of fluid and getting into a cool environment. Symptoms should rapidly improve, making the other options unlikely.

Chapter 10

Metabolic pathways and abnormalities

Questions

For each question, select the single best answer from the five options listed.

1. A 75-year-old woman with non-insulin dependent diabetes mellitus is on long-term diuretic therapy. She has had a difficult postoperative period after a partial colectomy, and is still on intravenous fluids. Recently, she has become increasingly confused and her blood osmolality is below normal.

    Which of the following is most likely to have caused her confusion?

    A   A blood glucose level of 10 mmol/L
    B   A blood urea level of 10 mmol/L
    C   A raised plasma sodium level
    D   Both blood urea and glucose elevated to 10 mmol/L
    E   Cerebral cellular overhydration

2. A 10-year-old boy with insulin-dependent diabetes mellitus has developed vomiting and is becoming drowsy and confused. His pulse is weak, with a rate of 100 beats per minute; blood pressure is 80/60 mmHg.

    Which of the following best explains his condition?

    A   Blood osmolality is rising due to increased sodium and chloride levels
    B   Cellular energy is derived from an excessive fat to carbohydrate ratio
    C   His pH is above 7.5 and is rising steadily
    D   Intracellular volume is falling, while extracellular volume is rising
    E   Vomiting is adding directly to his acid–base disturbance

3. A 55-year-old man undergoes a transfusion with 15 units of blood, following catastrophic bleeding from a gastric ulcer. He develops pulmonary damage and is transferred to the intensive care unit for ventilation with an increased oxygen concentration. His PO_2 is 8 kPa, PCO_2 4 kPa and pH 7.31.

    Which of the following is most likely to have caused these results?

    A   Anaemic hypoxia
    B   Brain damage causing under ventilation
    C   Ketoacidosis
    D   Hypoxic hypoxia with lactic acidosis
    E   Widespread haemolysis

4. A 20-year-old man presents following a car crash and is in a relatively stable state after initial resuscitation.

    Which of the following is most likely to maintain life after this severe physical stress?

    A   A negative sodium balance
    B   A positive nitrogen balance
    C   Depression of adrenocorticotrophic hormone secretion
    D   Glucocorticoid induced gluconeogenesis
    E   Hormonal reduction of breakdown of muscle proteins

5. A 40-year-old man presents with established hepatic disease and a preoperative coagulation screen shows an INR of 2.0.

    Which of the following metabolic disturbances is most likely to have caused this result?

    A   Decreased cholesterol in the bile
    B   Decreased conjugation of bilirubin
    C   Decreased formation of prothrombin
    D   Increased formation of bile acids
    E   Increased formation of fibrinogen

6. A 40-year-old woman is advised to lose 30 kg of body weight prior to surgery.

    Which of the following is the most effective dietary management of this woman?

    A   Energy intake equal to metabolic requirements plus 10%
    B   Her present food intake plus weight-losing drugs
    C   Less energy intake than metabolic requirements
    D   Most of her energy should be derived from fat
    E   She should eat only carbohydrate and protein

7. A 30-year-old woman presents with a fractured femur after a road traffic accident. For some years previously she had been receiving parenteral nutrition following surgical removal of a large portion of small bowel.

    Which is the most appropriate management of her parenteral nutrition?

    A   Decreased amino acid content
    B   Decreased lipid content
    C   Increased energy content
    D   Increased sodium content
    E   No change in her usual nutrition

8. A 50-year-old man with chronic liver failure presents with bleeding oesophageal varices, which is treated successfully. Next day he is stable, apart from moderate drowsiness. His outstretched arms show irregular flapping.

    Which of the following is most likely to have caused his drowsiness?

    A   Absorption of altered blood from the gut
    B   An increased blood urea level
    C   Cerebral damage related to hypotension
    D   Continued oesophageal bleeding
    E   Hypoglycaemia

Answers

1. E Cerebral cellular overhydration

The disturbances in blood glucose (A), urea (B), plasma sodium (C) and blood glucose and urea combined (D) all cause increased blood osmolality. A decreased blood osmolality implies an excess of body water in relation to dissolved components. This applies in all body fluids, since cell membranes and capillary walls in general are freely permeable to water. The most serious effects are experienced in the brain, because swelling of brain cells raises intracranial pressure, progressive and potentially fatal loss of brain function. This woman has had prolonged treatment with intravenous fluids and diuretics leading to over-dilution of body fluids. Low sodium and chloride levels make a major contribution to the low blood osmolality.

2. B Cellular energy is derived from an excessive fat to carbohydrate ratio

This boy is suffering from diabetic ketoacidosis. Insulin is required to promote the uptake of glucose into most energy-consuming cells, (brain cells are an exception). Cells must then derive most of their energy from fat and this leads to ketoacidosis which involves production of a huge excess of hydrogen ions.

Acidosis implies that the pH has fallen below 7.35 (C). Blood osmolality (A) is rising due to increased blood glucose. Glucose normally contributes about 5 mmol but this rises typically to 20–30 mmol because glucose is not entering the cells. The greatly increased blood glucose level causes an osmotic diuresis, which depletes all compartments of body water (D), resulting in hypotension and compensatory tachycardia. Vomiting, by loss of gastric acid, compensates in a minor way for the acidosis (E) which is overwhelmed by further serious loss of body fluid requiring immediate intravenous fluids and insulin replacement.

3. D Hypoxic hypoxia with lactic acidosis

This man developed pulmonary damage secondary to severe blood loss and massive blood transfusion (defined as a volume of transfusion equal to or greater than the patient's blood volume). Oxygen transport is severely impaired and this is one cause of hypoxic hypoxia (the other being a reduced inspired oxygen level). With severe hypoxia, mitochondrial oxygenation and generation of ATP may be inadequate, so anaerobic glycolysis can increase ATP to a just adequate level for survival. Anaerobic glycolysis produces lactic acidosis, a metabolic (or nonrespiratory) acidosis. A 5- to 10-fold increase in blood lactic acid is typical. There is no suggestion of residual anaemia (A) or of brain damage with under ventilation (B). Ketoacidosis (C) and widespread haemolysis (E) also are not supported by information given.

4. D Glucocorticoid induced gluconeogenesis

A major component of the stress response is a surge of cortisol. This is produced by release from the hypothalamus of corticotrophin releasing hormone which in turn releases adrenocorticotrophic hormone from the anterior pituitary (C). This releases cortisol from the adrenal cortex. If this mechanism fails at any point survival after severe physical stress depends on the administration of exogenous glucocorticoid.

The cortisol surge favours survival in various ways, but a major component is mobilisation of glucose for energy by diverting amino acids from protein repair to glucose synthesis in the liver. Thus body protein, particularly in skeletal muscle, is broken down (E). The excess nitrogen is excreted in the urine, giving a negative rather than a positive nitrogen balance (B). High levels of cortisol also contribute by their secondary mineralocorticoid action on the kidneys to retain sodium and chloride (A) and secondarily water, thus helping to maintain the circulation.

5. C Decreased formation of prothrombin

A major cause of a prolonged coagulation time and hence excessive bleeding in patients with liver disease is inadequate synthesis of prothrombin and other vitamin K dependent coagulation factors. Bilirubin metabolism (A) does not affect coagulation, nor does cholesterol (C). In liver disease formation of bile acids may be reduced, not increased (D) and this may hinder vitamin K absorption and prothrombin synthesis. This is also a problem in obstructive jaundice where bile acids as well as bilirubin may fail to reach the gut. Fibrinogen deficiency, not excess (E) is also a cause of bleeding.

6. C Less energy intake than metabolic requirements

It is essential for weight loss that energy use should exceed energy intake. The extent of the reduction can be related to the urgency of the situation. During dieting, all of the basic nutrients – fat, carbohydrate, protein, vitamins, trace elements and fibre are required for health. Energy for metabolic requirements, plus an additional 10% (A) would lead to weight increase; weight-losing drugs (B) also breach the requirement for decreased energy intake, and there are many and serious side effects of using such drugs. A high fat diet (D) does not allow the normal Krebs cycle to take place in mitochondria and carries the danger of ketoacidosis. The other unbalanced intake (E) would lead to deficiency of fat-soluble vitamins and an unpalatable and unhealthy diet. Normally energy is derived from a blend of fat and carbohydrate.

7. C Increased energy content

During the stress reaction the resting metabolic rate increases due to the various energy-consuming activities associated with survival. This requires a corresponding increase in the overall energy content of her diet, with increased, rather than decreased amino acids (A). Decreasing the lipid content (B) would risk inadequate total energy content.

8. A Absorption of altered blood from the gut

With bleeding oesophageal varices a variable amount of the blood proceeds along the gut and is absorbed. This constitutes a high protein load from broken down haemoglobin and plasma proteins. People with liver failure have impaired ability to deal with the products of a high protein meal, due to impaired conjugation and metabolism of toxins derived, with the help of bacteria, from protein. Urea formation from ammonia tends to be one of the detoxification functions that are depressed, so increased blood urea level (B) is inappropriate. No evidence is given to support the other options.

Chapter 11

Fluid balance

Questions

For each question, select the single best answer from the five options listed.

1. A 5-year-old boy presents to the paediatric surgery department with a 24-hour history of abdominal pain. His history and examination findings are consistent with a diagnosis of acute appendicitis. He is dehydrated with an estimated fluid deficit of 15%.

    Which of the following is the most appropriate resuscitation fluid?

    A   Packed red blood cells
    B   5% dextrose and 0.45% sodium chloride
    C   10% dextrose and 0.18% sodium chloride
    D   0.9% sodium chloride
    E   3% sodium chloride

2. A 67-year-old woman weighing 50 kg undergoes mastectomy for breast cancer. Intraoperative blood loss is 525 mL.

    This blood loss is what percentage of her estimated blood volume?

    A   5%
    B   10%
    C   15%
    D   20%
    E   25%

3. A 43-year-old man who has been involved in a road traffic accident is hypotensive and tachycardic in the resuscitation area of the emergency department. A CT scan shows a ruptured spleen with an estimated 1500 mL blood in the abdominal cavity.

    In the response to acute hypovolaemia, which of the following acts to restore an adequate circulating volume?

    A   Decreased antidiuretic hormone release
    B   Increased activation of the carotid bodies
    C   Increased activation of the parasympathetic nervous system
    D   Increased renin release
    E   Redistribution of blood from the renal medulla to the renal cortex

4. A 34-year-old man presents to the surgical admissions department with a history suggestive of acute gallstone pancreatitis. Intravenous rehydration with Hartmann's solution is commenced.

    Which of the following is the most likely ionic composition of Hartmann's solution?

    A   Calcium 20 mmol/L
    B   Chloride 111 mmol/L
    C   Lactate 10 mmol/L
    D   Potassium 15 mmol/L
    E   Sodium 154 mmol/L

5. A 64-year-old man presents with symptoms of a perforated gastric ulcer. He was dehydrated on admission and received 3 L of 0.9% sodium chloride for fluid resuscitation.

    Which of the following is the most likely biochemical derangement in this patient?

    A   Hyperchloraemic metabolic acidosis
    B   Hyperchloraemic metabolic alkalosis
    C   Hypernatraemic metabolic acidosis
    D   Hypochloraemic metabolic acidosis
    E   Hypochloraemic metabolic alkalosis

6. A 24-year-old healthy man weighing 70 kg is awaiting elective circumcision. The theatre list has been delayed so he has been given 1000 mL of 5% dextrose on the ward whilst he was waiting.

    Which of the following volumes is the interstitial fluid compartment most likely to increase?

    A   80 mL
    B   250 mL
    C   330 mL
    D   670 mL
    E   1000 mL

Answers

1. D 0.9% sodium chloride

The most appropriate choice of fluid is 0.9% sodium chloride. In the past, fluid prescribers have been advised to limit the sodium load in children, but the National Patient Safety Agency issued an alert in 2007 highlighting the dangers of hyponatraemia in children resulting from the administration of large volumes of hypotonic fluids, e.g. 0.18% and 0.45% sodium chloride. Packed red cells would not be indicated when there is only a 15% fluid deficit.

Although 4%/0.18% dextrose/saline and 5% dextrose are important sources of free water for maintenance, these should be used with caution in children because of the risk of dangerous hyponatraemia with excessive amounts, and that with some provisos they are not appropriate for replacement therapy.

2. C 15%

In this patient, estimated blood volume should be calculated using 70 mL/kg, i.e. 3500 mL, so 525 mL is 15% of the patient's estimated blood volume. In obese patients, this method would lead to an overestimate of blood volume so a value of 45–55 mL/kg of actual body weight would be used. Young children have a higher blood volume by weight approximately 80–90 mL/kg.

This should be judged in its clinical context because intraoperative blood loss is difficult to estimate, so heart rate, blood pressure, capillary refill time, peripheral perfusion, urine output, etc. should be considered in conjunction with any estimated blood loss. Postoperatively a drain can be useful in gauging ongoing blood loss but remember that drains can become blocked or be dislodged so they may not fill even in the context of significant bleeding.

3. D Increased renin release

The decreased venous return and cardiac preload seen in acute hypovolaemia cause a reduction in cardiac output and blood pressure falls. The first response is an increase in sympathetic activity in order to attempt to maintain perfusion of vital structures and restore cardiac output. The increase in sympathetic discharge is mediated by a decrease in the afferent activity of the carotid sinus baroreceptors to the dorsal hypothalamus.

The hypothalamo-pituitary-adrenal response is slower. Renin release is triggered by decreased renal blood flow and ultimately leads to the formation of angiotensin II within the lung. Renin is not only a potent arteriolar vasoconstrictor but also stimulates release of antidiuretic hormone from the posterior pituitary and aldosterone from the adrenal cortex. Antidiuretic hormone and aldosterone both enhance water and sodium reabsorption at the distal renal tubule. Redistribution of blood from the cortex to the medulla enhances sodium and water reabsorption.

4. B Chloride 111 mmol/L

Hartmann's is a balanced crystalloid electrolyte solution, which is isotonic with plasma. As shown in **Table 11.1**, it has a lower chloride and sodium content than 0.9% sodium chloride so helps to avoid problems with hyperchloraemic acidosis when large volumes are infused.

Lactate is metabolised by the liver to produce bicarbonate. Some groups advocate avoiding Hartmann's solution in patients with diabetes because of the risk of metabolism of one of the lactate isomers to glucose, but in clinical practice this effect is minimal. In addition, patients in hepatic failure may be at risk of lactate accumulation and acidosis if hepatic lactate metabolism is impaired. Potassium may accumulate in patients with significant renal failure.

Table 11.1 Comparison of the ionic composition of 0.9% sodium chloride and Hartmann's solution						
	Ionic composition (mmol/L)					
	Sodium	Potassium	Calcium	Chloride	Lactate	pH
0.9% sodium chloride	154	0	0	154	0	5.0
Hartmann's solution	131	5	2	111	29	6.5

5. A Hyperchloraemic metabolic acidosis

After the administration of a large volume of 0.9% saline, the most likely biochemical derangement is hyperchloraemic metabolic acidosis. This can be avoided by using a more balanced salt solution, such as Hartmann's solution (except when there is hypochloraemia, e.g. from vomiting). Stewart's theory of acid–base balance states that the strong ion difference, the total concentration of weak acids in the plasma and $PaCO_2$ are the three independent variables which determine acid–base balance. Strong ion difference can be calculated by subtracting the sum of the chloride and lactate concentrations from the sum of the sodium and potassium concentrations. An increase in the concentration of chloride ions as seen after infusion of 0.9% sodium chloride will decrease the strong ion difference and cause a metabolic acidosis to develop.

6. B 250 mL

Dextrose 5% is a way of administering free water because the glucose is rapidly taken up into cells. Dextrose 5% can be used for rehydration of the intracellular compartment, but will have negligible effect on the intravascular volume. As shown in **Figure 11.1**, in men 60% of body weight (3/5) is water, so in a 70 kg male total body water is approximately 42 L; two-thirds of this is intracellular and one-third extracellular. Dextrose 5% will equilibrate throughout all of the fluid compartments so two-thirds or approximately 670 mL will enter the intracellular space and one-third or approximately 330 mL will enter the extracellular space.

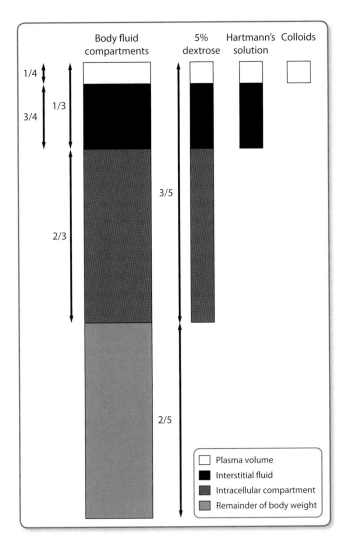

Figure 11.1 The relative sizes of body fluid compartments and distribution of three infusion fluids.

The extracellular space comprises the interstitial fluid, which accounts for 75% by volume, and the intravascular space, which accounts for 25% by volume. Therefore, approximately 250 mL will enter the interstitial fluid, leaving only 80 mL in the intravascular compartment.

Chapter 12

Sepsis and shock

Questions

For each question, select the single best answer from the five options listed.

1. A 32-year-old man is in the resuscitation bay of the emergency department. He is complaining of abdominal pain after being a restrained passenger in a road traffic accident. His heart rate is 128 beats per minute, blood pressure is 91/72 mmHg and respiratory rate is 38 breaths per minute. There are no obvious signs of head injury, but he appears confused. He has passed 10 mL of urine in the last hour via the urinary catheter

   How much blood loss is likely as a percentage of blood volume?

   A   Up to 15%
   B   15–30%
   C   30–40%
   D   At least 40%
   E   Not enough information to determine this

2. A 49-year-old woman with known rheumatoid arthritis on immunosuppression therapy presents with a 2-day history of a painful, red and swollen knee joint. Urgent gram staining of fluid aspirated from the knee reveals gram-positive cocci. The patient is developing septic shock.

   Which of the following factors is most closely associated with lower mortality in septic shock?

   A   Advanced age
   B   Gram-positive sepsis
   C   Presence of three or more organ failures
   D   Prior immunocompromise
   E   Unidentified source of sepsis

3. A 24-year-old man has fallen two storeys from the roof of a house. He has a Glasgow coma scale of 15 and is complaining of pain in his back. On arrival in the emergency department, he is hypotensive with warm peripheries despite 2 L of Hartmann's solution. Following primary and secondary survey, the only injury identified on a CT scan is a burst fracture of T10 with significant impingement of the spinal canal.

    In neurogenic shock, which is the most important contributor to hypotension?

    A   Decreased circulating volume
    B   Decreased parasympathetic tone
    C   Increased sympathetic tone
    D   Increased systemic vascular resistance
    E   Increased venous capacitance

4. An 84-year-old man is in the surgical high dependency unit the morning following laparotomy for a perforated duodenal ulcer. He had an episode of chest pain and dyspnoea overnight and is now hypotensive and tachycardic with cool peripheries and a raised jugular venous pressure. He is thought to be in cardiogenic shock and is awaiting transfer to the intensive care unit.

    Which is the most common postoperative cause of cardiogenic shock?

    A   Hypovolaemia
    B   Myocardial infarction
    C   Pericardial tamponade
    D   Pulmonary embolus
    E   Ventricular fibrillation

5. A 23-year-old woman is under general anaesthesia for tonsillectomy. The anaesthetist requests that surgery does not commence, since the patient is tachycardic and hypotensive, and the anaesthetist is concerned that the patient is in anaphylactic shock.

    Which is the most common cause of anaphylaxis under anaesthesia?

    A   Antibiotics, e.g. co-amoxiclav
    B   Colloids, e.g. gelofusine
    C   Induction agent, e.g. thiopentone
    D   Latex, e.g. surgical gloves
    E   Muscle relaxants, e.g. suxamethonium

6. A 67-year-old man presents to the emergency department with abdominal pain, jaundice and pyrexia suggestive of acute cholangitis. He is tachycardic and hypotensive. The consultant asks for the Surviving Sepsis Resuscitation bundle to be commenced.

    Which of the following is the most appropriate initial management?

    A   Administer broad spectrum antibiotic within 24 hours of admission
    B   Blood cultures are not essential if broad spectrum antibiotics are used
    C   Consider vasopressors if hypotension does not respond to minimum 20 mL/kg initial fluid resuscitation
    D   Maintain central venous pressure >12 mmHg
    E   Measure lactate on an arterial blood sample

Answers

1. C 30–40%

Shock is a term used to describe a state in which organ and tissue perfusion is inadequate. Hypovolaemic shock can be haemorrhagic or non-haemorrhagic in aetiology. Causes of non-haemorrhagic hypovolaemic shock include pancreatitis and intestinal obstruction. Haemorrhagic shock can follow rupture of an abdominal aortic aneurysm or trauma. The source of bleeding may not always be obvious – remember to think about a femoral fracture, chest injury, abdominal injury and blood loss onto the floor or at the scene. A significant percentage of blood volume can be lost before a young fit patient is no longer able to compensate and displays abnormal physiology. **Table 12.1** helps to estimate the percentage of circulating volume lost based on the physiological parameters observed.

Table 12.1 Recognising different classes of hypovolaemic shock				
	Class I	Class II	Class III	Class IV
Percentage blood volume	< 15	15–30	30–40	>40
Heart rate (beats per minute)	<100	>100	>120	>140
Blood pressure	Normal	Normal	↓	↓
Pulse pressure	Normal or ↑	↓	↓	↓
Respiratory rate (breaths per minute)	14–20	20–30	30–40	>35
Urine output (mL/h)	>30	20–30	5–15	Negligible
Cognitive state	Slight anxiety	Mild anxiety	Anxiety, confusion	Confusion, lethargy
Fluid response	Good response	Good response	Transient responder	No response

2. B Gram-positive sepsis

Overall mortality from septic shock is approximately 50%. Gram-negative sepsis, multi-organ failure, advancing age, co-morbidity and immunosuppression all increase mortality.

In septic shock, hypotension persists despite adequate fluid resuscitation and there is evidence of inadequate end organ perfusion, e.g. lactic acidosis or oliguria. Initially the circulation may be hyperdynamic and cardiac output increased but in latter stages hypotension with vasoconstriction may be seen especially in cases where the myocardium becomes ischaemic or there is hypovolaemia.

Septic shock is characterised by increased endothelial and capillary permeability, decreased systemic vascular resistance with relative hypovolaemia, impaired oxygen extraction and utilisation despite normal oxygen delivery and decreased myocardial contractility.

Management is largely supportive and efforts should be made to identify and treat the underlying cause. Few specific therapies exist, activated protein C had shown promise in recent years, but recently has been withdrawn as there is insufficient evidence to support its safe use.

3. E Increased venous capacitance

Neurogenic shock results from the loss of sympathetic outflow. Sympathetic tone and systemic vascular resistance are decreased, and venous capacitance is increased leading to hypotension. If the spinal cord injury is above the cardiac sympathetic supply (T1–T4) severe bradycardia and hypotension can occur. However, both bradycardia (resulting from unopposed vagal activity or hypoxia) and tachycardia (from relative intravascular depletion) may be seen. Spinal cord injury, severe head injury and high spinal anaesthesia are all potential causes of neurogenic shock. The terms spinal and neurogenic are not interchangeable; spinal shock describes a neurological deficit with no haemodynamic embarrassment characterised by flaccidity and loss of reflexes.

Neurogenic shock should be suspected in patients who behave as transient responders to fluid challenges with no source of bleeding and an appropriate mechanism of injury. Spinal cord injury should be managed in the same way as any trauma using ATLS principles. Intubation and mechanical ventilation may be required if the injury is above C3–C5 or if there is an associated head injury for airway protection or manipulation of PaO_2 and $PaCO_2$ if there are concerns regarding raised intracranial pressure.

4. B Myocardial infarction

Cardiogenic shock occurs when the heart fails to generate adequate cardiac output to maintain tissue perfusion due to failure of the ventricles to function effectively. Causes can either be intrinsic, e.g. acute myocardial infarction, or extrinsic, e.g. massive pulmonary embolism, tension pneumothorax and pericardial tamponade. In this case, myocardial infarction is most likely.

Treatment is generally supportive whilst the cause of ventricular failure is treated, e.g. percutaneous coronary intervention or drainage of a tamponade. Cardiogenic shock is a low cardiac output state with high cardiac filling pressures and high systemic vascular resistance. Supportive management of cardiogenic shock includes optimising preload, cardiac contractility, and afterload.

5. E Muscle relaxants, e.g. suxamethonium

The most common cause of anaphylaxis under anaesthesia is neuromuscular blocking agents. Other common causes include latex, antibiotics and colloids. Anaphylaxis is a Type 1 IgE-mediated immune response, which leads to release of histamine and other compounds from mast cells and basophils. Its onset is acute and causes life-threatening compromise of airway, breathing and circulation. An anaphylactic reaction is as a result of non-specific histamine release without prior sensitisation.

The approach to a patient with suspected anaphylaxis should be in an ABC manner. Whilst histamine mediates many of the clinical signs and symptoms, initial treatment should be with adrenaline; either 0.5–1 mg intramuscularly or 50–100 μg increments intravenously, with an antihistamine and steroid being administered as part of ongoing management. A fluid challenge should also be given but colloid should be stopped as this may be the cause of anaphylaxis. Consideration should be given to securing the airway with an endotracheal tube early because of worsening laryngeal oedema, but this should not delay administration of adrenaline.

Working Group of the Resuscitation Council (UK). Emergency treatment of anaphylactic reactions. Guidelines for healthcare providers. London: Resuscitation Council (UK), 2012.

6. C Consider vasopressors if hypotension does not respond to minimum 20 mL/kg initial fluid resuscitation

The Surviving Sepsis Campaign is a global initiative, which aims to reduce mortality from sepsis. The first 6-hour resuscitation bundle includes obtaining blood cultures prior to antibiotic administration, the measurement of serum lactate (from either a venous or arterial sample) and the administration of broad-spectrum antibiotics, administered within 2 hours of admission/diagnosis. For every hour antibiotic therapy is delayed after the onset of septic shock, the patient's chance of survival is reduced by almost 8%.

A large, randomised study demonstrated that early resuscitation with clear targets including central venous pressure, central venous oxygen saturation, lactate and mean arterial pressure achieved a reduction in in-hospital mortality from 44% to 29%.

The early goal directed therapy component of the resuscitation bundle is required if mean arterial pressure <65 mmHg or lactate >4 mmol/L.

Rivers E, Nguyen B, Havstad S, et al. Early goal-directed therapy in the treatment of severe sepsis and septic shock. NEJM 2001; 345:1368–77.

Chapter 13

Central nervous system

Questions

For each question, select the single best answer from the five options listed.

1. A 34-year-old man is admitted to the intensive care unit. He has been assaulted and sustained a significant head injury. He is normally fit and well.

   Which of the following parameters is most likely to increase cerebral blood flow?

   A   Central venous pressure 18 mmHg
   B   Core temperature 37.4°C
   C   Mean arterial pressure 90 mmHg
   D $PaCO_2$ 4.0 kPa
   E PaO_2 6.7 kPa

2. An 18-year-old woman with a ventriculoperitoneal shunt, which was inserted in childhood for hydrocephalus, presents with acute onset confusion. A sample of cerebrospinal fluid is taken from the device for sending to the laboratories for analysis.

   Which of the following results is abnormal?

   A   Glucose: 4.4 mmol/L (plasma value is 4.7 mmol/L)
   B   Opening pressure: 22 mmHg
   C   Protein: 0.3 g/L
   D   Red blood cell count: 2×10^6/L
   E   White cell count: 2×10^6/L

3. A 49-year-old man presents to the emergency department. The patient's history is unclear but he was found to be unresponsive by his wife when she awoke this morning so she called an ambulance. He has a recent history of worsening headache. His heart rate is 43 beats per minute, blood pressure is 170/90 mmHg and respiratory rate 14 breaths per minute. On examination, there are no localising signs but papilloedema is present.

   Which systemic effect is most commonly seen in patients with severely raised intracranial pressure?

   A   Decreased blood pressure
   B   Decreased heart rate
   C   Decreased pulse pressure
   D   Increased respiratory rate
   E   Nausea but no vomiting

4. A 63-year-old woman is admitted with a Gustilo grade III open fracture of her right ankle. She is taken to theatre that evening for debridement of the wound and definitive fixation under spinal anaesthesia. She returns to theatre 48 hours later for wound inspection and delayed closure. On the evening ward round, she is found to be agitated and confused.

    Which of the following is the most likely cause of her postoperative cognitive dysfunction?

    A   Higher level of education
    B   Perioperative hypotension
    C   Preoperative benzodiazepine use
    D   Regional rather than general anaesthetic technique
    E   Repeat surgery

5. A 77-year-old man is in the surgical ward one day following laparoscope-assisted anterior resection for bowel cancer. His family report that he seems confused. On review of the patient's drug chart, it is observed that he has received a number of drugs in the previous 24 hours.

    Which of the following drugs is the most likely cause of his postoperative cognitive dysfunction?

    A   Atropine
    B   Donepezil
    C   Levobupivacaine
    D   Paracetamol
    E   Remifentanil

6. A 64-year-old woman presents to the emergency department with a 2-week history of headache, fluctuating conscious level and slurred speech. She has a history of alcohol excess and hypertension for which she is not compliant with treatment. A CT scan reveals a subacute subdural haematoma.

    How is cerebral blood flow autoregulation most likely to be affected by chronic hypertension?

    A   Autoregulation curve is shifted to the left
    B   Autoregulation curve is shifted to the right
    C   Impaired at high mean arterial pressures
    D   Impaired at low mean arterial pressures
    E   Unchanged

7. A 24-year-old man is admitted to the intensive care unit following a bicycle accident where he sustained an isolated head injury. There has been some concern regarding raised intracranial pressure so a monitor has been inserted. Current observations show: blood pressure 115/78 mmHg (MAP 90 mmHg), heart rate 78 beats per minute, SpO_2 98% with FiO_2 0.35, central venous pressure +10 mmHg and intracranial pressure 20 cmH$_2$O (15 mmHg).

What is his cerebral perfusion pressure?

A 60 mmHg
B 65 mmHg
C 70 mmHg
D 90 mmHg
E 100 mmHg

Answers

1. E PaO$_2$ 6.7 kPa

The brain receives 14% of cardiac output, with the grey matter receiving twice as much blood flow as the white matter. When intracranial pressure is raised, it can be helpful to reduce cerebral blood volume to provide a temporary reduction in intracranial pressure.

Cerebral blood flow (CBF) is determined by a number of factors:

- PaCO$_2$: a reduction in CO$_2$ reduces cerebral blood flow. There is a linear relationship between PaCO$_2$ and CBF between 4 and 12 kPa (**Figure 13.1**)
- PaO$_2$: when PaO$_2$ decreases below 8 kPa there is a rapid increase. In the patient in this scenario, efforts should be made to increase PaCO$_2$ (**Figure 13.1**)
- Mean arterial pressure (MAP): a MAP of 90 mmHg falls well within the limits of cerebral autoregulation, so CBF is independent of MAP in a normal brain. However, in head injury this may be disrupted
- Temperature: CBF drops by 5% per degree Celsius drop in temperature hence the interest in therapeutic hypothermia in head injury
- Central venous pressure: helps to determine cerebral perfusion pressure but this will not directly affect CBF

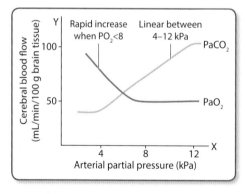

Figure 13.1 Effect of arterial oxygen and carbon dioxide tension on cerebral blood flow. When hypoxaemia (PaO$_2$ < 8 kPa) occurs, cerebral blood flow markedly increases in an attempt to maintain cerebral oxygenation. There is a linear relationship between PaCO$_2$ and cerebral blood flow between 4 and 12 kPa. When PaCO$_2$ is <4 kPa, maximal vasoconstriction has occurred so cerebral blood flow is independent of PaCO$_2$. When PaCO$_2$ is >12 kPa maximal vasodilatation has occurred, so no further increase in cerebral blood flow is seen.

2. B Opening pressure: 22 mmHg

Hydrocephalus refers to an increased cerebrospinal fluid (CSF) volume due to increased production (rare) or impaired drainage. To relieve hydrocephalus, ventriculoperitoneal shunts can be inserted into the lateral ventricle to drain CSF into the peritoneum via a catheter tunnelled under the skin. The shunt can become blocked or infected leading to symptoms and signs of raised intracranial pressure or central nervous system infection. There is usually a valve through which a sample can be obtained using a needle and the opening pressure of the system can be measured to aid diagnosis. Normal CSF parameters are shown in **Table 13.1**.

Cerebrospinal fluid occupies the space between the arachnoid mater and the pia mater and also is contained within the ventricles, cisterns and sulci of the brain and the central canal of the spinal cord.

It serves several main purposes:

- **Buoyancy:** the mass of the human brain is approximately 1.4 kg; however, the effective weight of the brain suspended in CSF is 50 grams.
- **Protection:** CSF cushions the brain tissue from injury when jolted or hit.
- **Chemical stability:** CSF maintains a constant ionic environment for the cells of the central nervous system and may act as a transport system for neurotransmitters and hormones. CSF flow facilitates provision of nutrients for neuronal and glial cells and clearance of metabolic waste from the central nervous system.
- **Prevention of brain ischemia:** CSF can partially buffer changes in intracranial pressure by redistribution from the intracranial to extracranial subarachnoid space.

Table 13.1 Normal cerebrospinal fluid values	
White cell count	0–5 x 10^6 cells/L (lymphocytes only, no neutrophils)
Red cell count	0–10 x 10^6 cells/L
Glucose	3.3–4.4 mmol/L or ≥60% of plasma
Protein	0.2–0.4 g/L
Opening pressure	7–18 cmH$_2$O

3. B Decreased heart rate

The Monro–Kellie hypothesis views the skull as a rigid box, which contains brain tissue, blood and cerebrospinal fluid. There is little scope for compensation but if one component increases in volume, there must be a corresponding decrease in another otherwise intracranial pressure increases. Once this increases above a certain threshold, perfusion will be compromised and critical ischaemia will eventually develop.

Symptoms and signs depend on whether the rise in intracranial pressure has occurred acutely or is a more chronic process. Systemic signs include hypertension and reflex bradycardia as part of Cushing's reflex. Pulse pressure is increased. Cushing's triad is constituted by papilloedema, bradycardia and abnormal respiration (usually a decrease in respiratory rate). Intracranial pressure can reach a critical point leading to brain herniation.

4. E Repeat surgery

In a cohort of 1200 postoperative patients of greater than 60 years of age, the incidence of postoperative cognitive dysfunction (POCD) was around 25% at 1 week and 10% at 3 months postoperatively. It is more common in patients with pre-existing cognitive dysfunction and a higher level of education seems to be protective. Surprisingly, preoperative benzodiazepine use is protective and perioperative hypotension and hypoxaemia have not been demonstrated to be risk factors. Types of surgery, which are higher risk, include cardiac, carotid and neurosurgery especially prolonged or repeat surgery.

In 40% of cases, there is no identifiable cause for POCD. Early causes within hours of surgery include residual anaesthetic agents, pain and opioid analgesia, hypoxaemia, hypotension, hypoglycaemia and intraoperative stroke. Causes which account for the development of POCD in the days following surgery include sepsis and organ failure, withdrawal from alcohol, nicotine or regular drugs and sleep deprivation or disruption.

5. A Atropine

Atropine crosses the blood–brain barrier (BBB) and has central anticholinergic actions, which have an adverse effect on cognitive function. The other drugs do not cross the BBB, making atropine the most likely cause.

6. B Autoregulation curve is shifted to the right

Autoregulation describes the process by which cerebral blood flow is maintained at a constant level in a normal brain despite fluctuations in blood pressure. This may be impaired by drugs, e.g. anaesthetic agents or disease states, e.g. head injury in the acute phase of subarachnoid haemorrhage.

In chronic hypertension, the whole curve is shifted to the right. In treated hypertension, with time the autoregulation curve returns towards normal values. This is important because in patients with chronic hypertension, a higher mean arterial pressure may need to be achieved to maintain adequate cerebral perfusion. Under general anaesthesia, the whole curve is shifted to the left as illustrated in **Figure 13.2**.

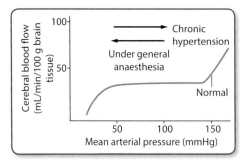

Figure 13.2 Effect of mean arterial blood pressure (MAP) on cerebral blood flow. Cerebral blood flow is independent of mean arterial pressure between 50 and 150 mmHg. Above 150 mmHg, cerebral blood flow increases passively with MAP. Below a MAP of 50 mmHg, the autoregulation mechanisms are unable to maintain normal cerebral blood flow so it decreases markedly.

7. B 65 mmHg

The equation used to calculate cerebral perfusion pressure is:

Cerebral perfusion pressure = mean arterial pressure – (intracranial pressure + central venous pressure).

- Normal cerebral perfusion pressure is 70–75 mmHg.
- Critical ischaemia occurs at a cerebral perfusion pressure of 30–40 mmHg
- Localised ischaemia may occur at a higher cerebral perfusion pressure than this
- The units should all be in mmHg.

It is important to maintain cerebral perfusion pressure after brain injury to prevent secondary brain insult occurring. This can be achieved by raising the mean arterial pressure or reducing the intracranial pressure. Once normovolaemia is achieved, agents such as noradrenaline can be used to augment mean arterial pressure. Mortality is increased by approximately 20% for each 10 mmHg reduction in cerebral perfusion pressure.

Chapter 14

Cardiovascular system

Questions

For each question, select the single best answer from the five options listed.

1. A 70-year-old man on surgical high-dependency unit has been admitted with a 2-day history of vomiting and upper abdominal pain. He is hypotensive and hypovolaemic, has cool peripheries and increased capillary refill. His hypotension is being treated by increasing cardiac preload with a fluid challenge of 500 mL crystalloid solution.

    Which of the following most accurately describes this patient's cardiac preload?

    A   Central venous pressure
    B   End-diastolic ventricular volume
    C   Pulmonary artery occlusion pressure
    D   Ventricular myocyte length
    E   Ventricular myocyte tension

2. A 65-year-old man on the surgical high-dependency unit has been complaining of chest pain for the past hour. Cardiac ischaemia is suspected since the patient has a history of angina and his ECG shows ST depression in the lateral leads.

    What is the main determinant of his coronary blood flow?

    A   Autonomic nervous system
    B   Blood viscosity
    C   Coronary artery diameter
    D   Diastolic blood pressure
    E   Myocardial oxygen demand

3. A 58-year-old man on the postoperative surgical ward has hypotension. He underwent a laparoscopic cholecystectomy earlier today. The patient has a history of ischaemic heart disease. To treat the hypotension his cardiac output will be optimised.

    To increase cardiac output with least impact on myocardial oxygen demand which of the following physiological variables should be optimised?

    A   Afterload
    B   Contractility
    C   Heart rate
    D   Preload
    E   Serum calcium

4. A 38-year-old woman underwent a laparoscopic biopsy of a vascular lesion. The biopsy results are being reviewed. On the histopathology report, there is no mention of the site of the biopsy, however, the biopsy is found to contain a large proportion of elastic tissue.

    Based on this report, where is the elastic tissue most likely to originate from?

    A   Aorta
    B   Arteries
    C   Arterioles
    D   Veins
    E   Vena cava

5. A 56-year-old man is being assessed for repair of a large aortic aneurysm. As part of his assessment he is going to undergo cardiopulmonary exercise testing.

    Which organ receives the greatest proportion of cardiac output before the start of the test?

    A   Brain
    B   Heart
    C   Liver
    D   Kidneys
    E   Skeletal muscle

6. A 65-year-old woman on the surgical high-dependency unit is peri-arrest. Her heart rate is 30 beats per minute, her SpO_2 is 80% and the monitor is unable to measure a systolic blood pressure. High–flow oxygen and IV fluids are being administered. The house officer asks if IV adrenaline should be given.

    Which one of the following adrenoreceptors causes vasoconstriction by adrenaline?

    A α_1
    B α_2
    C β_1
    D β_2
    E β_3

7. A 21-year-old man is brought in by ambulance to the emergency department with an abdominal stab wound. He is in class 3 hypovolaemic shock and is being resuscitated by the emergency team. The carotid baroreceptors are some of the main sensors of intravascular volume status.

    What is the afferent nerve supply of the carotid baroreceptors?

    A   Glossopharyngeal nerve
    B   Phrenic nerve
    C   Recurrent laryngeal nerve
    D   Sympathetic chain
    E   Vagus nerve

Answers

1. D Ventricular myocyte length

The initial length of a cardiac myocyte determines its contractility. It is, however, usually impossible to measure this directly in vivo and therefore surrogate measurements, such as left ventricular end-diastolic pressure (LVEDP), are used. It is assumed, providing ventricular compliance is normal, that LVEDP reflects ventricular volume and hence myocyte length. Classically a Frank–Starling curve is drawn with central venous pressure on the x-axis and stroke volume or cardiac output on the y-axis. Increasing preload (i.e. central venous pressure) leads to increased cardiac output until the myocyte becomes overstretched and cardiac output falls as occurs in cardiac failure. The position of the Frank–Starling curve is influenced by inotropic status (**Figure 14.1**).

In order for the heart to eject against the total peripheral resistance, tension needs to be generated in the myocytes. Myocyte tension therefore relates more closely to the concept of afterload.

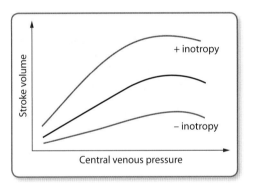

Figure 14.1 The Frank–Starling curve.

2. C Coronary artery diameter

The Hagen–Poiseuille equation (in a straight tube the value of resistance is inversely proportional to the fourth power of the radius) describes laminar flow through tubes. Flow is proportional to the pressure gradient along the tube (i.e. the gradient between aortic pressure and ventricular pressure). During systole left ventricular pressure is greater than aortic pressure and there is no blood flow to the left ventricle.

The cross sectional area of the tube is of greatest importance as flow is proportional to the fourth power of the radius. The radius of coronary arteries is matched to myocardial oxygen demand; as oxygen demand increases vessel radius increases. The mediators for this are adenosine and nitric oxide and the process is an example of autoregulation. Flow is inversely proportional to the length of the tube and viscosity of the fluid. The autonomic nervous system has little influence on coronary artery diameter.

3. D Preload

The main determinant of myocardial oxygen demand is the amount of myocardial work performed. Myocardial work is increased by increasing heart rate, contractility and afterload. Preload also increases contractility but, because of the Laplace relationship it produces a much smaller increase in O_2 demand than the other factors. Laplace's law applies for spheres, when applied to a human ventricle, gives the following equation: ventricular wall tension = pressure x $\sqrt[3]{volume}$. Doubling the intraventricular pressure by increasing contractility or afterload will double myocardial wall tension and therefore double myocardial work. Doubling the heart rate will also roughly double the myocardial work. If preload is increased by doubling end-diastolic ventricular volume however, the tension generated is only increased by approximately 26%.

4. A Aorta

One of the key functions of the aorta is to maintain blood flow and pressure during diastole. It achieves this by acting as an elastic reservoir. During systole it expands to accommodate the blood ejected from the ventricle. One-third of the stroke volume flows through the arteries to perfuse tissues but most remains in the aorta, stretching the vessel wall and storing potential energy. During diastole this energy is used as the aorta contracts due to elastic recoil and blood flow is thus maintained. For this to work effectively a nonregurgitant aortic valve and the presence of a peripheral resistance are required. As the aorta ages it loses elastic tissue and therefore becomes less compliant. A consequence of this is that there will be greater pressure variations during the cardiac cycle. This is one of the contributing factors to hypertension.

5. C Liver

Regional blood flow is regulated by the arterioles which contain a large proportion of smooth muscle in their walls. During exercise local metabolites produced in muscle and stimulation of β_2-adrenoreceptors cause vasodilatation in skeletal muscle vascular beds. Simultaneously sympathetic nervous system activation leads to vasoconstriction of splanchnic and renal arterioles. Myocardial oxygen supply increases primarily by increasing coronary blood flow as oxygen extraction is already 80% in the resting heart. Skin blood flow initially increases to promote heat loss from exercising muscle but at high cardiac outputs cutaneous vasoconstriction occurs in order to maintain muscle blood flow. This will lead to an increase in body temperature. **Table 14.1** below demonstrates the changes in distribution of blood flow in a patient going from rest to heavy exercise.

6. A α_1-receptors

Adrenoreceptors exert their effects via intracellular secondary messenger systems. They have widespread effects on the human body and can be grouped into α- and β-receptors. Adrenaline at low doses primarily affects β-receptors but in higher

Table 14.1 Distribution of blood flow in a 70 kg person during rest and exercise. The percentage in parentheses is the proportion of the cardiac output received by the organ at the given level of exercise.

	Resting blood flow (mL/min)	Light exercise blood flow (mL/min)	Vigorous exercise blood flow (mL/min)
Cerebral	650 (13%)	650 (7%)	650 (2.5%)
Coronary	250 (5%)	450 (5%)	1250 (5%)
Renal	1000 (20%)	900 (10%)	250 (1%)
Splanchnic/liver	1250 (25%)	1100 (12%)	250 (1%)
Skeletal muscle	1000 (20%)	4200 (47%)	22,000 (88%)
Skin	300 (6%)	1350 (15%)	500 (2%)
Other	550 (11%)	350 (4%)	100 (0.5%)
Total cardiac output	5000	9000	25,000

Table 14.2 Effects of adrenoreceptor subtypes

Receptor	Effect
α_1	Vasoconstriction
α_2	Inhibition of noradrenaline release from nerve endings Platelet aggregation
β_1	Increased chronotropy and inotropy Increased renin secretion
β_2	Bronchodilatation Vasodilatation
β_3	Lipolysis in fat cells

doses, including the dose used in cardiac arrest it has α effects also. Its onset is around 30 seconds and duration of effect a few minutes. **Table 14.2** details some of the effects of the adrenoreceptor subtypes.

β_2-receptors increase chronotropy and inotropy but to a lesser extent than β_1-receptors. They assume greater importance in heart failure when β_1-receptors are downregulated.

7. A The glossopharyngeal nerve

Carotid and aortic baroreceptors are stretch receptors that are stimulated by increased distention of the vessel. Following acute blood loss venous return decreases and due to the Frank–Starling mechanism blood pressure falls. Decreased intra-arterial pressure causes less vessel wall stretch and hence reduced activation of the baroreceptors. Afferent neurones from the carotid baroreceptors travel in the glossopharyngeal nerves and from the aortic baroreceptors via the vagus. These afferent neurones synapse with cardiovascular control centres in the brainstem. Decreased firing of these afferent neurones will lead to inhibition of central parasympathetic outflow and increased central sympathetic outflow. Increased sympathetic outflow causes vasoconstriction and an increase in heart rate and myocardial contractility thereby maintaining perfusion to vital organs.

Other components of the early phase include an increase in antidiuretic hormone and activation of the renin–angiotensin–aldosterone system (with an inhibition of atrial natriuretic peptide secretion). Increased erythropoiesis returns haemoglobin levels to normal over a few weeks.

Chapter 15

Respiratory system

Questions

For each question, select the single best answer from the five options listed.

1. A 33-year-old woman is admitted to the surgical high-dependency unit with acute pancreatitis. She is breathing 15 L/min of oxygen through a standard face mask. Her oxygen saturation reading is 91%.

   What most affects the actual oxygen percentage inspired by the patient?

   A   Inspiratory flow rate
   B   Oxygen consumption
   C   Respiratory rate
   D   Tidal volume
   E   Ventilation–perfusion matching

2. A 72-year-old man presents for elective repair of unilateral inguinal hernia associated with pain. He has a history of chronic obstructive pulmonary disease with long standing type 2 respiratory failure and poor exercise tolerance. A venous blood gas taken by the house officer shows a $PaCO_2$ of 8.5 kPa.

   In this patient's venous blood, how is most of the carbon dioxide (CO_2) transported?

   A   As bicarbonate
   B   As carbamino compounds
   C   As carbonic acid
   D   Bound to haemoglobin
   E   Dissolved in solution

3. A 70-year-old man has been admitted to the intensive care unit for invasive ventilation. He aspirated gastric contents during upper GI endoscopy for investigation of dyspepsia. The working diagnosis is acute respiratory distress syndrome secondary to aspiration pneumonitis. The family are asking about something they read on the internet called pulmonary surfactant treatment.

   What is the main constituent of pulmonary surfactant?

   A   Apolipoprotein
   B   Carbohydrate
   C   Cholesterol
   D   Lipid
   E   Protein

4. A 52-year-old woman on high-dependency unit has undergone open repair of
    aortic aneurysm 2 hours ago. She has sickle cell trait but is otherwise healthy.
    She received 14 units of blood intraoperatively and is now adequately resuscitated.

    What is the most likely factor impairing liberation of oxygen from haemoglobin for
    delivery to her tissues?

    A   Alkalosis
    B   Hypothermia
    C   Presence of haemoglobin S
    D   Reduced 2, 3-diphosphoglycerate activity
    E   Residual fetal haemoglobin

5. A 42-year-old woman on a surgical ward 36 hours post-laparoscopic
    cholecystectomy presents with breathlessness. She was previously fit and well. On
    examination, she has a painful and swollen left calf. There are no other abnormal
    clinical findings. Her partial pressure of oxygen (PaO_2) is 6.1 kPa (46 mmHg).

    What does the PaO_2 signify?

    A   Hypoxaemia
    B   Insufficient haemoglobin to carry oxygen
    C   The patient is on oxygen
    D   Tissue hypoxia
    E   Type 1 respiratory failure

6. A 62-year-old man on the surgical high-dependency unit is recovering following
    a paraumbilical hernia repair. There is a history of chronic obstructive pulmonary
    disease. He is breathing humidified oxygen 60% with a rate of 34 breaths per
    minute and has a PaO_2 of 7.4 kPa and $PaCO_2$ of 7.4 kPa.

    What is the most likely cause of his hypoxia?

    A   Excess oxygen administration
    B   High $PaCO_2$
    C   Humidification
    D   Impaired lung diffusion
    E   Pulmonary shunting

Answers

1. A Inspiratory flow rate

The inspired concentration of oxygen depends on the relative contributions of oxygen from the mask (100% oxygen) and entrained room air (21% oxygen). Inspiratory flow rate at rest can be estimated by thinking about the tidal volume (500 mL) and the respiratory rate. With a respiratory rate of 15 breaths/min and equal inspiratory and expiratory times (in reality inspiration time is normally about half of expiration time), the time for each inspiration would be 2 seconds. This gives a flow rate of 0.25 L/sec or 15 L/min. Although 15 L/min oxygen flow could theoretically deliver 100% oxygen to a patient breathing at rest, room air is inevitably entrained. If either respiratory rate or tidal volume increases, the inspiratory flow rate will exceed the maximum oxygen flow rate and room air must be entrained. In fact, maximum breathing capacity can be up to 170 L/min. This is why a tight-fitting face mask with a reservoir bag (e.g. 'trauma mask') using high flow oxygen (15 L/min) will deliver more oxygen to the patient.

2. A As bicarbonate

Venous blood carries the CO_2 from cellular respiration back to the lungs for excretion. Around 60% is in the form of bicarbonate (HCO_3^-) through the reaction with water ($H_2O + CO_2 \rightleftharpoons H_2CO_3 \rightleftharpoons H^+ + HCO_3^-$), the first part of which being catalysed by carbonic anhydrase. Amino groups in proteins in the blood (mainly haemoglobin) combine with CO_2 to form carbamates which account for around 5% in arterial blood and 30% in venous blood. Deoxygenated haemoglobin in the venous blood carries more CO_2 which is part of the Haldane effect. CO_2 is more soluble than oxygen but only accounts for around 10% in venous blood (5% in arterial). This patient has raised $PaCO_2$ and is at increased risk of postoperative respiratory complications. If the patient decides to go ahead with the surgery, he may benefit from having the procedure carried out under local or regional anaesthesia.

3. D Lipid

Surfactant is produced by type 2 alveolar cells and consists mainly of the lipid dipalmitoylphosphatidylcholine (DPCC) and other phospholipids. The pathophysiology of respiratory distress syndrome involves alveolar cell dysfunction and therefore inadequate surfactant production. Surface tension of the fluid lining the alveolar air spaces acts as a collapsing force. The law of Laplace tells us that the pressure (force) required to keep the alveolus open is proportional to the surface tension, and indirectly proportional to the radius of the alveolus (pressure = 2 x surface tension/radius). This means that as the alveolus reduces in size as expiration occurs, the pressure required to prevent collapse increases. Surface tension of water is around 70 dyn/cm (70 nM/m) whereas surfactant is between 0–20 dyn/cm (0–20 nM/m). The effect of surfactant is more pronounced at lower lung volumes (<1 dyn/cm, or <1 nM/m, at <40% total lung capacity). Surfactant therefore increases lung compliance, particularly at low lung volumes, and minimises atelectasis. Surface tension also draws fluid into the lungs, and so surfactant helps to keep the lungs dry.

4. D Reduced 2, 3-diphosphoglycerate activity

A left shift in the oxygen–haemoglobin dissociation curve equates to increased affinity for oxygen. The P_{50} (the oxygen partial pressure whereby haemoglobin is 50% saturated) moves further to the left, i.e. haemoglobin is less likely to release oxygen for any given PaO_2. This is caused by alkalosis, reduced 2,3-diphosphoglycerate activity, hypothermia, fetal haemoglobin and carbon monoxide. She is adequately resuscitated which implies adequate blood oxygenation, circulating volume, normothermia and absence of acidosis (a marker of hypoperfusion). She may have some haemoglobin S but this causes a right shift in the curve. Transfused blood has reduced 2,3-diphosphoglycerate activity and it takes time to replenish this by glycolysis following transfusion.

5. A Hypoxaemia

A decreased partial pressure of oxygen (PaO_2) in the blood is generally described as hypoxaemia. PaO_2 is not a measure of the total content of oxygen in the blood, which is largely dependent on haemoglobin. Normal PaO_2 (breathing room air) would be 10–14 kPa (75–105 mmHg). For a normal adult breathing oxygen it should be considerably higher than this. PaO_2 6.1 kPa is very concerning and oxygen should be applied if it has not already. There is a possibility that this could be an inadvertent venous blood gas, but other values such as pH and $PaCO_2$ would indicate whether this was possible and compatible. We need to know the $PaCO_2$ to distinguish type 1 (normo- or hypocapnic) from type 2 (hypercapnic) respiratory failure. This patient may have a pulmonary embolism and should be resuscitated and then investigated accordingly.

6. E Pulmonary shunting

Breathing room air, the inspired gas must be fully humidified by the time it reaches the lung. This accounts for a 1 kPa drop in the inspired partial pressure of oxygen. The inspired gas is then mixed with the alveolar gas, which contains CO_2, further reducing the oxygen concentration. Normal lungs have a negligible diffusion barrier, accounting for a small drop in oxygen, although this is increased in lung disease. Blood shunting through unventilated parts of the lung leads to a further drop in oxygen, which in the healthy lung is <2 kPa but can account for large differences in inspired and arterial oxygen. This oxygen cascade explains why a normal PaO_2 is 12–14 kPa when breathing room air at 21 kPa. This patient is probably breathing between 40–60 kPa of oxygen and pulmonary shunting is the only one of these factors that can explain the situation. This may be due to atelectasis or consolidation. Although the patient has chronic obstructive pulmonary disease and type 2 respiratory failure, the respiratory rate is high and supplementary oxygen is vital. The patient needs ventilatory support urgently.

Chapter 16

Gastrointestinal system

Questions

For each question, select the single best answer from the five options listed.

1. A 66-year-old man presents with severe widespread tooth decay. This began some 6 months ago when he developed generalised disease of his salivary glands.

   Which of the following best explains the rampant decay?

   A   Decreased aqueous secretion from the sublingual salivary glands
   B   Increased acid secretion from the parotid salivary glands
   C   Loss of calcium-rich watery salivary secretions
   D   Loss of potassium-rich watery salivary secretions
   E   Reflex sympathetic vasoconstriction

2. A 20-year-old man, a motorcyclist, is being nursed in the semi-prone recovery position to prevent regurgitated acid gastric contents from entering his lower airways while he is in coma (Glasgow coma scale 9).

   Which of the following neurological reflexes prevents regurgitation during vomiting?

   A   Reflex bronchoconstriction with centre in the medulla oblongata
   B   Reflex bronchoconstriction with centre in the pons
   C   Reflex elevation of the larynx with centre in the medulla oblongata
   D   Reflex elevation of the larynx with centre in the pons
   E   Reflex pyloric constriction with centre in the hypothalamus

3. A 35-year-old man presents with a duodenal peptic ulcer.

   Which of the following best explains how his pain can be relieved?

   A   Changing the pH of the fluid bathing the ulcer from 5 to 2
   B   Changing the pH of the gastric contents from 2 to 5
   C   Changing the pH of the gastric contents from 5 to 2
   D   Severing the nerve supply to the duodenum
   E   Stimulating gastric H_2 receptors.

4. A 62-year-old woman with difficulty swallowing and a tendency to choke has a percutaneous endoscopic gastrostomy inserted for enteral feeding.

    Which of the following best describes the fluid to be used in this feeding?

    A   Carbohydrate nutrition should be in the form of glucose only
    B   Daily energy content should be around 400 kcal (1.68 MJ)
    C   Fat content should be as low as possible
    D   Milk would be an appropriate constituent
    E   Protein nutrition should be in the form of a mixture of essential amino acids

5. A 58-year-old man presents with obstructive jaundice, the cause of which has been diagnosed as cancer in the head of the pancreas.

    Which of the following best explains the reason for his jaundice?

    A   Bile salts are failing to reach the duodenum
    B   Duodenal pH has changed due to a failure of pancreatic bicarbonate to reach the duodenum
    C   The bile duct and the pancreatic duct have a common opening into the duodenum
    D   The pancreatic duct is obstructed
    E   There is failure of excretion of conjugated bilirubin

6. A 48-year-old woman presents with a high jejunal fistula.

    Which of the following best describes why her condition is not a low (terminal) ileal fistula?

    A   Fistula content has a much greater acidity
    B   Fistula content has a higher amount of bile acids
    C   Fistula content has a higher concentration of nutrients
    D   Fistula has a lower vitamin B_{12} content
    E   Fistula has a lower volume

7. Two 34-year-old men have a stoma – one a colostomy in the left iliac fossa after rectal surgery, and the other an ileostomy in the right iliac fossa after a panproctocolectomy for ulcerative colitis. Contents of the colostomy bag in the left iliac fossa are relatively small in volume and consist of well-formed stools. Contents of the ileostomy bag in the right iliac fossa are relatively copious non-smelly fluid.

    What is the best explanation for the difference?

    A   More than 75% of fluid absorption from the entire gut takes place in the colon
    B   Random variation
    C   The caecum absorbs more fluid than the small intestine
    D   There is net secretion of fluid in the left (descending) colon
    E   The colon absorbs a small but significant proportion of ingested plus secreted fluid in the gut

8. A 50-year-old man presents with a 6-month history of projectile vomiting. For over 30 years he has suffered from indigestion for which he has self-medicated with drugs across the chemists counter. On examination, he is extremely dehydrated, with visible gastric peristalsis and succussion splash. His blood results are as follows:

pH	7.50
PCO_2	4 mmHg (5.3 kPa)
Bicarbonate	30.1 mmol/L
Haemoglobin	170 g/L
Urea	18 mmol/L
Creatinine	190 µmol/L

Which of the following is most likely to have caused this condition?

A   A metabolic alkalosis due to gastric outlet obstruction
B   Chronic renal failure leading to vomiting
C   Chronic respiratory failure with secondary polycythaemia
D   Compensated respiratory alkalosis
E   Renal failure as a side effect of medication for his indigestion

Answers

1. C Loss of calcium-rich watery salivary secretions

A healthy oral cavity depends on a steady flow from the serous (watery) secreting parotid glands, with some contribution from the seromucous submandibular glands. Saliva has antiseptic properties, helping to control pathogenic bacteria. However, the copious watery output from the parotid glands, being rich in calcium and phosphate ions, is particularly important in countering erosion of the teeth by acid-forming bacteria and healing minor surface abrasions in the enamel.

The sublingual glands (A) are mucous. The parotid secretions help to buffer acid (B). Like gastric and intestinal secretions generally, saliva is relatively rich in potassium (D), but this is not significant in preventing tooth decay. Neither is reflex sympathetic vasoconstriction (E) a contributory factor.

2. C Reflex elevation of the larynx with centre in the medulla oblongata

During swallowing and also during vomiting, the entrance to the larynx and hence the airways is reflexly closed by elevation of the larynx so that its entrance (which faces obliquely upwards and backwards) is jammed firmly against the base of the tongue. Thus swallowed material must pass from pharynx to oesophagus. The epiglottis is not an essential part of this mechanism (if the epiglottis is removed, the reflex still works). Reflexes for swallowing and vomiting have their centres in the medulla oblongata, not the pons (D).

Bronchoconstriction (A, B) narrows the airways during coughing, thus increasing air velocity for expulsion of mucus. Pyloric constriction (E) is part of the vomiting reflex, whereby gastric contents pass into the oesophagus rather than into the duodenum.

3. B Changing the pH of the gastric contents from 2 to 5

Peptic ulcers become more painful the greater the acidity of the fluid bathing them. The acid comes from the acid/pepsin secretion of the stomach. Normal gastric pH is around 2 (and normal urine around 4–5). Each unit of pH indicates a 10-fold change in hydrogen ion concentration. A change in pH from 2 to 5 (B) indicates a 1000-fold decrease in hydrogen ion concentration (pH is the negative log of the hydrogen ion concentration and pH 7 is neutrality, with blood pH around 7.4).

A reduction in gastric acidity is directly and effectively produced by blocking the hydrogen ion pump which pumps hydrogen ions from the parietal cells to the gastric lumen. H_2 receptors mediate stimulation of the parietal cells to produce acid, so blockade of these receptors reduces ulcer pain (E). Cutting the vagal nerve supply of the parietal cells (vagotomy) also reduces acid secretion, therefore cutting the nerve supply of the duodenum (D) is not an option. Changing the pH of both the fluid bathing the ulcer (A) and the gastric contents (C) from 5 to 2 would increase hydrogen ion content and hence acidity.

4. D Milk would be an appropriate constituent

Enteral nutrition is essentially a good oral diet in liquid form; milk is a good starting point. Advantages of enteral rather than parenteral nutrition are that the fluid is administered into the gut; normal digestion takes place, elemental diets are not required and the gut remains in use and healthy rather than suffering atrophy. The daily energy content should be related to the recipient's daily requirements – in the sedentary state 4–5 times the value given in B would be appropriate. Elemental diets containing glucose (A) and amino acids (E) (plus fat, minerals, vitamins) are not required here. Fat content (C) should not be restricted to low levels.

5. E There is failure of excretion of conjugated bilirubin

Obstructive jaundice implies an obstruction to the excretion of conjugated bilirubin into the gut for elimination in the faeces. In this man's case the cancer in the head of the pancreas is causing the obstruction by compression of the nearby duodenum including the bile duct which conveys bile into the duodenum.

In this condition bile salts may also fail to reach the duodenum (A), but they are colourless so do not contribute to jaundice (where the pigment bilirubin causes the typical spectrum of skin colour abnormalities). Failure of pancreatic bicarbonate reaching the duodenum (B), a common opening of the bile and pancreatic ducts into the duodenum (C) and obstruction of the pancreatic duct (D) do not themselves interfere with excretion of bilirubin.

6. B Fistula content has a higher amount of bile acids

Bile acids are required for emulsification in the jejunum and are reabsorbed and recycled to the liver via portal venous blood draining the terminal ileum. This reduces the metabolic cost to the body of synthesising all the bile acids required for emulsification and hence digestion of fats. Vitamin B_{12} is also absorbed actively, rather than secreted (D) in the terminal ileum.

The upper jejunum, rather than the upper ileum, is the main site of final digestion into amino acids and monosaccharides (C) and also the main site of absorption of these nutrients and also fat. Gut contents have to be around neutrality (pH 7) for the final digestion and absorption, rather than acidic (A). Bicarbonate is added in the duodenum via the pancreatic duct and from local duodenal glands (E).

7. E The colon absorbs a small but significant proportion of ingested plus secreted fluid in the gut

In 24 hours 500 mL of intestinal contents pass through the ileocaecal valve and this is reduced to 150 mL after water absorption in the colon (the volumes are influenced by dietary fibre content).

By the time the gut contents reach the start of the colon in the right iliac fossa, most of the ingested plus secreted fluid has been absorbed (A). Most of this is absorbed in the small intestine, mainly in the jejunum (not the caecum (C)). There is net absorption (not secretion) as the fluid passes along the colon (D) so by the time the contents reach the left iliac fossa they have changed from the fluid to the formed faecal state. This effect hugely exceeds random variations (B) in colostomy and ileostomy bag contents.

Patients with an ileostomy are liable to have electrolyte disturbances in the long run because of the electrolyte content of the relatively large amount of fluid lost.

8. A A metabolic alkalosis due to gastric outlet obstruction

This man's pH is raised, indicating an alkalosis; the bicarbonate is also raised, indicating that the alkalosis is metabolic in origin. For a respiratory alkalosis the PCO_2 would be low (D). This man gives a clear picture of gastric outlet obstruction from a long-standing peptic ulcer. Large amounts of relatively concentrated hydrochloric acid produced in the stomach are lost in the vomitus. Loss of hydrogen ions leads to alkalosis. Loss of chloride ions leads also to hypochloraemia. Like all intestinal fluids, gastric contents have a relatively high potassium content, hence hypokalaemia may also be present. His raised bicarbonate could be due in part to bicarbonate-containing medications for his dyspepsia.

With loss of fluid by vomiting, and inability to take oral fluids, the man is suffering from severe dehydration. This is confirmed by the raised haemoglobin concentration [haemoconcentration, rather than secondary polycythaemia (C)]. Dehydration would also account for the raised urea and creatinine levels (so no need to postulate chronic renal failure (B) or as a side-effect of the antacid medication (E).

This man requires urgent resuscitation with intravenous fluids prior to surgery to relieve the gastric outlet obstruction.

Chapter 17

Genitourinary system

Questions

For each question, select the single best answer from the five options listed.

1. A 48-year-old man underwent an emergency laparotomy for multiple trauma when a partial hepatectomy and splenectomy was carried out. Significant bleeding occurred during the operation.

    What is the most likely finding on his urine analysis?

    A   Decreased osmolality
    B   Decreased sodium
    C   Decreased specific gravity
    D   Increased specific gravity
    E   Increased urinary pH

2. A 40-year-old window cleaner fell from a height sustaining multiple musculoskeletal injuries with fracture pelvis. He was taken to theatre for emergency fracture fixation and external fixation of his pelvis. The estimated total blood loss was 1500 mL. Postoperatively he has reduced urine output.

    Which mechanism is most likely to be the cause of his oliguria?

    A   Aldosterone reduction
    B   Antidiuretic hormone reduction
    C   Angiotensin II increase
    D   Nitric oxide increase
    E   Renin reduction

3. A 66-year-old man undergoes a transurethral resection of the prostate (TURP). The procedure was prolonged by up to 2 hours but was performed successfully. Shortly after returning to the ward, the patient develops a seizure.

    What is the most likely blood profile of this patient?

    A   Hypernatremia and decrease in blood ammonia
    B   Hypernatremia and hypoglycaemia
    C   Hyponatremia and increase in blood ammonia
    D   Hyponatremia and decrease in blood ammonia
    E   Hyponatremia and hypoglycaemia

4. A 66-year-old woman presents with minimal urine output for 2 days and suprapubic discomfort. She has a bladder ultrasound scan which shows 650 mL of urine in her bladder. Pelvic and neurological examinations are normal. Pelvic and renal tract ultrasounds are both normal.

   What is the most likely cause of this woman's urinary retention?

   A   Bladder cancer
   B   Fibroids
   C   Multiple sclerosis
   D   Rectal cancer
   E   Urethral stenosis

5. A 78-year-old man is referred as an emergency with a 3-day history of minimal urine output, nocturnal incontinence and a palpable bladder. After reviewing the patient, a urethral catheter is inserted, which drains 1650 mL of urine initially and thereafter 200–400 mL hourly following insertion. An ultrasound of the renal tract immediately following catheterisation shows bilateral hydroureter and hydronephrosis. His renal function is shown below.

Test	Result (mmol/L)	Reference range (mmol/L)
Urea	23	2.5–6.6
Creatinine	696	60–120
Sodium	134	135–145
Potassium	6.7	3.6–5.0

   What is the most likely diagnosis?

   A   Bilateral ureteric stones
   B   High pressure chronic urinary retention
   C   IgA nephropathy
   D   Low pressure chronic urinary retention
   E   Upper tract urothelial carcinoma

6. A 30-year-old man presents to the emergency department with a 3-day history of left loin pain, nausea and vomiting. He has no fever. He denies urinary or bowel symptoms. His abdomen is soft and urinalysis shows microscopic haematuria only. He has no past medical history and takes no regular medication.

    His blood results are detailed in the table below. A CT of kidneys, ureters and bladder (CTKUB) shows normal kidneys bilaterally with a 5 mm left ureteric calculus with minimal proximal dilatation.

Test	Result (mmol/L)	Reference range (mmol/L)
Urea	14.3	2.5–6.6
Creatinine	173	60–120
Sodium	140	135–145
Potassium	4.0	3.6–5.0

    Which of the following is the most likely cause of his renal failure?

    A   Contrast nephropathy
    B   Dehydration
    C   Glomerulonephritis
    D   Obstructive nephropathy
    E   Reflux nephropathy

7. A 36-year old woman, a mother of four, presents to the urology clinic with a 6-month history of nocturia, urgency and occasional incontinence. She does not complain of any bowel symptoms. She is not on any medication. On examination, her abdomen is soft and non-tender. Urinalysis is negative. She has not had any further investigations.

    What is the most probable diagnosis?

    A   Bladder outflow obstruction
    B   Mixed incontinence
    C   Overactive bladder
    D   Stress incontinence
    E   Urge incontinence

8. A 36-year-old diabetic man in a wheelchair attends the emergency department with an intense headache. On examination, his blood pressure is 200/120 mmHg. He is profusely sweating. Abdominal examination reveals a distended bladder.

    What is the most likely cause of these symptoms?

    A   Anaphylactic shock
    B   Autonomic dysreflexia
    C   Diabetic neuropathy
    D   Malignant hypertension
    E   Spinal shock

Answers

1. D Increased specific gravity

The most likely diagnosis is increased specific gravity. The blood loss during the operation is likely to reduce renal blood flow. This will result in an increase in the urine specific gravity as water retention occurs in an attempt to maintain circulating volume. To prevent damage to the glomerular capillaries, the kidney has an ability to autoregulate renal blood flow compensating for fluctuations in blood pressure (within certain parameters). This is also necessary for the clearance of metabolic waste and the recovery of filtered electrolytes.

Urine specific gravity is a measure of the urinary solute concentration. It is a measure of urine density relative to water density and the normal reference range is between 1.005 to 1.03. It is elevated in dehydration/blood loss as the kidney attempts to conserve water, concentrating urinary solutes.

2. C Angiotensin II increase

The most likely cause of this patient's oliguria is an increase in angiotensin II. The juxtaglomerular cells of the kidney detect a reduced blood pressure secondary to the blood loss. In response, renin is secreted into the circulatory system and the renin–angiotensin–aldosterone system is activated (**Figure 17.1**) to maintain the patient's blood pressure and compensate for the loss of intravascular volume.

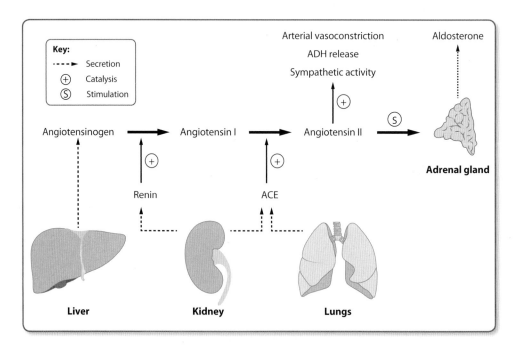

Figure 17.1 The renin–angiotensin–aldosterone system.

Angiotensin II simulates the release of ADH which in turn increases collecting duct permeability to water by stimulating aquaporin receptors, resulting in an increase in water reabsorption. Angiotensin II also causes arterial vasoconstriction and an increase in sympathetic activity. Aldosterone indirectly increases blood pressure through sodium and water retention.

3. C Hyponatraemia and increase in blood ammonia

The diagnosis in this patient is TURP syndrome where hyponatraemia and an increase in blood ammonia would be expected. TURP syndrome occurs when large amounts of fluid are absorbed into the prostatic venous sinuses during the procedure particularly when it is prolonged and large glands are resected. Fluid absorption ranges from 10 to 30 mL/min, and therefore the risk of TURP syndrome is proportionate to the length of the operation, especially for operations lasting longer than 60 minutes. Other risk factors for TURP syndrome include the size of the opened venous sinuses, the amount of irrigation fluid used, and the use of excess amounts of hypotonic intravenous fluids. Glycine 1.5% is universally used as the irrigation fluid during a TURP. It has the advantage of being non-conductive, non-haemolytic and transparent as well as economical. It does, however, have the disadvantage of being hypoosmolar. Glycine is metabolised in the liver into ammonia, resulting in a rise in blood ammonia levels. If this level is dangerously high, it will result in encephalopathy.

Excessive fluid absorption leads to an acute rapid volume expansion, which causes hypertension and reflex bradycardia. This will dilute the serum osmotic gradient and potentially cause cerebral oedema which will result in a lowered Glasgow Coma Score and rarely seizures. These symptoms are also exacerbated by the raised blood ammonia level.

4. E Urethral stenosis

This patient's urinary retention is due to urethral stenosis. Urinary retention is much less common in women than men. **Table 17.1** illustrates some of the common causes of retention in men and women.

Table 17.1 Summary of the causes of urinary obstruction in men and women	
Male	**Female**
Meatal stenosis	Prolapse
Phimosis	Uterine masses
Prostate enlargement	
Both	
Bladder masses	
Congenital	
Drugs	
Iatrogenic	
Neurological	
Urethral strictures	
Urinary tract infection	

As neurological and clinical examination of the pelvis are normal, as well as ultrasound of the pelvis and renal tract, the cause of urinary retention in this patient is urethral stenosis. Other methods for investigating urinary retention, besides detailed history and examination, include flexible cystoscopy, CT-urethrogram and urodynamic studies. Treatment for ureteral stenosis is urethral dilatation.

5. B High pressure chronic urinary retention

This man is in chronic urinary retention as he has a non-painful bladder, which remains palpable or percussible after passing urine. In association with this, the patient has renal dysfunction which is likely to be caused by high pressure in his bladder causing back pressure on to his kidneys. This is known as high pressure chronic retention as opposed to low pressure chronic retention where there would be normal renal function. The patient is in diuresis and therefore should be admitted to replace the loss intravenously. The most common cause for this presentation of urinary retention is benign prostatic hyperplasia for which he should be offered a transurethral resection of the prostate. This should only be carried out after his renal failure has been treated which may take a few days, sometimes weeks depending upon the duration of the problem.

6. B Dehydration

Note the 3-day history of nausea and vomiting which is the cause of his dehydration. Renal failure can be prerenal, renal or postrenal. The degree of dilatation is not indicative of the degree of obstruction in the collecting system. However, in the presence of bilateral normal kidneys a single obstructed kidney would not normally result in acute renal failure as the other kidney would compensate. A CT of kidneys, ureters and bladder is a non-contrast imaging modality used for the diagnosis of urinary tract calculi, and therefore contrast nephropathy is not possible. With 3 days of nausea and vomiting, dehydration (prerenal failure) is the most likely cause. In the presence of kidney stones, one should also consider infection and nonsteroidal anti-inflammatory drugs as contributing factors.

7. D Overactive bladder

Lower urinary tract symptoms can be broadly categorised into obstructive or storage symptoms (see **Table 17.2**). This patient complained of storage symptoms of which overactive bladder is the most likely cause. Symptoms of overactive bladder are urgency (hallmark symptom), with or without urge incontinence, and usually with frequency and nocturia. In most cases, the cause of overactive bladder is not known, however it can be caused by neurological disease.

The presumed diagnosis would be detrusor over activity, which is a urodynamic diagnosis characterised by involuntary detrusor contractions during the bladder filling phase.

Table 17.2 Obstructive and storage lower urinary tract symptoms	
Obstructive	**Storage**
Straining	Frequency
Hesitancy	Urgency
Weak stream	Nocturia
Intermittent stream	Incontinence
Terminal dribbling	
Incomplete bladder emptying	

8. B Autonomic dysreflexia

Autonomic dysreflexia is a phenomenon typically seen in patients with spinal cord injuries. It is caused by imbalanced sympathetic activation, leading to life threatening hypertension. If not treated promptly, the exceedingly high peripheral blood pressure can result in seizures, retinal haemorrhages and cerebral haemorrhage.

In those with a spinal cord injury, a stimulus below the level of injury results in an unbalanced physiological response due to loss of inhibitory impulses below the level of injury. The stimulus causes an excessive sympathetic response resulting in vasoconstriction below the level of injury.

The greater splanchnic vascular beds are one of the largest reserves of circulatory volume and are supplied from T5–T9. Injuries above T6 will result in uninhibited sympathetic tone to constrict the splanchnic vascular beds resulting in systemic hypertension. Autonomic dysreflexia is therefore more common in patients with spinal injury above T6 but can also occur below this level.

In this scenario, the patient has loss of bladder function due to his spinal cord injury and is in acute urinary retention. The urinary retention results in a strong sensory impulse travelling up the spinal cord and results in a sympathetic surge. A catheter should be inserted in this patient to drain the bladder as well as medical management to control the blood pressure.

Chapter 18

Endocrine system

Questions

For each question, select the single best answer from the five options listed.

1. A 35-year-old woman with features of Grave's disease is on the waiting list for subtotal thyroidectomy. She has been on antithyroid treatment for 2 months. At her preoperative assessment in the outpatient clinic, she complains of feeling too hot and is found to be sweating, with a sinus tachycardia of 90 beats per minute and an arterial blood pressure of 170/90 mmHg.

   Which of the following is the most effective management?

   A   Postpone operation for further stabilisation
   B   Referral to a cardiologist for management of hypertension
   C   Reiterate that antithyroid drugs and surgery are the way forward
   D   Turn down the thermostat in the outpatient department
   E   Urgent treatment for early atrial fibrillation

2. A 75-year-old man is undergoing emergency closure of a perforated duodenal ulcer. There was difficulty in obtaining a detailed history of his previous condition due to a degree of memory loss and confusion. He mentioned having taken tablets for pains in his hands, which showed features of rheumatoid arthritis. Relatively early in the operation his blood pressure begins to drop despite apparently adequate fluid administration. Several pressor agents are tried without benefit. His pressure becomes satisfactory again after an intravenous injection of hydrocortisone.

   Which of the following is most likely to have caused this condition?

   A   Nonspecific age-related effects
   B   Preoperative paracetamol affecting clotting factors in the bone marrow
   C   Preoperative paracetamol affecting clotting factors in the liver
   D   Preoperative steroids interfering with adrenocortical function
   E   Preoperative steroids interfering with the immune system

3. A 57-year-old woman is referred to the surgical outpatient clinic for a thyroidectomy. The patient has been complaining of flu-like symptoms for the last 3 weeks. She has also been complaining of heat intolerance and reduced appetite. On examination of her neck, the thyroid gland appears enlarged and tender. Blood tests reveal the following:

Test	Result	Reference range
TSH	0.2 mU/L	0.4–4 mU/L
T$_3$	10 pmol/L	3.5–8 pmol/L
T$_4$	30 pmol/L	9–25 pmol/L

Which of the following is the most likely diagnosis?

A   De Quervain's thyroiditis
B   Early hypothyroidism
C   Grave's disease
D   Hashimoto's thyroiditis
E   Secondary hyperthyroidism

4. A 25-year-old man on insulin injections for diabetes mellitus (present since childhood) has had total colectomy with an ileoanal pouch procedure for familial adenomatous polyposis. Postoperative progress has been satisfactory, and he is now receiving oral nutrition and fluids. Several days after surgery a nurse reports that he is behaving out of character – he became unpleasant when she arrived to take his observations and would not allow these to proceed. He is sweating and his hand is shaking when you take his pulse rate. His pulse rate is 90 beats per minute and his blood pressure is 160/70 mmHg.

Which of the following is the most effective management?

A   Cool patient down with a bedside fan
B   Determine blood glucose measurement and give oral glucose
C   Immediate injection of the due dose of insulin
D   Immediate intravenous infusion of 5% dextrose
E   Prescribe a mild oral sedative

5. A 40-year-old man presents following repeated episodes of renal colic and is being investigated for an underlying cause. His only other complaint is of vague abdominal discomfort. Investigations show no evidence of underlying renal disease. Blood tests reveal an increased calcium level and a reduced phosphate level. His plasma proteins are normal.

Which of the following is the most likely diagnosis?

A   Hyperthyroidism
B   Hypoparathyroidism
C   Hypothyroidism
D   Primary hyperparathyroidism
E   Secondary hyperparathyroidism

6. A 57-year-old woman underwent a total thyroidectomy for medullary carcinoma of the thyroid.

Which of the following tumour markers is used clinically to screen for recurrence?

A   Serum calcitonin levels
B   Serum parathyroid hormone levels
C   Serum T$_3$ levels
D   Serum thyroglobulin levels
E   Serum thyroid stimulating hormone levels

7. A 52-year-old diabetic woman presents with a history of unintentional weight loss, diarrhoea and a widespread skin rash with erythematous blisters involving the abdomen and legs suggesting migratory necrolytic erythema.

Which of the following is the most likely diagnosis?

A   Adenocarcinoma of the colon
B   Adenocarcinoma of the pancreas
C   Carcinoid syndrome
D   Insulinoma
E   Malignant glucagonoma

8. A 55-year-old man attends the preoperative assessment clinic for an elective cholecystectomy. The patient is currently on furosemide and ramipril for his heart failure. He has smoked 40 cigarettes a day for the last 30 years. On examination no abnormality was detected. Blood and urine analysis are performed and show the following:

Test	Result	Reference range
Urea	5.3 mmol/L	2.5–6.6 mmol/L
Creatinine	80 µmol/L	60–120 µmol/L
Sodium	125 mmol/L	135–145 mmol/L
Potassium	4.8 mmol/L	3.6–5.0 mmol/L
Serum osmolality	Low	
Urine osmolality	High	

Which of the following is the most likely explanation for these results?

A   Excessive water intake by the patient
B   Hypertonic hyponatremia
C   Hypotonic hypervolemic hyponatremia
D   Pseudohyponatremia
E   Syndrome of inappropriate ADH release

9. A 48-year-old woman attends her GP clinic complaining of fatigue and muscle pain. She is currently taking ramipril and bisoprolol for hypertension. On examination her blood pressure is 170/110 mmHg. Blood tests reveal the following:

Test	Result	Reference range
Sodium	150 mmol/L	135–145 mmol/L
Potassium	3.0 mmol/L	3.6–5.0 mmol/L
Renin	Low	

Which of the following is the most likely diagnosis?

A   Addison's disease
B   Cushing's disease
C   Primary hyperaldosteronism
D   Secondary hyperaldosteronism
E   Syndrome of inappropriate ADH secretion

Answers

1. C Reiterate that antithyroid drugs and surgery are the way forward

This woman still has marked features of hyperthyroidism. They are caused by increased activity in mitochondria whereby energy (and heat) production is increased. The overall basal metabolic rate is raised and the associated increased heat production. Body temperature starts to rise and this leads to reflex stimulation of sweat glands. Cardiac activity increases, partly from a direct action of excess thyroid hormones, and partly due to reflex activity to increase peripheral blood flow and dissipate the excess heat. Since the adverse effects stem from excessive thyroid activity, antithyroid drugs and subtotal thyroidectomy should eventually control the unpleasant symptoms.

2. D Preoperative steroids interfering with adrenocortical function

This man developed hypotension which was not responsive to adequate fluid administration and pressor agents. This is the picture seen with an inadequate cortisol response to the stress of major surgery. The prompt response to intravenous hydrocortisone confirms the previous deficiency of the adrenal glucocorticoid, cortisol (hydrocortisone is also a potent glucocorticoid). Long-term glucocorticoid therapy (e.g. prednisone) disrupts the release of hormones from the hypothalamus and anterior pituitary and hence the adrenal secretion of cortisol. As a result, the cells forming these hormones suffer disuse atrophy and so cannot respond to the stress of major surgery. Without adequate cortisol replacement treatment during the peri-operative phase, morbidity and mortality risks are high.

Although steroids also suppress the immune system, this would not account for the hypotensive crisis observed (B).

3. E De Quervain's thyroiditis

This patient is suffering from De Quervain's thyroiditis (sub-acute thyroiditis) and therefore was wrongly referred for a thyroidectomy, as it is a self-limited condition that does not require thyroid medications or surgery. The 'flu-like' symptoms and a tender thyroid gland on examination is a classical presentation of De Quervain's thyroiditis. It is usually precipitated by a viral illness. De Quervain's thyroiditis can also present with symptoms of hypothyroidism as well as hyperthyroidism. The prognosis is generally excellent.

4. B Determine blood glucose measurement and give oral glucose

Episodes of hypoglycaemia are relatively common in diabetic patients on insulin, especially during restabilisation post-operatively. An early cerebral sign of hypoglycaemia is out-of-character behaviour. Increasing drowsiness and impairment of consciousness develop as the blood sugar falls appreciably below the 5 mmol/L level and a severe fall can lead to coma and death. The brain has no energy stores and relies on uptake of glucose from a normal extracellular level (insulin does not influence this uptake). This man was still relatively cooperative (allowed his pulse and blood pressure to be taken) so it should not be difficult to persuade him to take a glucose-rich drink or sweet snack.

His sweating is not due to excessive heat (A) but is part of a reflex sympathetic response which also causes the tremor and hyperdynamic circulation. Sympathetic activity helps to combat hyperglycaemia, adrenaline being particularly effective with its β-adrenoceptor action. Intravenous glucose (D) is not necessary when oral glucose or sucrose can be taken; if the patient is unconscious, intravenous 10% glucose (2–5 mL/kg) must be given immediately.

5. D Primary hyperparathyroidism

The major role of parathyroid hormone is to maintain the extracellular calcium ion level. This is important because interstitial extracellular fluid bathes nerves, muscles, bones, and also the (normally four) parathyroid glands. If extracellular calcium ion level falls, nerves and muscles become hyper-excitable leading to tetany. However, a fall in calcium ions stimulates release of parathyroid hormone; this increases phosphate excretion into the urine, lowering extracellular phosphate. Parathyroid hormone also favours the activation of vitamin D, thereby absorbing more calcium into the body from the gut (**Figure 18.1**).

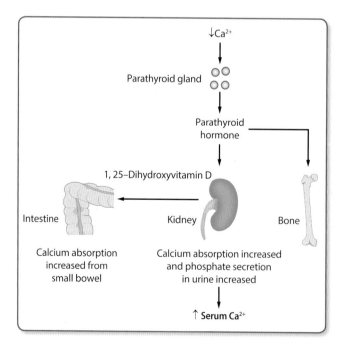

Figure 18.1 The calcium homeostasis pathway.

Secondly, in the urine, the level of phosphate rises because more is being excreted as mentioned above. In addition, because plasma calcium has increased, more filters into the urine. Thus, the calcium and phosphate ions in urine increase; when the maximal solubility product increases, solid calcium phosphate is deposited and grows into renal stones. Vague abdominal pains are a feature of hypercalcaemia, which hyperparathyroidism induces.

6. A serum calcitonin levels

This patient has medullary thyroid carcinoma for which serum calcitonin levels are used to screen for the recurrence of the disease. Medullary thyroid cancer originates from the para-follicular (C) cells, which produce the hormone calcitonin. Medullary thyroid cancer is the fourth most common type of thyroid cancer (after papillary, follicular and anaplastic). It is associated with multiple endocrine neoplasia syndrome (MEN), specifically MEN 2A and MEN 2B.

Tumour markers are commonly tested in the MRCS part A.

7. E Malignant glucagonoma

This patient is suffering from malignant glucagonoma. This is a type of pancreatic neuroendocrine tumour (PanNETs). Glucagonoma is a rare, slow growing tumour of the alpha cells of the pancreas. The rash is classical migratory necrolytic erythema and is commonly seen in patients with malignant glucagonoma. Symptoms are non-specific and slow in onset. To summarise the syndrome consists of; diabetes, migratory necrolytic erythema, anaemia, diarrhoea and patients are more prone to thromboembolic disease. Psychiatric disturbances also occur.

Glucagonomas comprise 8% to 13% of all functioning PanNEts occurring between the ages of 40 and 70 years, women being more commonly affected. Those with an alpha cell tumour, plasma glucagon levels may be up to 30 times above normal. Like other functioning PanNETs these tumours are malignant in 50–70% of cases.

8. E Syndrome of inappropriate ADH release

This patient is suffering from a paraneoplastic syndrome. He has a lung tumour producing ectopic release of antidiuretic hormone (ADH) causing a low sodium in his blood biochemistry. The patient has a significant smoking history and a lesion in his chest X-ray making the syndrome of inappropriate antidiuretic hormone (SIADH) the most likely cause. SIADH is most commonly associated with small cell carcinoma of the lung. Patients with SIADH have an elevated urine osmolality and a low serum osmolality due to the excess water reabsorption from the collecting ducts.

The hyponatremia is caused by an excess in water rather than a reduction in sodium in the plasma. If the patient had been drinking excessive amounts of water (A) the urine would be low in osmolality as the kidneys will be eliminating the excess fluid. Hypotonic hypervolemic hyponatremia (C) would typically present with signs of fluid overload e.g. pitting oedema of the limbs and a raised JVP.

9. B Primary hyperaldosteronism

This woman is suffering from primary hyperaldosteronism which is evident by the fact that her hypertension is refractive to treatment, with hypokalaemia and a low renin level. Primary hyperaldosteronism, also known as Conn's syndrome, results in excessive production of aldosterone from the adrenal glands. The aldosterone acts on the collecting ducts of the kidney to stimulate potassium secretion and sodium reabsorption (**Figure 18.2**). Aldosterone also promotes hydrogen loss in the collecting ducts resulting in a metabolic alkalosis. This is the opposite to Addison's disease (A) where a high potassium and a low blood pressure would be expected due to the lack of aldosterone production.

Hyperaldosteronism can be primary where the excess aldosterone is a result of an adrenal adenoma or adrenal hyperplasia, or secondary (D) where the adrenal gland is stimulated by high renin levels to produces excess aldosterone. The way to differentiate between primary and secondary hyperaldosteronism is by checking the serum renin levels which would be low in the former and high in the latter.

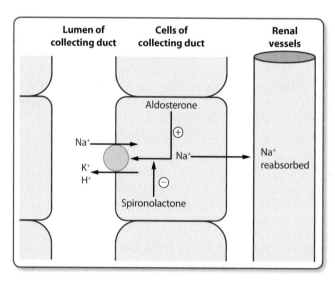

Figure 18.2
Aldosterone release stimulates the absorption of potassium secretion and hydrogen loss. Spironolactone inhibits the actions of aldosterone in cells of the collecting duct.

Chapter 19

The liver

Questions

For each question, select the single best answer from the five options listed.

1. A 45-year-old man suffering from chronic liver failure presents with bilateral ankle swelling and ascites.

   Which of the following is most likely to have caused both these conditions?

   A   A low circulating albumin level
   B   A low circulating fibrinogen level
   C   A raised albumin/globulin level in the circulation
   D   Hepatic encephalopathy
   E   Portosystemic anastomoses

2. A 64-year-old woman with obstructive jaundice is being evaluated for non-urgent surgery within the next few weeks. Her coagulation screening shows an INR of 1.8 with normal values for fibrinogen and platelets.

   What is the most appropriate management of this patient?

   A   Arrange surgery as soon as possible
   B   Commence regular injections of vitamin C
   C   Commence regular injections of vitamin K
   D   Give factor VIII intravenously over the perioperative period
   E   Infuse fresh frozen plasma over the perioperative period

3. A 66-year-old man has been admitted with severe vomiting of fresh blood and has required rapid transfusion of six units of blood. He is known to have long-standing hepatic cirrhosis with evidence of liver failure and ascites.

   What is most likely source of the bleeding?

   A   A duodenal ulcer related to coagulation problems
   B   Oesophageal varices related to deficiency of vitamin B_{12}
   C   Oesophageal varices related to gastric acid reflux
   D   Oesophageal varices related to portal venous hypertension
   E   Stress-related gastric ulcers

4. A 35-year-old woman with jaundice presents with a raised bilirubin level in which both conjugated and unconjugated forms are above normal. The blood urea and creatinine are both increased, and haemoglobin is decreased. The patient also has several (asymptomatic) gallstones in the gallbladder.

    What is the most appropriate management of this patient?

    A   Commence vitamin B$_{12}$ injections to treat the anaemia
    B   Ignore the raised urea and creatinine because liver failure may be present
    C   Investigate a possible haemolytic anaemia
    D   Investigate a possible hepatic failure of bilirubin conjugation
    E   Proceed to removal of the gallstones

5. A 45-year-old man presents with mild abdominal discomfort and is subsequently found to have several small gallstones. He is otherwise well.

    What is the most appropriate management of this patient?

    A   Consider elective cholecystectomy after full informed consent
    B   Investigate for impaired absorption of bile salts and bile pigments
    C   Scan his liver for hepatic secondary tumours
    D   Treat the gallstones medically with bile pigments
    E   Treat the gallstones medically with bile acids

Answers

1. A A low circulating albumin level

Synthesis of circulating albumin is a major liver function. A low albumin level (together with a low albumin/globulin ratio, C) is a major indicator of liver failure. Since albumin is the major contributor to plasma oncotic pressure which retains fluid in the circulation, deficiency increases fluid filtration from the capillaries. Thus, the low albumin leads to dependent oedema – manifested in the ankles in the upright posture and around the sacrum in those confined to bed. Ascites is related to a combination of increased filtration pressure in the peritoneal capillaries due to portal hypertension (often found in liver failure) and decreased opposing oncotic pressure. Thus both his conditions are strongly related to the low circulating albumin level.

Hepatic encephalopathy is impaired brain function related to toxins accumulating in liver failure and portosystemic anastomoses are enlarged venous channels which, in the oesophagus can rupture, causing sudden severe haemorrhage.

2. C Commence regular injections of vitamin K

With obstructive jaundice, bile is not reaching the gut. Absence of bile salts in the gut impairs absorption of fat and fat-soluble vitamins. Of these vitamin K is essential for formation of prothrombin in the liver. Prothrombin deficiency increases clotting time so INR (patient's clotting time divided by standard normal value) is elevated to 1.8 and there is a clear danger of excessive haemorrhage at operation due to impaired clotting. The vitamin K deficiency can be reversed by injections of the vitamin, bypassing the gut. Advancing the time of non-urgent surgery (A) would increase risks inappropriately. Factor VIII (D) is used during surgery in patients with haemophilia, and fresh frozen plasma (E) is used when there are multiple or uncertain abnormalities of clotting.

3. D Oesophageal varices related to portal venous hypertension

Hepatic cirrhosis, by the scarring it causes, often impedes flow of portal blood through the liver, hence causing portal venous hypertension. The presence of ascites supports the diagnosis of portal hypertension, as does the severity of the bleeding. Increased pressure in the portal veins leads to diversion of blood through distended, weak-walled portosystemic anastomoses. These are common in the lower oesophagus and are prone to catastrophic bleeding.

Deficiency of vitamin B_{12} and gastric acid reflux are not significant contributory factors (B, C).

4. C Investigate a possible haemolytic anaemia

With both unconjugated and conjugated bilirubin raised, a haemolytic anaemia is suggested. The liver is conjugating more bilirubin than usual and yet is not keeping pace with the build-up of freshly released unconjugated bilirubin from broken-down red cells. The haemolytic anaemia needs to be investigated and treated before dealing with asymptomatic gallstones (E), which in this case may be pigment stones from the increased biliary content of conjugated bilirubin.

There is no suggestion of liver failure in this case and even if present it would not explain the raised urea and creatinine (B) which also need investigation (urea is normally formed in the liver, so its value may fall slightly in liver failure).

5. A Consider elective cholecystectomy after full informed consent

This is a young patient with gallstones who is otherwise well. Although he has minimal symptoms, as he is young, cholecystectomy should be considered after full informed consent. Although a case can be made to leave things alone, he may develop complications later in life when he might have developed co-morbid disease. Laparoscopic cholecystectomy is one of the safest operations in good hands and eliminates the dreadful possibility, although rare, of cancer of the gallbladder which carries a dismal prognosis.

Investigating the patient for impaired absorption of bile salts and bile pigments (B) and hepatic secondaries (C) is not necessary as he remains otherwise well. Bile pigments are not a method of treatment (D).

Chapter 20

Inflammation

Questions

For each question, select the single best answer from the five options listed.

1. A 40-year-old woman is admitted for surgery having been diagnosed with autoimmune thyroid (Grave's) disease. Damage to the thyroid causing diffuse hyperplasia and high vascularity is caused by mechanisms similar to a type II hypersensitivity reaction.

   What is the most likely mechanism for this reaction?

   A Activated T cells sensitised to nickel compounds
   B Antibody binding to antigens
   C Antigens becoming trapped inside macrophages
   D Bacterial infection in the gland
   E Circulating immune complexes deposit in the gland

2. A 55-year-old man presents with severe respiratory problems after elective cardiac surgery. He is diagnosed with acute respiratory distress syndrome triggered by endotoxin liberation.

   What are the most likely immunological effects of endotoxin liberation?

   A Activation of CD8+ cytotoxic T cells
   B Decreased vascular permeability and prevention of vasodilation
   C Induction of B cells and the antibody response.
   D Macrophage activation and initiation of the cytokine cascade
   E Sensitisation of mast cells by antigen specific IgG

3. A 43-year-old man has received a renal transplant after kidney failure. Three weeks after his transplant, he starts showing symptoms of acute rejection.

   What is the most likely immunological mechanism involved in acute rejection?

   A Alloreactive T cells infiltrate the graft
   B Immune complexes producing an inflammatory response
   C Immunosuppressive drug related toxicities
   D Pre-existing antibodies to major histocompatibility class I or ABO antigens
   E Reoccurrence of the original disease.

4. A 65-year-old man, recently retired, has taken up bee-keeping. After being stung several times, his most recent sting causes him to collapse with anaphylactic shock. His symptoms were very similar to the anaphylactoid reactions he had occasionally seen previously when handling the bees.

   What is the most likely difference in mechanism between the anaphylactic and the anaphylactoid reaction?

   A   Anaphylactoid reactions are allergic reactions to milk proteins
   B   Anaphylactoid reactions are caused by direct activation of mast cells and are not immune mediated.
   C   Anaphylactoid reactions require high circulating levels of immunoglobulin E
   D   Anaphylactoid reactions require primary sensitisation of mast cells by the immune response
   E   There is no difference – they are both the same

5. A 45-year-old man presents with a wound infection for investigation. The wound contains high levels of phagocytic (pus) cells. Elimination of infection by phagocytic cells is a major mechanism in the prevention of sepsis and inflammation.

   What is their most likely mechanism of action?

   A   Provide the main defence against virus infected cells
   B   Inhibit complement activation
   C   Ingest and kill invading bacteria
   D   Provide 'help' for B-cells in primary adaptive immune response
   E   Secrete antibodies during the immune response

6. A 36-year-old woman with systemic lupus erythematosus is admitted for a kidney transplant after her own organ has ceased to function.

   What is the most likely immunological mechanism that initiated the damage to her kidney?

   A   Activation of the alternative complement pathway
   B   Antibody binds to antigens immobilised on kidney cells and tissues
   C   Antigen binds directly to proximal tubule cells causing cell sensitisation
   D   Circulating immune complexes deposit in the tissues
   E   Damage to the tissues is caused by activated T cells

7. A 30-year-old woman sustained a leg injury while gardening and was admitted to hospital. Dirt and soil in the wound caused an infection, initiating an acute inflammatory response. Activation of the alternative complement pathway is central to this process.

   What is the most likely mechanism of complement activation by this pathway?

   A   Complement attaches to IgE antibody on mast cells
   B   Complement attaches to immune complexes bound to phagocytic cells
   C   Complement coated bacteria bind directly to CD8+ cytotoxic T cells
   D   Complement components in blood are activated by bacteria
   E   T lymphocytes bind to bacterial peptides complexed with MHC class II molecules

Answers

1. B Antibody binding to antigens

The inflammatory response is a normal, necessary part of the immune response (**Figure 20.1**). Hypersensitivity reactions occur when an antigenic stimulus cannot be removed (e.g. chronic infection, autoimmune disease). In type II reactions, antibody is formed against antigen on the surface of cells in individual organs (**Table 20.1**). When the antigen is a cell receptor, antibody binding can either initiate or inhibit stimulation by the natural ligand. In Grave's disease autoantibody binds to the thyroid stimulating hormone receptor on the thyroid gland, permanently stimulating the production of thyroxine. Normally this is controlled by feedback regulation when high levels of thyroxine inhibit release of thyroid-stimulating hormone from the pituitary gland, but will have no effect on autoantibody production.

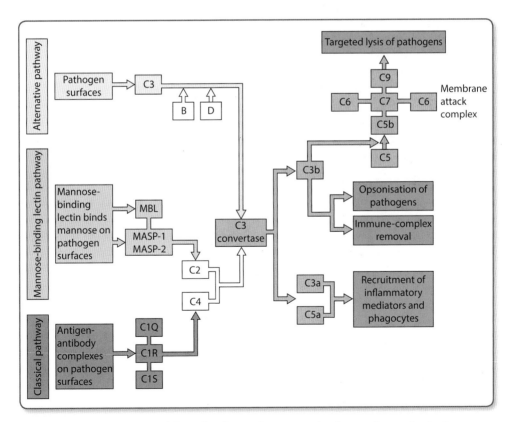

Figure 20.1 An overview of the role of complement activation pathways in the immune response.

Table 20.1 Comparison of the immune mechanisms which lead to the initiation of the four types of hypersensitivity reaction	
Hypersensitivity reaction	**Mediated by**
Type I (immediate)	Allergen-specific IgE bound to mast cells is cross-linked by initiating allergen leading to mast cell degranulation
Type II	Antigen-specific IgG or IgM antibody binds to antigen on tissues and organs
Type III	Antigen-specific IgG or IgM antibody forms complexes with circulating antigen which then deposit in a range of tissues
Type IV (delayed)	Three variants: contact, tuberculin, granulomatous mediated by T lymphocytes

2. D Macrophage activation and initiation of the cytokine cascade

Endotoxins are structural components of Gram-negative bacterial cell walls made up of polysaccharides and lipids called bacterial lipopolysaccharides. Their active component, responsible for most toxic effects, is lipid A. Picogram quantities of lipopolysaccharides entering the circulation will rapidly stimulate macrophages (through TLR4 receptors) to release tumour necrosis factor-α. This initiates an inflammatory cascade through release of IL-1, IL-6, platelet activating factor and eicosanoids. Neutrophils activate, aggregate and adhere to endothelial cells. Endotoxins also directly activate coagulation, fibrinolytic and contact dependant pathways. Classical and alternative complement pathways are also activated (**Figure 20.1**). This results in vasodilation, hypotension and poor organ perfusion.

3. A Alloreactive T-cells infiltrate the graft

Major histocompatibility (MHC) molecules on the cell surface have a major role in immune recognition, presenting antigen to either CD8+ T cells (MHC class I) or CD4+ T cells (MHC class II). Most of the rejection response is to these molecules which show wide genetic variability between individuals. Rejection involves different immune effector mechanisms and timing is important in determining which is occurring. Acute rejection occurs in days to weeks and is initiated when donor dendritic cells (passenger leucocytes) migrate out of the transplanted kidney to recipient lymph nodes and stimulate a primary allogeneic response. Activated T-cells return to the kidney where they generate cytotoxic T-cells and induce delayed type hypersensitivity reactions (type IV (**Table 20.1**). Both CD4+ and CD8+ T cells can cause graft rejection.

4. B Anaphylactoid reactions are caused by direct activation of mast cells and are not immune mediated

In type I hypersensitivity reactions, adjacent allergen-specific IgE molecules on mast cells, cross-linked by their specific allergen, activate the mast cell to release its pharmacological mediators (**Table 20.1**). Pollen, house dust mite, animal dander elicit local responses, but food, bee stings, drugs can cause a systemic response (anaphylactic shock) when all the mast cells release their pharmacological mediators at the same time. Anaphylactoid reactions are also caused by systemic release of mast cell mediators but here there is no immune involvement, no sensitisation phase and no IgE production. The agent acts directly on the mast cells or by activating the alternative complement pathway (**Figure 20.1**). Nonsteroidal anti-inflammatory drugs, radio-opaque organic iodines and intravenous anaesthetic induction agents may do this.

5. C Ingest and kill invading bacteria

Phagocytic cells (macrophages and neutrophils) are the main immune mechanism for removal of invading microbes, and act by ingesting and killing them. Toll-like receptors, C-type lectins and 'scavenger receptors' have been identified as pathogen-associated molecular patterns (PAMPs) recognised by phagocytes on microbial surfaces. Intracellular PAMPs such as unmethylated guanosine cytosine (CpG) sequences of bacterial DNA and double-stranded RNA from RNA viruses also act in this way. The organism is phagocytosed into a vacuole which fuses with cytoplasmic granules which release their contents to kill and digest the organism by oxygen-dependent and independent mechanisms. Uptake by the phagocyte is significantly enhanced by coating the organism (opsonisation) with complement, antibody or both (**Figure 20.1**).

6. D Circulating immune complexes deposit in the tissues

Systemic lupus erythematosus is the classic systemic or non-organ-specific autoimmune disease and is characterised by chronic production of large numbers of small immune complexes which overwhelm normal disposal mechanisms (**Table 20.1**). They deposit in the walls of small blood vessels in the renal glomerulus, joints and other organs leading to complement fixation by the classical pathway and migration of inflammatory cells to the site (type III hypersensitivity reaction) (**Figure 20.1**). The consequent tissue damage causes more immune complexes to form and the inflammation induced can cause sufficient damage for the organ to cease functioning and require transplantation.

7. D Complement components in blood are activated by bacteria

Microorganisms activate the alternative complement pathway (**Figure 20.1**). Once activated, C3b binds to the surface of the organism opsonising it for phagocytosis. C3a and C5a act on mast cells to release mediators that affect vascular permeability and also neutrophil chemotactic factors. Their combined effects allow fluid and plasma components including more complement to move to the site of infection. Upregulation of adhesion molecules allows neutrophils (which have a C3b receptor) to adhere to capillary walls (margination), move along a chemotactic gradient to the infection site and phagocytose the C3b coated bacteria which started the process. This is the acute inflammatory response, an important mechanism in innate immunity. Macrophages can also initiate this response independently of mast cells through activation by endotoxin, C5a, and C3b coated bacteria.

Chapter 21

Cellular injury and infection

Questions

For each question, select the single best answer from the five options listed.

1. A 28-year-old woman is concerned that her breasts fluctuate in size according to the stage of her menstrual cycle. It is explained to her that this is in response to changes in the hormone levels in her body causing the cells of her breast tissue to proliferate and regress each month.

    What is the name given to the process whereby cells proliferate and regress under hormonal influence?

    A   Atrophy
    B   Apoptosis
    C   Avascular necrosis
    D   Degeneration
    E   Dysplasia

2. A 35-year-old woman is informed that the result of her cervical smear test shows dysplastic changes of the cervical epithelium.

    Which description most accurately describes dysplasia?

    A   All different types of cells mixed together
    B   Cells showing changes which look malignant
    C   Cells which are failing to become fully mature
    D   Cells which are looking primitive and not differentiated
    E   Cells with lightly coloured large nuclei

3. A 55-year-old woman has developed the clinical and biochemical features of chronic renal failure. A CT-guided renal biopsy shows signs of swelling with clear vacuoles appearing in the cytoplasm. There are also some fatty globules in the cytoplasm.

    Which process is most likely to explain these microscopic changes?

    A   Defence against viral infection
    B   High intracellular potassium levels
    C   Permanent cell damage
    D   Rapid repair and division of cells
    E   Reversible cell injury

4. A 59-year-old man has been complaining of gastro-oesophageal reflux symptoms which has not improved despite being started on a proton pump inhibitor. An endoscopy is performed which showed a red velvety mucosa over the gastro-oesophageal junction. Biopsies were taken which shows changes in keeping with Barrett's oesophagus.

    Which word accurately describes this process?

    A   Atrophy
    B   Metaplasia
    C   Dysplasia
    D   Hyperplasia
    E   Hypertrophy

5. A 25-year-old man, an intravenous drug user, has died of a fulminating chest infection. At postmortem the lungs look like a piece of cheese when viewed macroscopically. Microscopically they show fragmented pieces of cells enclosed within a clear inflammatory border.

    What is the underlying pathology?

    A   Abscess formation
    B   A carbuncle
    C   Caseous necrosis
    D   Coagulative necrosis
    E   Liquefactive necrosis

6. A 60-year-old man underwent a femoropopliteal bypass using an artificial graft. Postoperatively the wound becomes infected and the graft is found to be infected with *Staphylococcus epidermidis*.

    What special mechanism is this organism using to protect itself from attack?

    A   Ability to produce collagenase
    B   Absorption of plasmids from other resistant bacteria
    C   Developing a glycoprotein biofilm in which it can lie dormant
    D   Lying dormant inside erythrocytes for part of its life cycle
    E   Rapid mutation to give it antibiotic resistance

7. A 47-year-old man is waiting on a decortication for treatment of his empyema. He is currently barrier nursed due to a contagious infection that he is being treated for. After reviewing the patient, an infection control officer asks that you wash your hands rather than use the alcohol gel.

    Which microorganism is not killed by alcohol gel?

    A   *Clostridium difficile*
    B   *Escherichia coli* O157
    C   Human immunodeficiency virus
    D   Methicillin-resistant *Staphylococcus aureus*
    E   *Streptococcus pneumonia*

8. A 56-year-old man has an oesophagogastroduodenoscopy. Following the procedure, a medical student questions how the endoscope is cleaned.

   Which of the following are used to clean endoscopes?

   A   Alcohol gel
   B   Ethylene oxide
   C   Formaldehyde
   D   Glutaraldehyde
   E   Povidone-iodine

Answers

1. B Apoptosis

The natural process of cell death occurs under the influence of hormone changes is called apoptosis. Unlike necrosis (C), which is a result of external or pathological agents, there is usually very little inflammation and no other tissues are involved. Apoptosis is a normal not a pathological part of the anatomy and physiology of the human body. Atrophy (A) denotes reduction in the size of cells or decreased function which is not the case here. Similarly, degeneration (D) is not the process here as it signifies change of tissue to a lesser functionally active form. Dysplasia (E) signifies abnormality of development in pathology and is precancerous and so is not the process here.

2. C Cells which are failing to become fully mature

Cells showing rapid division but failing to become fully mature are dysplastic. It is a response by cells to stress. The cells start to divide more rapidly and fail to mature into their fully differentiated state. They have a higher nuclear to cytoplasmic ratio. They also lose the normal architecture of the nucleus. They are not malignant cells, but in some cases, such as the cervix, the dysplastic changes can indicate that malignant change is likely to occur in future. The other possibilities (A, B, D, E) are not the changes occurring here – A shows mixed cellularity, B shows malignancy, D denotes undifferentiated cells and E are just cells with hyperchromatic nuclei.

3. E Reversible cell injury

Swelling is a cardinal sign of temporary cell injury. In those injured cells, which normally metabolise actively, this may be accompanied by the accumulation of triglycerides because these cells are not able to metabolise fatty acids properly. In irreversibly damaged cells, there will also be coagulation of proteins and disruption of cell membranes. The nucleus becomes small and dense (pyknotic) and may even start to fragment.

4. C Metaplasia

Metaplasia refers to the reversible change in one fully differentiated cell type to another. This patient has metaplastic change in his lower oesophagus due to acid reflux changing the normal squamous cell epithelium to columnar epithelium with goblet cells. The importance of Barrett's oesophagus is that it can progress to adenocarcinoma of the oesophagus.

5. C Caseous necrosis

The features in the history here point to tuberculosis. *Mycobacterium tuberculosis* which produces a very characteristic necrotic lesion with contents the consistency of cheese. Liquefactive necrosis (E) would be more characteristic of a staphylococcal infection, which produces an abscess. Coagulative necrosis (D) is characteristic of non-infective causes of death such as ischaemia. A carbuncle (B) is a subcutaneous collection of pus so it is not found in the lung.

6. C Developing a glycoprotein biofilm in which it can lie dormant

Staphylococcus epidermidis is a normal skin commensal and so it is not normally a pathogen. However, it has an unexpected ability to form a glycoprotein biofilm on the surface of implants which is impervious to antibodies and antibiotics. So long as it remains dormant in the matrix of this biofilm, it can survive in the human and wait for an opportunity to break out. Other pathogenic organisms employ a variety of methods to protect themselves from their host. Many bacteria, especially *Escherichia coli,* gain resistance to antibiotics by rapidly mutating to new strains which have resistance (E). Some of these bacteria can transfer resistance to antibiotics to other species of bacteria by the direct transfer of naked DNA in plasmids. Again *Escherichia coli* is commonly implicated. Collagenase (A) destroys collagen and is implicated in the rapid spread of *Clostridium* through tissues. *Plasmodium* spends part of its life cycle within the erythrocyte (D).

7. A *Clostridium difficile*

Clostridium difficile spores are not killed by alcohol gel. All the other organisms listed are killed by the use of alcohol gel. When in contact with a patient with *Clostridium difficile* infection it is important to wear gloves, and use soap and water to wash hands properly after taking the gloves off.

8. Glutaraldehyde

2% glutaraldehyde is the most commonly used chemical agent to clean endoscopes, following a manual clean. However, glutaraldehyde has been reported as a sensitising and irritating agent with side effects including nausea and vomiting, rhinitis, asthma and headaches. This is why the exposure time to the chemical should be kept to a minimum. Alternative agents are currently under investigation to replace glutaraldehyde. Formaldehyde is traditionally used to sterilise surgical instruments. Povidone–iodine is used to disinfect skin, wounds and mucous membranes pre-operatively. Alcohol gel is used for hand sanitisation.

Chapter 22

Wounds and wound healing

Questions

For each question, select the single best answer from the five options listed.

1. A 20-year-old healthy student is caught in a bomb blast and sustains an injury to her right leg. There is skin loss with abrasions, and a wood splinter hidden deep beneath a laceration on the outside of her thigh.

    What is the most likely cause for the delay in wound healing?

    A   Diabetes mellitus
    B   Foreign body
    C   Malnutrition
    D   Site of wound
    E   Smoking

2. A 36-year-old man underwent an emergency conventional open appendicectomy for acute appendicitis and was discharged after 48 hours. He returns 3 days later with a high swinging pyrexia and severe pain in the stitch line. There were signs of inflammation and a yellowish discharge from the wound.

    Which of the following is the most appropriate management of this patient?

    A   CT scan of the abdomen
    B   Open the wound on the ward
    C   Re-exploration in operating theatre
    D   Start antibiotics
    E   Start intravenous fluids and antipyretics

3. A 45-year-old woman presents with bouts of right upper abdominal pain associated with fatty meals. She is diagnosed as has having multiple gallstones with chronic cholecystitis and undergoes an elective laparoscopic cholecystectomy with a conventional four-port approach.

    Which of the following terms best describes the wounds created for the ports?

    A   Clean
    B   Clean contaminated
    C   Contaminated
    D   Dirty
    E   Dirty infected

4. A 55-year-old man, who is a smoker and an alcoholic, presents to the emergency department with acute upper abdominal pain and shock. He is diagnosed as having peritonitis with free gas under the dome of diaphragm. He undergoes emergency laparotomy with repair of a duodenal ulcer perforation and thorough peritoneal lavage. The abdominal fascia is closed with polypropylene but the skin is left open due to extensive contamination of the wound during surgery. The wound is dressed daily and the skin is closed after 72 hours.

   Which of the following best describes the procedure carried out above?

   A   Primary closure (healing by first intention)
   B   Secondary closure (healing by secondary intention)
   C   Delayed primary closure
   D   Delayed secondary closure
   E   Tertiary closure

5. A 35-year-old man was admitted with a sebaceous cyst on the front of the sternum which was excised and the incision was closed primarily. The patient presents 6 months later with local itchiness and nodular swelling at the incision site. The swelling is firm in consistency and extended into the adjoining skin beyond the incision. Intralesional triamcinolone therapy improved the lesion symptomatically.

   Which of the following is the most likely diagnosis?

   A   Cylindroma
   B   Fibroma
   C   Hypertrophic scar
   D   Keloid
   E   Recurrent sebaceous cyst

6. A 66-year-old diabetic man sustained an unstable pelvic fracture after a fall from height. He was initially treated with several weeks of bed rest. Upon transfer to a tertiary care centre, examination of the sacral region revealed a 10 × 12 cm area of full thickness skin loss with exposed sacral bone.

   Which of the following stages of pressure bed sore best describes the above ulcerated wound?

   A   Stage 1
   B   Stage 2
   C   Stage 3
   D   Stage 4
   E   Stage 5

Answers

1. B Foreign body

Wound healing depends on local and systemic factors. Some important local factors which can hinder healing are the presence of a foreign body, blood clot or dead/devitalised tissue in the wound, infection, tissue hypoxia, and vascular compromise, e.g. due to poor blood supply/vascular insufficiency or tight sutures in a wound. The vascularity in the wound may be reduced from previous irradiation or diabetes leading to microangiopathy or atherosclerosis. The presence of any foreign body in the wound leads to the persistence of infection and should be suspected as a cause of delayed healing when other local or systemic factors are absent. Systemic factors include advancing age, insufficiency of vitamins A and/or C, zinc and proteins, systemic malignancy, chemotherapy, radiotherapy, immunosuppressive illness, venous oedema, diabetes, malignancy, uraemia, obesity and peripheral vascular disease.

2. B Open the wound on the ward

Signs suggestive of surgical site infection are increasing local pain at the surgical site with signs of inflammation (redness, shiny skin, a discharge, induration of the surrounding tissue and tenderness to palpation). This is usually accompanied by a swinging pyrexia. The most appropriate management is to open the wound and collect any discharge for gram stain, culture and sensitivity. The wound should then be washed out and a non-stick, absorbent dressing applied. Starting antibiotics alone would convert the wound abscess into an antibioma, prolong the illness, postpone local wound healing and increase the risk of septicaemia. Any collection of pus needs to be found and drained. If there had been signs of peritonitis (abdominal distension, bowel ileus, widespread tenderness and rebound tenderness beyond the midline) or an intra-abdominal collection visible on ultrasound or CT scan, then formal exploration in the operating theatre would be more appropriate.

3. B Clean contaminated

One classification of wounds is based on the degree of contamination. There are the following classes of wounds:

- **Class I or clean wound:** This refers to all elective surgical wounds which are uninfected and where the respiratory, gastrointestinal, hepatobiliary or genitourinary systems are not entered e.g. varicose vein.
- **Class II or clean contaminated wound:** This refers to a surgical wound created when the respiratory, gastrointestinal, hepatobiliary or genitourinary systems are entered under controlled conditions and without any significant contamination e.g. appendicectomy.
- **Class III or contaminated wound:** Wounds involving significant contamination from the gastrointestinal tract or a major breach in the sterile technique are included in this category e.g. operations on the colon or rectum with spillage.

- **Class IV or dirty/infected wound:** Contamination of the wound with purulent material from an existing source of infection like perforation of a hollow viscus, severe inflammation e.g. peritonitis or gangrenous appendicitis.

The above classification is valuable in deciding on antibiotic management. Prophylactic antibiotics are given either as a single dose at induction or three doses over the first 24 hours and are used for Class I and II wounds. Therapeutic antibiotics are given to patients with Class III and IV wounds and may need to be continued for 5 or more days.

4. C Delayed primary closure

Class I and Class II category wounds which have been created in elective surgery, such as those after an incised traumatic wound with little or no contamination, or after elective surgical procedures as described in Question 3, may be closed by primary closure. This leads to primary healing or 'healing by first intention'. It is now a standard practice to irrigate the wound with saline before approximating the skin with sutures or staples. Closure of the subcutaneous tissue separately is no longer thought to be necessary. However, presence of infection at the surgical site or significant contamination of the wound to pus, intestinal contents or faecal matter is best managed by leaving the wound open with daily return to the operating theatre for cleaning and redressing. Once the wound is clean (2–5 days later) it is closed by delayed primary closure. In cases where there is heavy contamination or presence of dead tissue requiring daily debridement or extensive tissue destruction, the wound is allowed to heal by granulation. Such a wound progressively contracts with the maturation of collagen and undergoes epithelialisation from the edges. It closes by the formation of a scar over several weeks or months. Such a form of healing is referred to as secondary healing or 'healing by secondary intention' and produces a scar which is usually wide and thick.

5. D Keloid

There is a delicate difference between hypertrophic and keloid scars:

Hypertrophic scars are usually raised above the skin level but stay within the confines of the original wound. They are more frequently seen when scars cross areas of tension or are located on flexor surfaces crossing the joints. Hypertrophic scars are particularly prone to occur after extensive burns which have healed by scarring. Hypertrophic scars can be prevented by meticulous approximation of skin edges without tension.

Keloid scars are raised above the skin level and also tend to invade the normal skin surrounding the initial scar. There is an autosomal dominant trait and are commoner in people with darker skin. Histologically, the collagen fibres are larger and thicker than normal. The first-line treatment of keloid is non-surgical with the use of intralesional injection of steroids like triamcinolone. Radiation, pressure garments and the topical application of silicone sheets may also be useful. Surgery combined with radiotherapy is the last option and is valuable for debulking very large lesions.

6. D Stage 4

Bed sores are pressure sores, defined as skin ulceration accompanied with tissue necrosis as a result of prolonged pressure. These are not uncommon in patients who are debilitated and on prolonged bed rest, immobilised for trauma or due to paraplegia. Elderly and immunocompromised people are particularly vulnerable. A pressure sore passes through the following stages:

Stage 1: non-blanching erythema or redness of the skin in the absence of any breach in the continuity of the overlying skin

Stage 2: partial thickness loss of skin involving the epidermis and dermis

Stage 3: full thickness skin loss with exposed subcutaneous tissue but intact fascia

Stage 4: the same as above but extending into deeper tissues like muscle, tendons, bones or joints

Figure 22.1 illustrates a typical Stage 4 bed sore. **Figure 22.2** shows the various stages in the formation of a bed sore. **Table 22.1** summarises the pathology and management of a bed sore.

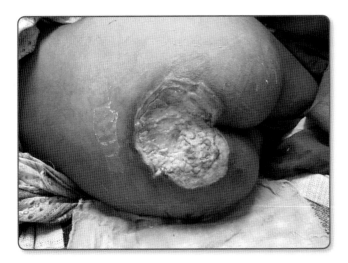

Figure 22.1 Stage 4 type of pressure bed sore with exposed sacral bone and deep muscles. Note the sloping type of edges consistent with healing ulcer. Such a patient needs to be nursed in the lateral position if possible and needs the help of a plastic surgeon to plan an appropriate wound cover.

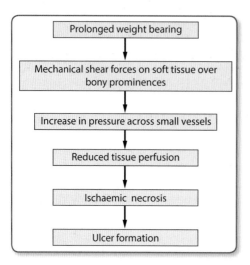

Figure 22.2 Stages in the formation of a bed sore.

Table 22.1 Summary of pathology and management of bed sore	
Definition	A chronic wound following tissue necrosis from pressure
Aetiology	Paraplegia Peripheral vascular disease Unconscious and confused bed-bound patients
Sites	Any bony prominences: • Sacrum • Ischium • Trochanter • Heel

Treatment	Supportive:
	    Improve tissue perfusion, oxygenation, correct anaemia and malnutrition, relieve pressure
	Surgery:
	    Consider only after careful and detailed assessment
	Prevention:
	    Multidisciplinary approach is necessary

Chapter 23

Disorders of growth and differentiation

Questions

For each question, select the single best answer from the five options listed.

1. A 72-year-old man presents with symptoms of bladder outflow obstruction. Ultrasound of the bladder shows a bladder diverticulum.

   Which of the following is most likely to have caused the formation of the diverticulum?

   A   Apoptosis of prostatic cells
   B   Hyperplasia of bladder musculature
   C   Hypertrophy of bladder musculature
   D   Inflammatory response in bladder neck
   E   Regeneration of transitional bladder epithelium

2. A 55-year-old woman has suffered from chronic renal failure for 10 years and has been on haemodialysis over the same period. During this 10-year period, she has developed renal osteodystrophy from secondary hyperparathyroidism.

   Which of the following is most likely to have caused the hyperparathyroidism?

   A   Carcinoma of parathyroid glands
   B   Combined pattern growth of parathyroid glands
   C   Hyperplasia of parathyroid glands
   D   Multiplicative growth of parathyroid glands
   E   Parathyroid adenoma

3. A 52-year-old man underwent an emergency left hemicolectomy for an annular carcinoma of the upper descending colon. The resected specimen showed huge dilatation and thickening of the bowel proximal to the growth.

   Which of the following is most likely to have caused this change in the macroscopic appearance of the proximal large bowel?

   A   Hyperplasia of the bowel musculature
   B   Hypertrophy of the bowel musculature
   C   Inflammatory response from the carcinoma
   D   Pseudomalignant epithelial hyperplasia
   E   Regeneration of columnar intestinal epithelium

4. A 45-year-old woman complained of a breast lump. After formal triple assessment, she underwent surgical removal of the lump. Histology showed no malignancy with fibrocystic changes.

   Which of the following is most likely to have caused these changes?

   A   Apoptosis
   B   Breast duct hypertrophy
   C   Dystrophic calcification
   D   Granulomatous mastitis
   E   Hyperplasia of breast epithelium

5. A 50-year-old man, a heavy smoker, suffers from long-standing gastro-oesophageal reflux disease. Histology of the lower one-third of the oesophagus shows a Barrett's oesophagus with an associated mucosal abnormality.

   Which of the following is the most likely abnormality?

   A   Accretionary growth
   B   Differentiation
   C   Dysplasia
   D   Heterotopia
   E   Metaplasia

6. A 30-year-old man who recently arrived in the UK from North Africa presents with haematuria. Cystoscopy reveals the presence of bilharzial nodules with papillomas. Histology does not show a carcinoma but does show a mucosal abnormality.

   Which of the following is the most likely abnormality in the mucosa?

   A   Dysplasia
   B   Granuloma
   C   Metaplasia
   D   Multiplicative growth
   E   Pseudotubercles

7. A 65-year-old woman, on medical treatment for ulcerative colitis for 10 years, has been on annual colonoscopic surveillance. This is combined with random colonic biopsies.

   Which of the following changes is the pathologist looking for in the biopsies?

   A   Auxetic growth
   B   Dysplasia
   C   Hyperplasia
   D   Metaplasia
   E   Regeneration

8. A 40-year-old woman sustained a blunt injury to her breast as a result of a road traffic accident where the steering wheel struck her chest wall. Two weeks later she presents in the breast clinic with a breast lump at the site of the injury.

    Which of the following is the most likely diagnosis?

    A Breast carcinoma
    B Duct ectasia
    C Fibroadenoma
    D Fat necrosis
    E Granulomatous mastitis

Answers

1. C Hypertrophy of bladder musculature

In this patient, there is hypertrophy of the urinary bladder musculature resulting in thickening. The stimulus to this change is mechanical. Because of bladder outflow obstruction, most commonly from an enlarged prostate, there is increased workload on the bladder to empty. The stimulus to overcome the obstruction results in increased cellular size without cell replication; and the bladder muscle hypertrophies. With continued obstruction, the intravesical pressure increases causing trabeculation. When the obstruction is not relieved, it results in sacculation which is herniation of the mucosa through the trabeculated musculature of the bladder. Ultimately, sacculation leads to formation of a diverticulum. The most common site of a diverticulum is next to the ureteric orifice as it is the site of maximum weakness. This common pathological outcome in bladder outflow obstruction can be summarised as:

Bladder outflow obstruction → hypertrophy of bladder musculature → trabeculation → sacculation → diverticulum formation (**Figure 23.1**).

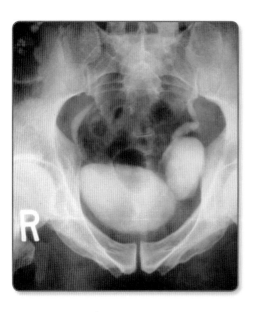

Figure 23.1 Intravenous urogram showing bladder diverticulum.

2. C Hyperplasia of parathyroid glands

This patient has parathyroid hyperplasia where all four parathyroid glands are enlarged. The increase in size of the glands is due to proliferation of the chief cells (specialised parathyroid C-cells) in response to the renal failure. This biochemical stimulus results in hyperphosphataemia, relative hypocalcaemia and disordered vitamin D metabolism, a clinical situation called secondary hyperparathyroidism, where there is an increased demand for function resulting in multiplication of the number of cells, and also resulting in diffuse enlargement of the glands. Rarely, one of the glands may become hyperplastic when it is called an adenoma. Such a clinical scenario is referred to as tertiary hyperparathyroidism. Microscopically the normal glandular adipose tissue is replaced by hyperplastic chief cells arranged in sheets or trabecular or follicular pattern. Scattered oxyphil cells are common with small foci of adipose tissue.

3. B Hypertrophy of bowel musculature

The growth disorder here is classical hypertrophy of the proximal large bowel. The stimulus here is mechanical, caused by prolonged obstruction from the annular colonic carcinoma (**Figure 23.2**) that has formed over a period of time. Obstructive features occur in cancer in the left colon where the lumen is narrow and the faecal contents more solid. As a result of the functional demand to overcome the obstruction, changes occur to adapt to the pathology in an attempt for the solid faecal matter to negotiate the narrowed lumen. When trophic signals or functional demand increases, adaptive changes to satisfy these needs lead to increased cell size. In organs made of terminally differentiated cells (e.g. heart, skeletal muscle and intestinal muscle) such adaptive response is accomplished by increase in cell size, i.e. hypertrophy. The stimulus to enlarge may be increased work load, as in this case, or an increase in endocrine and neuroendocrine mediators.

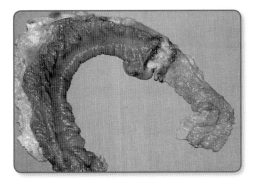

Figure 23.2 Carcinoma of the descending colon.

4. E Hyperplasia of breast epithelium

The underlying pathology here is hyperplasia of the breast epithelium, aptly called epithelial hyperplasia (epitheliosis). Fibrocystic (non-proliferative) breast change may represent an exaggerated physiological response. This includes gross and microscopic cysts. There is proliferation of epithelial cells which occurs in the interlobular and intralobular ducts and the acini resulting in a mass obliterating the lumina, which is filled by hyperplastic epithelium. Cysts of various sizes are dispersed in dense, fibrous connective tissue. Some of the cysts are large and contain old blood-tinged proteinaceous debris.

Atypical hyperplasia can be a sinister finding. Here, there is disordered orientation of cells: nuclear pleomorphism with occasional mitotic cells. This is termed atypical ductal or lobular hyperplasia which has a 4- to 5-fold increased risk of developing invasive cancer, a risk further enhanced by a strong family history.

5. C Dysplasia

The abnormality here is dysplasia, a pre-malignant change occurring in the presence of Barrett's oesophagus which is columnar-lined lower oesophagus. Barrett's oesophagus occurs as a result of metaplasia from long-standing chronic gastro-oesophageal reflux disease. The condition is usually confined to the lower one-third of the oesophagus but may extend higher. The squamous epithelium is replaced by a 'specialised epithelium' which consists of a mixture of intestine-like epithelium of well-formed goblet cells, gastric foveolar cells and Paneth cells. In dysplasia, this specialised epithelium is altered by variation in size and shape of the cells, nuclear enlargement, irregularity, hyperchromatism, larger nucleus-to-cytoplasm ratio and disorderly arrangement. The dysplasia may be mild, moderate or severe, the latter being considered by some as carcinoma in situ. The risk of cancer in such a situation is 25 times higher than in the general population, this risk being enhanced by the increased length of the involved oesophagus.

6. C Metaplasia

This patient has metaplasia of the bladder from long-standing bilharzial infestation with *Schistosoma haematobium*. Presence of ova in the bladder submucosa results in cystitis glandularis and cystitis cystica. In due course pseudotubercles form, which coalesce to form nodules. In long-standing cases, areas of transitional cell epithelium transform into squamous metaplasia which is also called leucoplakia. This will ultimately give rise to squamous cell carcinoma which is not the usual type of bladder cancer (normally transitional cell carcinoma) and has a poor prognosis. A similar type of change may occur anywhere in the urinary tract infested with this parasite, with an equally sinister outcome. In the urinary tract metaplasia can also occur in the presence of a long-standing stone in the renal pelvis or the urinary bladder with a similar outcome. Metaplasia is conversion of one type of cell type to another. It is an adaptive response to a chronic persistent injury.

7. B Dysplasia

In this instance, dysplasia is the change that the pathologist is particularly looking for. Ulcerative colitis is a diffuse mucosal disease with acute and chronic inflammatory cells. Crypt abscesses are a typical feature where aggregates of polymorphs are seen within distended crypts. There is lack of mucin in the epithelium with mucosal atrophy. In long-standing cases, there is epithelial dysplasia which is precancerous. Microscopically, there is alteration in mucosal architecture and epithelial abnormalities showing hypercellularity with variation in the size, shape and staining qualities of the nuclei. High-grade dysplasia will soon result in colorectal cancer which may occur in more than one site, known as synchronous cancer. Therefore, this is an indication for panproctocolectomy. The longer the duration of the disease, the greater is the chance of developing cancer. Hence, all patients with the disease longer than 10 years should be on annual colonoscopic surveillance.

8. D Fat necrosis

This woman classically has developed fat necrosis, a condition that can easily be confused with breast carcinoma. The condition results from direct trauma to adipose tissue resulting in extracellular liberation of fat. Here the release of intracellular fat produces a brisk inflammatory response with phagocytosis by polymorphs and foamy macrophages, ultimately leading to fibrosis and calcification. This results in a palpable mass in the breast as in this patient. Sometimes the mass can be hard often with skin tethering lending credence to a diagnosis of carcinoma. Necrotic fat cells, an acute inflammatory cell infiltrate, cholesterol clefts and haemorrhage are seen early in the course of fat necrosis. The clinician should be aware that fat necrosis may bring the patient's notice to a lump not previously felt which may turn out to be a carcinoma.

Chapter 24

Neoplasia

Questions

For each question, select the single best answer from the five options listed.

1. A 35-year-old woman presents with a lump in the region of her right femoral triangle. This has gradually been growing in size over 2 years. It is 8 cm in diameter, neither painful nor tender, easily mobile and slips under the finger.

    What is the most likely diagnosis?

    A   Aneurysm of femoral artery
    B   Secondary metastasis
    C   Lipoma
    D   Lymphoma
    E   Soft tissue sarcoma

2. A 70-year-old man undergoes an anterior resection for rectal cancer. The histology from the specimen is reported as Dukes' stage B cancer.

    Which statement describes this stage?

    A   Confined to the bowel wall
    B   Metastasised to liver
    C   Metastasised to regional lymph nodes
    D   Penetrating mucosa
    E   Spread to perirectal (extra-rectal) tissues

3. A 60-year-old man undergoes a total gastrectomy for carcinoma of the stomach. The histology of the surgical specimen shows a well-differentiated carcinoma.

    Which of the following does this pathological feature indicate?

    A   Anaplastic growth
    B   Fibrous infiltration
    C   Increased mitosis
    D   Marked nuclear pleomorphism
    E   Original intestinal type epithelium

4. A 16-year-old boy has recently arrived in the UK for treatment of a Burkitt's lymphoma which is affecting the jaws.

    Which of the following is most likely aetiology of this malignant neoplasm?

    A   Aromatic amines
    B   Bacteria
    C   Genetically inherited
    D   Ultraviolet radiation
    E   Virus

5. A 60-year-old man, who had a malignant tumour excised 5 years ago, presents with a painful, warm, pulsatile lump in the middle of his upper thigh. An X-ray of his femur shows a solitary lytic lesion on the upper shaft of the femur.

    Which of the following is the most likely malignant tumour that was resected 5 years ago?

    A   Colorectal carcinoma
    B   Gastric carcinoma
    C   Prostatic carcinoma
    D   Renal cell carcinoma
    E   Testicular teratoma

6. A 56-year-old man, who has tested positive for AIDS, presents with a slightly painful, non-itchy, reddish-brown ulcerative skin lesion, 4 cm in diameter, on the dorsum of his left foot. This has been gradually increasing in size over 6 months. There is marked swelling of the foot and distal leg.

    What is the most likely diagnosis?

    A   Angiosarcoma
    B   Kaposi's sarcoma
    C   Lymphangiosarcoma
    D   Secondary skin metastasis
    E   Soft tissue sarcoma

7. A 3-year-old boy is brought to the emergency department by his mother, who says that while bathing her son she noticed asymmetry of her child's abdomen, with the right side looking much larger. He also had three episodes of haematuria over the previous 4 months. On examination, there is a mass in the right side of the abdomen and loin. The right iris is absent.

    What is the most likely diagnosis?

    A   Ganglioneuroma
    B   Hepatoblastoma
    C   Neuroblastoma
    D   Rhabdomyosarcoma of the urinary bladder
    E   Wilms' tumour (nephroblastoma)

Answers

1. C Lipoma

This patient has a lipoma on the front of her thigh, a benign tumour arising from the subcutaneous fat. The classical clinical features of the condition are: a slow-growing painless lump, non-tender, mobile and easily slips under the finger; referred to as the 'slipping' sign (**Figure 24.1**).

A neoplasm, also called a tumour, is a lesion that results from the autonomous growth of cells which persist after the initiating cause has ceased. According to their biological behaviour, neoplasms are classified as benign and malignant. The latter can be a carcinoma arising from epithelial tissues or sarcoma arising from connective tissues. Any tumour, benign or malignant is named by its cell or tissue of origin with the suffix '-oma'. A benign tumour replicates the parent cell of origin, is slow-growing and remains localised (non-invasive) and well-circumscribed by a surrounding capsule; it never spreads to distant organs (metastasis).

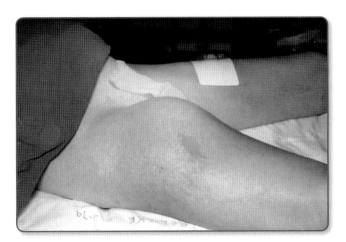

Figure 24.1 A fatty swelling that slips easily under the finger tip: lipoma.

2. E Growth spread to perirectal (extra-rectal) tissues

Dukes' stage B denotes the spread of cancer to perirectal tissues beyond the rectal wall. In 1932 Cuthbert Dukes described the post-operative staging of rectal carcinoma in three stages (A to C) according to the spread. In stage A, the cancer is confined to the rectal wall, i.e. involving mucosa, submucosa and muscle; in stage B, the cancer has gone beyond the muscle into the perirectal tissues without lymph node involvement; when there is lymph node metastasis, it is stage C. In some quarters stage C is subdivided into C1 and C2, the latter denoting involvement of the apical lymph node at the origin of the inferior mesenteric artery. Later, a 4th stage (stage D) was added to a growth that had spread to the liver. At the time of resection, 15% belong to stage A, 35% to stage B and the remaining 50% to stage C.

3. E Original intestinal type epithelium

When a carcinoma is reported as being well differentiated, it signifies that the cells have a strong resemblance to the parent structure. Differentiation is a term used to mean the degree to which the tumour histologically resembles its cell of origin; the more the cancer cell is akin to its original cell, the better differentiated the tumour is, and therefore the prognosis is better. Thus, tumours may be graded as well-differentiated (good prognosis), moderately differentiated (intermediate prognosis) and poorly differentiated (bad prognosis).

In the case of the stomach, intestinal type gastric cancers originate from sites of intestinal metaplasia which are typically well-differentiated adenocarcinoma and form polypoid tumours or ulcers. Biologically, these types of gastric cancers, referred to as early gastric cancer, behave in a more benign manner with a much better prognosis than advanced gastric cancer which carries a dismal prognosis.

4. E Virus

The carcinogen in Burkitt's lymphoma is a virus discovered in 1964 by Michael Epstein, a pathologist, and Yvonne Barr, a virologist, and hence called Epstein–Barr virus (EBV). The tumour is named after Denis Burkitt who first brought attention to this condition in Uganda in 1958. Epstein–Barr virus is a human herpesvirus which is so common all over the world that the vast majority of adults have antibodies to it. Epstein–Barr virus was the first virus to be confirmed as a causal agent for a human malignant tumour. Burkitt's lymphoma is a B-cell tumour in which EBV is within the DNA of the lymphocytes. Normally suppressor T cells keep the B-cell proliferation under control. However, in chronic malaria, there is a lack of T-cell response. This results in uncontrolled B-cell proliferation going on to the formation of a lymphoma. Nasopharyngeal carcinoma is another tumour caused by EBV.

5. D Renal cell carcinoma

The primary tumour would have been a renal cell carcinoma (adenocarcinoma of the kidney). It is also known as Grawitz's tumour, hypernephroma or clear cell carcinoma. Renal cell carcinoma most often metastasises via the blood stream to the lungs and bones, particularly long bones. Secondary bone cancer is typically very vascular, hence the pulsatile lump in the thigh. This bone secondary is lytic, and therefore eventually, a pathological fracture will result. If a fracture is imminent then surgical stabilisation with an intramedullary nail should be planned as soon as the vascularity of the tumour has been reduced with arterial embolisation. Histologically, the bone secondary replicates the clear cell cancer of the kidney. The cancer arises from cells of the proximal convoluted tubule and is an adenocarcinoma in a mixed form containing clear and granular cells. Macroscopically it is yellow in colour because of the high lipid content.

6. B Kaposi's sarcoma

As this patient is known to have AIDS, a vascular, ulcerative skin lesion in a limb is likely to be Kaposi's sarcoma which occurs in immunocompromised patients.

It was described in 1872 by Moritz Kaposi. This is a malignant proliferative tumour arising from vascular endothelial cells. It occurs in immunocompromised patients. The lesion commences as a reddish-brown or purple cutaneous nodule that ulcerates and may be solitary or multiple. Lymphatic obstruction may give rise to swelling of the limb from lymphoedema. Histologically there is granulation tissue with proliferation of vessels with poorly differentiated, spindle-shaped, neoplastic endothelial cells and extravasation of red blood cells and inflammatory cells.

Since the arrival of the human immunodeficiency virus (HIV) infection, Kaposi's sarcoma is most commonly seen in patients with AIDS. Human herpes virus 8 (HHV-8) is the causative organism. 75% of patients with AIDS who have HHV-8 in the blood will develop Kaposi's sarcoma within 5 years.

7. E Wilms' tumour (nephroblastoma)

This child has a right Wilms' tumour, the most common abdominal solid tumour in children. Haematuria, a rare symptom, denotes that the growth has invaded the renal pelvis and is therefore at a locally advanced stage. Absence of the iris and hemi-hypertrophy of the body are associated with this condition. An intravenous urogram may show a soft tissue shadow with irregular pelvicalyceal pattern (**Figure 24.2**). Macroscopically the tumour is a soft solid mass of whitish tissue with cystic cavities, haemorrhage and necrosis. Histologically the tumour consists of normal fetal tissue of primitive mesenchyme cells of embryonic nephrogenic blastema. Hence there are highly cellular areas of undifferentiated mesenchymal cells, immature tubules, striated muscle fibres, cartilage and bone.

Stage 1 – Tumour confined to kidney

Stage 2 – Tumour extending beyond the kidney

Stage 3 – Tumour incompletely excised with positive lymph nodes

Stage 4 – Distant metastases

Stage 5 – Bilateral tumours

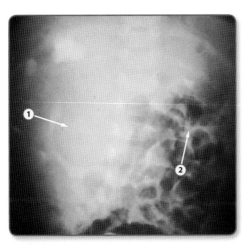

Figure 24.2 Nephrotomography showing: huge soft tissue shadow on the right (1) with normal excretion on the left (2).

Chapter 25

Surgical immunology

Questions

For each question, select the single best answer from the five options listed.

1. A 17-year-old man is admitted to hospital following a road accident. His spleen is removed because it is ruptured.

   Which role of the spleen will be lost with its removal that may affect the patient's future health?

   A   Deletion of immature autoreactive T cells
   B   Major site of insulin producing cells
   C   Primary lymphoid organ where immature lymphocytes arise
   D   Removal of encapsulated bacteria by phagocytic mechanisms
   E   Responds to the pituitary gland to produce thyroxine

2. A 55-year-old man scheduled for surgery was found to be HIV positive at pre-assessment.

   What is the most likely effect of this infection on his immune response to infection?

   A   His ability to phagocytose and kill bacteria will be lost
   B   Activation of an effective adaptive immune response will be impaired
   C   Activation of the alternative complement pathway will be prevented
   D   None; HIV infection does not affect the immune response
   E   Innate immune defences will be impaired

3. A 60-year-old man with septicaemia due to an antibiotic resistant infection was admitted to hospital. In septicaemia, uncontrolled activation of inflammatory cytokines can lead to acute respiratory distress syndrome and multiorgan failure.

   What are cytokines?

   A   Antigen-specific molecules produced by B lymphocytes
   B   Part of an enzyme cascade activated by immune complexes
   C   Small signalling proteins that regulate immune activation
   D   Subtype of cytotoxic T cells
   E   Ultracellular enzymes which kill bacteria within phagocytic cells

4. A 70-year-old woman is admitted for hip replacement. She had suffered for many years from chronic rheumatoid arthritis, an autoimmune disease with progressive joint destruction.

What is the most likely mechanism causing autoimmune disease?

A   The body mounts an immune response against itself
B   Chronic activation of allergen specific IgE sensitised mast cells initiates the disease
C   A deficient immune response due to the action of an external agent
D   A genetic defect causing a deranged immune response
E   T cell activation is inhibited

5. A 21-year-old woman is admitted to hospital for the removal of her wisdom teeth. Investigations reveal that she has high levels of circulating IgM antibody.

What statement below best describes IgM antibodies?

A   Antibodies that can survive on mucosal surfaces
B   Antibodies which bind to mast cells during allergic reactions
C   Antibodies which can confer protection to newborn infants
D   Long-lived antibodies that provide long-term protection against infection
E   Short-lived antibodies produced during the early stages of ongoing infection

6. A 30-year-old man is going to work in Uganda for 6 months. As a precaution he has a Heaf (six-needle) test, and this gives a positive reaction.

What is the most likely immunological significance of this result?

A   Determines exposure to Lyme disease
B   Determines protective antibody responses to vector-borne infections
C   Determines T-cell responses to the tubercle bacillus
D   Measures allergic responses to grass and flower pollens
E   No immunological significance

7. A 70-year-old woman, admitted for a corneal graft, will not require immunosuppressive therapy after surgery because the anterior chamber of the eye is considered to be 'immunologically privileged'.

What is the most likely immunological mechanism involved?

A   Adaptive immune responses do not occur there.
B   All immune cells are destroyed immediately upon arrival
C   Beneficial responses are promoted while damaging ones are suppressed.
D   Immune cells arrive but are prevented from entering
E   Immune cells become functionally inactive on entering the site

Answers

1. D Removal of encapsulated bacteria by phagocytic mechanisms

The spleen is a secondary lymphoid organ composed of red pulp and white pulp and a marginal zone. In white pulp, lymphoid tissue forms a periarteriolar sheath composed of B-cell follicles and a T-cell area. B-cell germinal centres (stimulated follicles) also contain follicular dendritic cells and phagocytic macrophages. Aged platelets and red cells are destroyed in the red pulp. Various antigen-presenting cell types and a distinct subset of long-lived B-cells are present in the marginal zone. The spleen filters foreign antigens present in the blood and provides a site where antigen presentation and activation of lymphocytes can take place. It has a unique role in the phagocytic removal of encapsulated bacteria.

2. B Activation of an effective adaptive immune response will be impaired

Human immunodeficiency virus (HIV) selectively targets and kills CD4+ T lymphocytes. Activated CD4+ T cells provide help to CD8+ cytotoxic T-cells and B-cells in activating an adaptive immune response. Repeated cycles of infection eventually eliminate all the CD4+ T-cells and their bone marrow precursors. AIDS is defined by a CD4+ T-cell count of less than 200 cells/μL and takes an average of 10 years to develop.

3. C Small signalling proteins that regulate immune activation

Cytokines are small soluble signalling molecules that enable all immune cells to regulate themselves, each other and any cell that expresses the requisite cytokine receptor. Chemokines are a cytokine subset that orchestrates immune cell movement to the optimal anatomical site to carry out their function. Once cytokine activation occurs, a cascade of inflammatory and regulatory cytokines is initiated which serves to self-regulate the system. In septicaemia, the cytokine tumour necrosis factor alpha (TNF-α) synergising with other cytokines such as IL-1 and interferon gamma can override these regulatory mechanisms.

4. A The body mounts an immune response against itself

Autoimmune disease occurs when a genetically susceptible individual comes in contact with an environmental trigger. Immune tolerance mechanisms, which prevent recognition of self proteins by the immune system, are bypassed by a number of mechanisms and an autoimmune response occurs. Diseases form a spectrum from organ-specific (e.g. Graves' disease) at one end to non-organ-specific or systemic (e.g. systemic lupus erythematosus) at the other end. Rheumatoid arthritis lies towards the systemic end of the spectrum and damage to the joints is caused by deposition of immune complexes in the joints (type III hypersensitivity reaction) leading to complement activation by the classical pathway and inflammation (**Figure 20.1**).

5. E Short-lived antibodies produced during the early stages of ongoing infection

Five classes of antibody are produced by activated B cells namely IgG (a monomer of the basic structure); IgM (a pentamer of the basic structure); IgA (a dimer of the basic unit); IgE (which circulates bound to mast cells) and IgD (monomeric surface receptor on B cells). IgM is the first antibody produced during the primary immune response. It is short-lived and eventually replaced by IgG. At second and subsequent exposure, the main antibody class produced is IgG which is long-lived and confers long-term protection against subsequent exposure to the same infection. High circulating IgM levels are indicative of an ongoing current infection.

6. C Determines T-cell responses to the tubercle bacillus

Type IV delayed type hypersensitivity reactions come in three variants – contact, tuberculin and granulomatous all mediated by T cells. The Heaf test employs the tuberculin reaction and can be used to determine previous exposure to *Mycobacterium tuberculosis* and efficacy of vaccination. On first exposure, either to the natural infection or vaccine, primary sensitisation of the adaptive immune response occurs and memory T-cells are formed. On second contact, when small amounts of organism are injected into subcutaneous tissue, memory cells are activated, and CD4+ T helper 1 lymphocytes move to the site of inoculation (**Table 20.1**). The response evolves over 24 or 48 hours.

7. C Beneficial responses are promoted while damaging ones are suppressed

'Privileged sites' were thought to be locations where immune responses did not occur. More extensive tests have revealed that these sites are not immunologically impaired but have differences in their self-regenerative capacity. The eye is poorly regenerative and can be completely destroyed by a pro-inflammatory cell-mediated adaptive response. It therefore promotes beneficial responses while suppressing those that would cause local damage. Anterior chamber epithelial cells express Fas ligand which preferentially leads to destruction of Th1 lymphocytes but allows Th2 responses. Tumour growth factor-β present in the fluid limits T cell proliferation and induces Th2 and T regulatory cells thus inflammatory responses are prevented.

Chapter 26

Surgical microbiology

Questions

For each question, select the single best answer from the five options listed.

1. A 70-year-old man, who is an insulin-dependent diabetic and a smoker, is due to undergo a below-knee amputation for gangrene of his foot that cannot be re-vascularised. He is not allergic to any antibiotic.

    What is the most appropriate antibiotic prophylaxis for this patient?

    A   Benzylpenicillin
    B   Cefuroxime
    C   Erythromycin
    D   Tetracycline
    E   Vancomycin

2. A 50-year-old man with severe acute pancreatitis is in the intensive care unit. A contrast-enhanced CT scan on the 3rd day in the intensive care unit showed pancreatic necrosis.

    What is the most appropriate next step in his management?

    A   Antibiotic treatment
    B   Fine-needle aspiration cytology of the pancreatic necrosis
    C   Intravenous nutrition
    D   Laparotomy
    E   Observe with daily ultrasound

3. A 15-year-old girl underwent an emergency splenectomy for trauma. She is now at increased risk of infection.

    Which one of the following organisms is most likely to be the causative agent?

    A   Clostridia
    B   Encapsulated bacteria
    C   *Klebsiella*
    D   *Pseudomonas aeruginosa*
    E   *Staphylococcus aureus*

4. A 45-year-old man underwent emergency surgery 2 weeks ago for severe soft tissue injury around an open comminuted fracture of his tibia and fibula. An external fixator was applied. He has now developed osteomyelitis of his tibia.

   Which of the following is the most likely organism causing his osteomyelitis?

   A *Clostridium tetani*
   B *Escherichia coli*
   C *Pseudomonas aeruginosa*
   D *Staphylococcus aureus*
   E *Streptococcus*

5. A 72-year-old man underwent aortobifemoral bypass graft. Following this he spent 2 days in the intensive care unit because he had medical complications. The right groin wound became infected on the 8th postoperative day. The swab report came back as methicillin-resistant *Staphylococcus aureus.* He had received the usual antibiotic prophylaxis according to the unit's protocol.

   Which of the following is the most appropriate antibiotic to be started?

   A Aminoglycoside
   B Carbapenems
   C Cephalosporins
   D Glycopeptides
   E Imidazoles

6. A 75-year-old woman underwent an emergency sigmoid resection and Hartmann's procedure for perforated diverticulitis. Postoperatively she is in the intensive treatment unit. On the 2nd day her readings are as follows:

   - Temperature: 39.8°C
   - Heart rate: 98 beats per minute
   - Respiratory rate: 28 breaths per minute
   - White cell count: 3×10^9 with immature neutrophils

   Which of the following conditions is she most likely to have?

   A Infection
   B Multiple organ dysfunction syndrome (MODS)
   C Sepsis
   D Severe sepsis
   E Systemic inflammatory response syndrome

7. A 45-year-old man, an insulin-dependent diabetic for 20 years, presents as an emergency with painful scrotal oedema, sloughing of a part of scrotal skin and a perianal abscess. A clinical diagnosis of Fournier's gangrene was made.

   Which organism is most likely to have caused this condition?

   A *Clostridium difficile*
   B *Clostridium perfringens*
   C Combination of organisms
   D Gonococci
   E Tubercle bacillus

8. A 52-year-old man underwent small bowel resection 4 weeks ago for Crohn's disease, this being his fourth resection in as many years. He has been left with only a few feet of small bowel. Therefore, it was felt necessary to give him parenteral nutrition for which he has a right subclavian tunnelled central venous line. For almost a week he has been pyrexial with a temperature ranging from 38°C to 39°C.

What is the most likely cause of his pyrexia?

  A Central line catheter
  B Deep wound infection
  C Pneumonia
  D Subphrenic abscess
  E Urinary tract infection

Answers

1. A Benzylpenicillin

Benzylpenicillin is the prophylactic antibiotic of choice as this patient has no history of drug allergy. 1.2 g is given intravenously during induction of anaesthetic and every 6 hours for the next 48 hours. This prophylaxis is against *Clostridia perfringens* to avoid gas gangrene. Bactericidal prophylaxis prevents intraoperative microbial contamination. All hospitals have a local policy which is followed except in exceptional cases of drug allergy.

Cefuroxime, a cephalosporin, is used when the patient is allergic to benzylpenicillin. Vancomycin is reserved for methicillin-resistant *Staphylococcus aureus*.

2. B Fine-needle aspiration cytology of the pancreatic necrosis

Fine-needle aspiration cytology should be carried out by the radiologist at the time of contrast-enhanced CT. If cytology confirms that the necrosis is infected, then the appropriate antibiotic is started after culture and sensitivities are obtained (**Figure 26.1**). More importantly in case of infected necrosis, the patient should undergo a laparotomy for thorough necrosectomy and lavage of the lesser sac under broad spectrum antibiotic cover. At the same time a feeding jejunostomy is

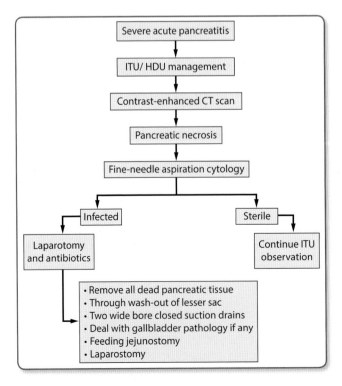

Figure 26.1 Management of severe acute pancreatitis. HDU, high-dependency unit; ITU, intensive care unit.

performed. The abdomen is closed by a laparostomy as second-look procedures are not uncommon. If the necrosed tissue is sterile, close observation is continued by repeated ultrasound or CT scan looking for the presence of gas. Surgical treatment of infected pancreatic necrosis can be carried out by laparoscopic approach depending upon the policy of the unit.

In some units, the presence of necrosed tissue in the lesser sac is an indication to start prophylactic antibiotics although this is controversial.

3. A Encapsulated bacteria

Patients who have undergone splenectomy are in danger of developing opportunist post-splenectomy infections (OPSI) in the form of septicaemia from encapsulated organisms such as *Streptococcus pneumoniae*, *Neisseria meningitidis* and *Haemophilus influenzae*. The risk is greater in children, the immunosuppressed, and those undergoing a splenectomy for haematological disorders, the incidence being highest during the first 3 years after splenectomy. In elective splenectomy, prophylactic vaccination should be given 2 weeks before surgery while in emergency splenectomy it should be given immediately after the operation.

After splenectomy, antibiotic prophylaxis should be given to all in the first 3 years, and then continued in children up to the age of 16 years and in immunocompromised patients. Prophylaxis should consist of twice daily penicillin in doses of 500 mg for adults and 250 mg for children; in those below 2 years the dose is 125 mg. Patients allergic to penicillin should be protected by erythromycin or chloramphenicol.

4. D *Staphylococcus aureus*

The most likely organism is *Staphylococcus aureus* which is the causative pathogen in more than 90% of patients. In children and neonates rarely *Haemophilus influenzae*, *Escherichia coli* and group B streptococci and in those with sickle-cell disease *Salmonella* may be the causative organism; very rarely gram-negative bacilli such as *Pseudomonas* may be responsible.

The cause in this patient is post-traumatic. There are no bone changes in the first 2 weeks. Therefore, an X-ray will only act as a baseline for future reference. Ultrasound-guided fluid aspiration and blood cultures will confirm the organism so that the appropriate antibiotic can be used. Prompt recognition and treatment prevents long-term complications of chronic osteomyelitis which may be seen in about 5%. In chronic osteomyelitis, there may be formation of dead bone (sequestrum) surrounded by normal bone (involucrum). The involucrum may have perforations (cloaca) through which parts of sequestrum may exude out as a sinus.

5. D Glycopeptides

This patient has a methicillin-resistant *Staphylococcus aureus* (MRSA). He should be started on a glycopeptide, such as vancomycin or teicoplanin. Vancomycin is the initial drug of choice, but some strains are developing resistance to it and in that case teicoplanin is the next choice. These drugs act by inhibiting peptidoglycan synthesis in the bacterial cell wall. MRSA is a type of nosocomial infection, a term used to signify infection acquired within the hospital.

The condition is easily transmissible and once acquired can be very difficult to eradicate. Therefore, prevention is highly important. Prevention strategies include: meticulous hand-washing, patient screening before high-risk major surgery, isolation of infected patients and postponement of elective surgery in carriers.

6. E Systemic inflammatory response syndrome

This patient has the typical parameters of systemic inflammatory response syndrome (SIRS) which can complicate a range of disorders such as:

- severe acute pancreatitis
- major trauma
- burns
- major emergency surgical procedures

SIRS is a hypermetabolic state where there is an exaggerated generalised manifestation of a local immune and inflammatory reaction. This massive inflammatory reaction with cell damage, results from systemic release of cytokines such as:

- tumour necrosis factor-alpha (TNF-α)
- interleukin-1 (IL-1)
- IL-6
- platelet activating factor

Several pathophysiological changes occur which are:

- loss of microvascular integrity
- increased vascular permeability
- systemic vasodilatation
- decreased myocardial contractility
- poor oxygen delivery to tissues that suffer from oxygen debt

The condition is associated with organ system dysfunction. Prompt intensive care unit management consists of:

- controlling the source of infection by surgery or interventional radiology
- prevention of tissue hypoxia which may require ventilation
- metabolic support by total parenteral nutrition
- prevention of nosocomial infections by appropriate antibiotics (**Figure 26.2**).

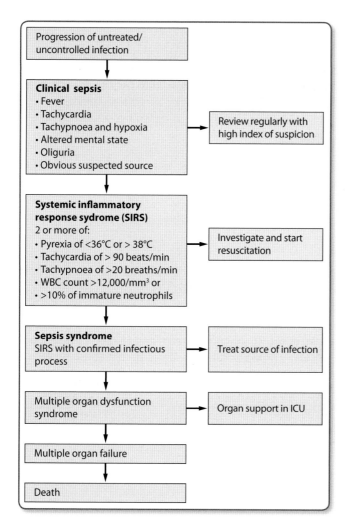

Figure 26.2 Steps in sepsis.

7. C Combination of organisms

This condition is caused by a mixed group of organisms which are coliforms, staphylococci, *Bacteroides,* clostridia and anaerobic streptococci. There is synergistic action between these organisms. The underlying pathology is necrotising fasciitis with spreading dermal gangrene. This may develop in devitalised tissues within areas of trauma. It is known to occur after relatively minor trauma. Patients, usually immunocompromised, are systemically ill and their pain is very severe, out of proportion to the clinical picture where signs may be minimal. Crepitus may be felt from underlying gas. This may be confirmed by ultrasound or CT scanning.

Management:

- early diagnosis
- vigorous resuscitation by circulatory support

- aggressive intravenous antibiotic therapy
- radical surgical debridement

Regular review under a general anaesthetic will be needed to ensure that all necrotic tissue is removed. Hyperbaric oxygen, not widely available, may have a role. In the long-term extensive plastic surgery will be required to cover the defects.

8. A Central line catheter

This patient's pyrexia is from central line catheter unless proven otherwise. Central line catheter infection occurs more commonly in lines used for parenteral nutrition. The pathogens responsible are:

- Skin commensals such as coagulase-negative *Staphylococcus*
- *Staphylococcus aureus*
- *Candida*
- Enterococci
- *Klebsiella*

Infection results from initial colonisation of the catheter hub from the hands of the carers; organisms establish themselves in the fibrin sheath of the intravascular part of the catheter thus gaining access to the bloodstream and cardiac valves. Lines with multiple lumens are particularly prone to catheter sepsis. Routine flushing with an anticoagulant, strict catheter handling protocols and a dedicated nursing team will reduce the incidence of this septic complication which carries a significant mortality and morbidity.

The diagnosis is confirmed by isolating the organism. In proven catheter infection, the line is removed and a new one inserted at a different site.

Chapter 27

Surgical haematology

Questions

For each question, select the single best answer from the five options listed.

1. A 35-year-old woman is having preoperative screening before laparoscopic cholecystectomy. She has had four children in the last 10 years, during which time she has suffered from heavy periods. For many years she has been on oral iron preparations intermittently. A full blood count shows haemoglobin of 105 g/L, mean cell volume is low, reticulocyte count is normal, red blood cells are pale.

   What is the most likely diagnosis?

   A Macrocytic anaemia due to failure of DNA replication
   B Macrocytic anaemia due to iron deficiency
   C Microcytic anaemia due to failure of DNA replication
   D Microcytic anaemia due to iron deficiency
   E Normocytic anaemia due to bone marrow failure

2. A 25-year-old man presents to day case surgery for a cervical lymph node biopsy. He has had persistent cervical lymphadenopathy for 1 month, with unexplained weight loss and profuse night sweating. He also reports being more lethargic than normal. His histology shows the presence of Reed–Sternberg cells.

   Which one of the following is the most likely diagnosis?

   A Acute leukaemia
   B HIV
   C Hodgkin's lymphoma
   D Non-Hodgkin's lymphoma
   E Tuberculosis

3. A 30-year-old man with thalassaemia major presents with recurrent episodes of right upper quadrant pain, which is worse after eating fatty food and associated with nausea. He is diagnosed with cholecystitis and undergoes a cholecystectomy.

   What would be the likely composition of gallstones found on histology?

   A Calcium oxalate stones
   B Cholesterol stones
   C Mixed gallstones
   D Pigment stones
   E Struvite stones

4. A 4-year-old Afro-Caribbean boy is referred to the general surgeons for an elective splenectomy. He has had two episodes of severe left upper quadrant pain in the last year, with a drop in haemoglobin requiring urgent blood transfusion. He was found to have a palpable mass in the left upper quadrant on examination. He also reports having swollen fingers and blood in the urine. Some of his siblings suffer from the same condition.

   What is the likely cause of his condition?

   A   Gaucher's disease
   B   Hodgkin's lymphoma
   C   Infectious mononucleosis
   D   Sickle cell anaemia
   E   Thalassaemia

5. A 35-year-old man is brought to the emergency department following a road traffic accident. On examination, he was found to have extensive bruising on the abdomen and a FAST (focused abdominal sonography in trauma) scan revealed free fluid in the perisplenic and pelvic spaces. His left leg was shortened and externally rotated. The patient underwent extensive surgery to fix a fractured neck of femur and a laparotomy was performed to investigate the free fluid further. He was found to have splenic rupture and a splenectomy was performed.

   Postoperatively he developed a widespread rash and is bleeding from his cannula sites.

   Blood tests were sent for analysis and the laboratory results are shown below:

Normal values	Result	Reference range
Platelet count	45×10^9/L	$150–450 \times 10^9$/L
Prothrombin time	15.1 seconds	9.5–13.5 seconds
APTT	130 seconds	70–120 seconds
Fibrinogen level	1.0 g/L	2.0–4.0 g/L
Fibrinogen degradation products	15 µg/mL	<10 µg/mL
D-dimer	250 ng/mL	<224 ng/mL

   Which one of the following is the most likely diagnosis?

   A   Allergic reaction
   B   Disseminated intravascular coagulopathy
   C   Incorrect heparin dose administration
   D   Meningitis
   E   Sepsis

Answers

1. D Microcytic anaemia due to iron deficiency

The history strongly suggests chronic iron deficiency due to increased loss of iron in her heavy periods; blood loss at the time of delivery would add to this. Iron deficiency is the major cause of microcytic anaemia. The cells are small and pale because of inadequate iron content. Normal red cells are in essence cellular bags filled with haemoglobin. In this case the anaemia should be corrected with oral iron before major surgery. A rising reticulocyte count during treatment with iron would confirm increased bone marrow activity and a response to the iron. The more active the bone marrow the greater is the percentage of circulating red cells showing the reticular pattern, which is lost during final maturation in the first day or so in the circulation.

In macrocytic anaemia (B), the cells are large because cell division in the red bone marrow is slowed. In normocytic anaemia (E), the cells are normal but the bone marrow is not able to maintain the required rate of production.

2. C Hodgkin's lymphoma

The presence of Reed–Sternberg cells on histology are characteristic of Hodgkin's lymphoma. Hodgkin's lymphoma is a malignancy affecting the lymphocytes in white blood cells. It commonly presents with axillary, cervical and inguinal lymphadenopathy. Epstein–Barr virus is a strong risk factor for Hodgkin's lymphoma. Night sweats, fever and weight loss in Hodgkin's lymphoma are poor prognostic indicators and are known as B symptoms.

Although HIV (B) increases the risk of Hodgkin's lymphoma there are no symptoms to suggest that this patient has underlying HIV. Non-Hodgkin's lymphoma and tuberculosis (D,E) presents with similar symptoms but the finding of Reed-Sternberg cells on histology excludes theses diagnoses.

3. D Pigment stones

The chronic haemolysis that occurs in thalassemia (and also other haemolytic condition like sickle cell anaemia) leads to an increase in unconjugated bilirubin, which predisposes to the development of pigment gallstones. Pigment stones are composed of calcium bilirubinate. Cholesterol stones (B) are the most common type of gallstones found on histology (B) but in this case the patient has a strong risk factor for developing the rarer type of pigment gallstone. Mixed gallstones can also be seen (C) but there is no information in the question to suggest a mixed picture, with pigment stones still being the most likely diagnosis. Calcium oxalate and struvite stones (A, E) are not seen in the gallbladder but are components of renal calculi.

4. D Sickle cell disease

This patient has signs and symptoms suggestive of sickle cell disease. Sickle cell disease occurs when a person inherits two copies of an abnormal haemoglobin gene from each parent. The two episodes of severe left upper quadrant pain are indicative of splenic sequestration crisis. In sickle cell disease, the red blood cells are fragile and an abnormal shape and due to the narrow vessels of the spleen intrasplenic sickling can occur as the spleen clears away the abnormal red blood cells. This can lead to sudden engorgement of the spleen and a drop in haemoglobin leading to a painful and life-threatening crisis, requiring an urgent blood transfusion. Recurrent splenic sequestration crisis is an indication for prophylactic splenectomy. The swollen fingers are a sign of dactilitis, a feature of sickle cell disease.

Gaucher's disease (A) is an autosomal recessive condition which causes anaemia and hepatosplenomegaly but the splenomegaly is painless in this condition. Although Hodgkin's lymphoma (B) and infectious mononucleosis (C) can cause splenomegaly it does not cause dactilitis or blood in the urine, and is not inherited; the history suggests that some of the boy's other siblings have the same condition. Thalassaemia (E) can present in a similar fashion to sickle cell anaemia and is an inherited condition. It may also require prophylactic splenectomy, but does not cause the dactilitis in this case.

5. A Disseminated intravascular coagulopathy

This patient has a combination of low platelets, low fibrinogen levels, with raised fibrinogen degradation products, raised d-dimers and prolonged prothrombin time and APTT, making disseminated intravascular coagulopathy (DIC) the most likely diagnosis. Major surgery is a risk factor for the development of DIC,

In DIC there is systemic activation of the coagulation cascade which results in both widespread clotting in small blood vessels and bleeding (as the platelets and clotting factors are consumed by the process). Tissue factor, a glycoprotein is one of the key mediators of this condition, which is released into the circulation after vascular damage and triggers the clotting cascade pathways. The resulting decrease in tissue perfusion can lead to organ damage and significant morbidity and mortality.

Chapter 28

Surgical biochemistry

Questions

For each question, select the single best answer from the five options listed.

1. A 50-year-old woman requires total parenteral feeding.

   Which of the following is the most appropriate management to meet her 24-hour energy requirements?

   A   5% dextrose and 10% amino acid solution
   B   20% dextrose and 10% lipid
   C   5% dextrose as the sole provider of energy
   D   50% dextrose as the sole provider of energy
   E   20% lipid as the sole provider of energy

2. A 60-year-old man with a long history of duodenal ulcer has the typical clinical features of gastric outlet obstruction with incessant non-bilious vomiting, visible gastric peristalsis and succussion splash. He has Chvostek's sign (tapping in front of the ear causes spasm of the facial muscles).

   Which of the following is most likely to have caused his spasm?

   A   Acidotic tetany from respiratory acidosis
   B   Acidotic tetany from respiratory alkalosis
   C   Alkalotic tetany from metabolic alkalosis
   D   Alkalotic tetany from respiratory acidosis
   E   Alkalotic tetany from respiratory alkalosis

3. A 25-year-old woman, who does not look after her type 1 diabetes well, has been brought into the emergency department with diabetic ketoacidosis. She has a high anion gap acidosis.

   Which of the following is most likely to have caused the acidosis?

   A   A decrease in bicarbonate concentration
   B   A decrease in chloride concentration
   C   An increase in potassium concentration
   D   An increase in sodium concentration
   E   Combined increase in sodium and decrease in chloride

4. A 50-year-old man with cancer of the pyloric antrum is severely malnourished with hypoalbuminaemia due to gastric outlet obstruction. He is to have parenteral feeding prior to radical gastrectomy.

Which of the following is the most effective feeding regimen?

A Amino acids, derived from animal and vegetable proteins
B Amino acids including essential amino acids
C Dextran
D Mixture of dextrose, intralipid and amino acids
E Mixture of dextrose, intralipid and dextran

5. A 20-year-old man has been admitted with multiple injuries after his car crashed. Several days after admission, he has to be taken to theatre for debridement of his wounds. A preoperative screen shows that he has developed a dangerously low circulating fibrinogen level.

Which of the following is most likely to have caused this condition?

A Congenital hypofibrinogenaemia
B Liver damage either pre-existing or due to the crash
C Loss of fibrinogen with the blood he lost
D Normal clotting to limit blood loss
E Widespread activation of clotting in regions of injury

6. A 60-year-old woman is being investigated prior to possible hip replacement for osteoarthritis. She has fairly well-controlled multiple myeloma, although she has increased circulating myeloma proteins. During her assessment she appears very tense, is hyperventilating and then develops carpopedal spasm. However, a plasma calcium measurement taken at this time is normal.

Which of the following is the most likely to have caused her spasms?

A Non-specific muscle cramps
B Respiratory acidosis combined with hyperproteinaemia
C Respiratory acidosis combined with hypoproteinaemia
D Respiratory alkalosis combined with hyperproteinaemia
E Respiratory alkalosis combined with hypoproteinaemia

Answers

1. B 20% dextrose and 10% lipid

As in normal life, this woman requires a blend of carbohydrate and lipid for daily energy. Carbohydrate is required for efficient functioning of the Krebs cycle in the mitochondria. However, lipid has the advantage of a high-energy content (around 9 kcal/g) compared with carbohydrate (and protein) which each delivers around 4 kcal/g. However, lipid alone (E) cannot be metabolised in the Krebs cycle efficiently and leads to increasing ketoacidosis. A litre of 5% dextrose (C) provides only 200 kcal of energy – just about one-tenth of the daily need. The higher the concentration of dextrose, the more energy it provides but the more irritant it is (hence the need to deliver into a large central vein for dilution). One litre each of 20% dextrose and 10% lipid provides 800 + 900 = 1700 kcal. Together with energy derived from the necessary amino acid infusion, this makes a reasonable contribution to her daily energy needs, and can be adjusted in relation to individual needs. Lipids are also vehicles for delivery of fat-soluble vitamins. Clearly the woman also requires appropriate amounts of minerals and other micronutrients.

Solution A provides inadequate energy, and Solution D is highly irritant.

2. C Alkalotic tetany from metabolic alkalosis

This man has alkalotic tetany due to incessant vomiting. The vomiting is non-bilious, consistent with gastric outlet obstruction. Thus, he is losing large amounts of gastric hydrochloric acid. The acid is produced in the parietal cells. These generate hydrogen ions in a process that involves combination of water and carbon dioxide:

$$H_2O + CO_2 \rightleftharpoons H^+ + HCO_3^-$$

The parietal cells secrete the hydrogen ions (together with chloride ions) into the gastric lumen and the bicarbonate ions pass into the circulation. Normally the hydrogen ions are reabsorbed in the small intestine but in this case, they are lost to the body in the vomit, so the bicarbonate level rapidly soars to give a metabolic alkalosis. An alkalosis, either respiratory or metabolic, alters the properties of the plasma proteins, so that they bind more of the circulating calcium ions, giving rise to a critical reduction in free calcium ions; this causes the tetany.

Acidosis protects against tetany, so A and C are wrong. There is no respiratory alkalosis in this case (D) and a respiratory acidosis cannot cause alkalotic tetany (E).

3. A A decrease in bicarbonate concentration

In diabetic ketoacidosis, the deficiency of glucose in cells causes them to rely on excessive lipid metabolism for energy. This generates ketoacids which liberate huge amounts of hydrogen ions. These swamp all the compensatory mechanisms and in the process reduce the bicarbonate level, which can fall to half or less than half of the normal value. The anion gap is a simple calculation of the combined sodium and potassium (ionic) blood levels, minus the combined chloride and bicarbonate levels, all in mmol/L. The normal gap is thus around $(140 + 5) - (105 + 25) = 15$. In severe cases of ketoacidosis the bicarbonate can slump to 10, doubling the gap in this case to 30. Other causes of a high anion gap acidosis are lactic acidosis and salicylate poisoning, where the bicarbonate is again depleted by buffering.

Changes in the other ions mentioned in B–E have little effect on the gap in this case.

4. D Mixture of dextrose, intralipid and amino acids

The aim is to improve this man's nutrition, and particularly his albumin level, promptly prior to urgent surgery. He requires a high-energy diet to maintain his metabolism and allow some restoration of lost weight, so amino acids alone would be inappropriate (C, D, E). In addition to a blend of carbohydrate and fat to provide energy, he requires an appropriate mix of essential amino acids to build up his circulating and muscle proteins. Essential amino acids are those which the body cannot synthesise. An appropriate mix of amino acids would be similar to those in plasma albumin. Dextran (B) is used to temporarily expand the blood volume but is of no nutritional value.

This man's survival and recovery from major surgery depend on an adequate stress response, which in turns depends on adequate reserves of energy and protein.

5. E Widespread activation of clotting in regions of injury

This young man has developed a low fibrinogen which must be corrected before surgery. The condition is consumptive coagulopathy due to disseminated intravascular coagulation. Extrinsic factors generated by widespread tissue damage initiate the widespread laying down of fibrin clot within blood vessels, depleting body levels of fibrinogen and other clotting factors. This is a relatively rare complication (C, D) and there is no evidence given in the question for options A and B.

6. D Respiratory alkalosis combined with hyperproteinaemia

This woman has two causes for hypocalcaemic tetany rather than non-specific muscle cramps (A) – her hyperventilation and her hyperproteinaemia (myeloma proteins adding to normal plasma proteins – E). Hyperventilation (due to stress) leads to a respiratory alkalosis (B, C). The mechanism of the alkalosis is lowering of the body's carbon dioxide level by increased excretion. This moves the equation below to the right, mopping up hydrogen ions:

$$H^+ + HCO_3^- \rightleftharpoons H_2O + CO_2$$

When body fluids are depleted of hydrogen ions, circulating proteins subtly alter their properties and mop up more free calcium ions in the plasma. We need to bear in mind that biochemistry laboratories measure total plasma calcium whereas it is the free calcium ions that determine whether or not there is tetany. Therefore, we would expect her total serum calcium to be normal in alkalotic tetany, and the ionized calcium to be low. Furthermore, in a patient with raised plasma proteins, the level of bound calcium ions will also sustain a compensatory rise.

A fall in free calcium ions changes the properties of proteins in excitable tissue membranes so that muscle spasms occur. Therefore, her total plasma calcium can be normal while the free ions are seriously reduced and the bound calcium is correspondingly elevated. A 'corrected' calcium level can be calculated by a formula involving plasma protein measurements.

Chapter 29

Central nervous system

Questions

For each question, select the single best answer from the five options listed.

1. A 25-year-old roofing contractor fell off a ladder on to a concrete floor and hit his temporal region. He was talking coherently as he came into the emergency department but rapidly became unconscious. He is found to have a dilated pupil reacting to light and a Glasgow Coma Score of 11.

    What is the most likely diagnosis?

    A   Acute subdural haematoma
    B   Brainstem injury
    C   Cerebral concussion
    D   Extradural haematoma
    E   Subarachnoid haemorrhage

2. A 65-year-old man, a heavy smoker, is being treated with radiotherapy for an inoperable bronchogenic carcinoma. He has attended with an intense early morning headache for 1 week which is associated with vomiting and loss of visual acuity.

    What is the most likely diagnosis?

    A   Acoustic neuroma arising from the 8th cranial nerve
    B   Cerebral metastasis
    C   Medulloblastoma
    D   Meningioma
    E   Pituitary adenoma

3. A 57-year-old man is admitted complaining of a sudden onset of intense occipital headache, which he describes as a 'hammer blow' to the back of his head. While giving his history he lapses into unconsciousness.

    What is the most likely diagnosis?

    A   Acute subdural haematoma
    B   Bleeding into a meningioma
    C   Extradural haemorrhage
    D   Subarachnoid haemorrhage from a ruptured berry aneurysm
    E   Transient ischaemic attack from internal carotid artery stenosis

4. A 45-year-old man complains of a 6-week history of throbbing early morning headache with vomiting. Recently he has noticed that he has lost lateral vision on both sides and is bumping into the sides of doorways and into people. His vision is blurred.

What is the most likely diagnosis?

A Bilateral optic neuritis
B Cerebellopontine angle tumour
C Glioma of the frontal lobe
D Migraine
E Pituitary adenoma

5. A 75-year-old woman on the medical ward has cognitive impairment with episodes of falling off to sleep. Her medication includes dipyridamole and warfarin. She accidentally fell out of bed a week ago, striking her head. At no time after this has her Glasgow Coma Score fallen below 14.

What is the most likely diagnosis?

A Acute subdural haematoma
B Cerebral infarction
C Chronic subdural haematoma
D Dementia
E Reversible intermittent neurological deficit from carotid artery stenosis

Answers

1. D Extradural haematoma

This patient has extradural haematoma. He has had a lucid interval followed by a deteriorating Glasgow Coma Score (GCS) and a dilated pupil. Extradural haematoma is caused by rupture of the middle meningeal artery which enters the middle cranial fossa through the foramen spinosum (see Chapter 1). As the haematoma enlarges in the confined space of the cranium, features of raised intracranial pressure (ICP) develop. The enlarging haematoma displaces the medial part of the temporal lobe against the midbrain which is displaced downward through the tentorial opening. This transtentorial herniation pushes the uncus against the 3rd cranial nerve (oculomotor) which is compressed by the sharp edge of the tentorium causing pupillary dilatation. Before this event occurs a protective response, called the Cushing reflex, sets in to improve cerebral circulation and oxygenation called cerebral autoregulation.

The patient requires an immediate CT scan followed by a craniotomy and evacuation of the haematoma.

2. B Cerebral metastasis

The classical clinical presentation of a brain tumour is early morning headache, vomiting and visual disturbance from papilloedema, all due to raised intracranial pressure (ICP). As the brain is contained within a closed box, any space-occupying lesion will cause a rise in ICP. According to the Monro–Kellie hypothesis, because of the non-compliant skull and dura, a small increase in intracranial volume results in a sharp increase in ICP. Sometimes focal neurological features may be a presenting feature, for example, bitemporal hemianopia in a pituitary tumour; seizures may be an emergency presentation. Metastatic tumours are the most common intracranial neoplasms. They spread to the brain in the bloodstream. In order of frequency, the tumours most likely to spread to the brain are:

- lung
- breast
- melanoma
- kidney
- colon

Overall, 25% of cancer sufferers will develop cerebral secondaries. In almost 15% of cerebral secondaries, the primary remains undetected.

3. D Subarachnoid haemorrhage from ruptured berry aneurysm

Berry (saccular) aneurysms are responsible for 75% of subarachnoid haemorrhages. The vast majority (90%) occur at the bifurcation of an artery in the circle of Willis at the base of the brain. This is because the tunica media is lacking at this point which weakens the vessel wall thus predisposing to turbulence of blood flow. This causes fragmentation of the internal elastic membrane resulting in aneurysm formation – the pathology being shaped like a berry, hence the name.

They occur with equal incidence at the junction of the anterior cerebral and anterior communicating arteries, the internal carotid complex and the trifurcation of the middle cerebral artery; in 20% they are multiple. Silent aneurysms are seen in 25% over the age of 55. Aneurysms at the bifurcation of the basilar artery account for 5% of cerebral aneurysms. The most common presentation is subarachnoid haemorrhage as an emergency.

4. E Pituitary adenoma

This patient has clinical features of raised intracranial pressure and bitemporal hemianopia, caused by pressure from the tumour on the optic chiasma. This is the characteristic presentation of a pituitary tumour, but in the case of large tumours the 3rd, 4th and 6th cranial nerves may also be involved. Some tumours may produce endocrine dysfunction; rarely a pituitary tumour may be a part of multiple endocrine neoplasia Type 1. This is a hereditary condition where there is pituitary adenoma, parathyroid adenoma, pancreaticoduodenal endocrine tumours.

Pituitary adenomas can be classified into three types:

- acidophil adenomas produce excessive quantities of growth hormone
- basophil adenomas produce excessive adrenocorticotrophic hormone
- chromophobe adenomas have no endocrine properties

Tumours under 10 mm are called microadenomas. They are only symptomatic if they produce a hormone; tumours over 10 mm are called macroadenomas. They can produce symptoms from pressure effects and from hormone overproduction.

5. C Chronic subdural haematoma

This patient has chronic subdural haematoma, a condition most common in the elderly. There is a typical history of minor head injury in the recent or distant past. Those on anticoagulants and antiplatelet drugs are particularly prone to bleeding after minor trauma. The cerebral hemispheres float in the cerebrospinal fluid being loosely fixed by blood vessels and cranial nerves. When the cerebral hemispheres strike the inside of the skull, the force of displacement causes the dura to move with the skull and the arachnoid to move with the cerebrum. This shearing effect causes the bridging and cortical veins in the subdural space to rupture and the haematoma to spread in the subdural space and hence is frequently bilateral.

Clinical features are variable: headaches, focal signs, seizures and cognitive impairment. A CT scan shows a hyperdense lesion which is diffuse and concave in appearance. The treatment is surgical evacuation.

Chapter 30

Cardiovascular system

Questions

For each question, select the single best answer from the five options listed.

1. A 70-year-old man, a heavy smoker, complains of cramp-like pain in both his calves after walking 400 metres when he has to stop. He can continue for a similar distance after a 10-minute rest.

   What is the most likely diagnosis?

   A   Bilateral varicose veins
   B   Intermittent claudication
   C   Morton's metatarsalgia
   D   Osteoarthritis of both knees
   E   Prolapsed intervertebral disc

2. A 35-year-old woman presents to her GP with headaches and general feelings of tiredness and lethargy. The GP did not find anything untoward except for a blood pressure of 140/90 mmHg. The GP heard a systolic bruit over the renal area.

   What is the most likely diagnosis?

   A   Malignant hypertension
   B   Nephrotic syndrome
   C   Pheochromocytoma
   D   Renal artery stenosis
   E   Renal cell carcinoma

3. A 33-year-old man returned home to the UK after a 6-week trekking holiday in the Amazon rainforests of Brazil. Twenty-four hours after the 13-hour flight, he developed gross swelling of his entire left lower limb from the groin distally; and the limb felt heavy and painful. He has a temperature of 38°C.

   What is the most likely diagnosis?

   A   Deep vein thrombosis
   B   Femoral artery embolism
   C   Filariasis
   D   Lymphangitis
   E   Acute thrombophlebitis

4. A 60-year-old man, of ASA 1 anaesthetic risk, underwent a total gastrectomy for stomach cancer. While in the intensive care unit, 12 hours after the operation, his blood pressure has dropped to 80 mmHg systolic with a pulse rate of 120 bpm; he has not put out any urine over the last 3 hours. He has an oxygen saturation of 92%.

    What is the most likely cause of this postoperative problem?

    A Acute respiratory distress syndrome (ARDS)
    B Hypovolaemic shock
    C Myocardial infarction
    D Pulmonary embolism
    E Septic shock

5. A 50-year-old man is admitted with increasing recurrent angina and severe dyspnoea. Six months ago, he had a fairly severe myocardial infarct of the left anterior descending and circumflex arteries. His present ECG shows persistent ST segment elevation and abnormal Q waves.

    What is the most likely diagnosis?

    A Cor pulmonale
    B Dressler's syndrome
    C Ischaemic cardiomyopathy
    D Myocardial rupture
    E Left ventricular aneurysm

Answers

1. B Intermittent claudication

This patient has intermittent claudication which is the result of atherosclerosis. The condition affects the aorta and medium-sized arteries and develops over several decades. Risk factors are male sex, obesity, increasing age, family history, hypertension, diabetes, increased C-reactive protein, smoking and the use of the contraceptive pill; environmental and genetic factors also play a part. An increased level of low-density lipoprotein cholesterol and a decreased level of high-density lipoprotein predisposes to atheroma formation.

The typical lesion in atherosclerosis is a fibroinflammatory lipid plaque which progressively enlarges to obstruct the vessel lumen. The plaques grow into and involve the tunica media. In coronary and cerebral arteries, the plaque is eccentric so that it obstructs only a part of the lumen. Over the following years complications arise. These include thrombus formation, plaque rupture and stenosis (frequently a problem in the carotids). Aneurysmal dilatation can also occur, especially in the aorta.

2. D Renal artery stenosis

This patient has renal artery stenosis causing renovascular hypertension. The most common cause is atherosclerosis, but in younger patients, especially women it may be fibromuscular hyperplasia (dysplasia). This leads to thickening of the walls of medium sized arteries, such as the renal, splanchnic, vertebral and internal carotid. Unlike atherosclerosis, the proximal part of the artery is less involved than the distal part where the tunica media causes stenosis. Macroscopically fibrous and muscular ridges project into the lumen where smooth muscle is replaced by fibrous tissue; intimal hyperplasia may also occur with connective tissue encircling the adventitia. When the condition is due to atherosclerosis, the entire vascular system will be affected with involvement of the origin of the artery from the aorta.

Clinically patients present with hypertension and a systolic bruit over the renal artery. A renal angiogram confirms the diagnosis. The treatment is percutaneous transluminal angioplasty, with or without stenting.

3. A Deep vein thrombosis (DVT)

Following a long flight, this man has developed iliofemoral deep vein thrombosis. Venous thrombosis results from any condition that predisposes to impaired venous return and stasis. The risk factors for DVT are prolonged immobility (as in this patient), pregnancy, oral contraceptives, long major surgical procedures, malignancy, haematological disorders and multiple traumas. More than 90% occur in deep veins of the legs beginning in the calf. The causative factors are endothelial injury, stasis and a hypercoagulable state. A thrombus in the vein may result in thrombophlebitis in which there is inflammation superimposed on bacterial infection. Here, the clot is adherent to the vein wall and is unlikely to get dislodged. In phlebothrombosis, on the other hand, there is no underlying inflammation or infection; the clot can get dislodged and cause pulmonary embolism. The diagnosis can be confirmed by a duplex scan, supplemented if necessary by a venogram.

4. B Hypovolaemic shock

This patient has the features of shock which can be defined as acute circulatory failure with inadequate tissue perfusion of vital organs resulting in generalised cellular hypoxia. Shock in the immediate postoperative period following a major operation in a patient who has no preoperative co-morbidities (ASA 1 anaesthetic category), is due to hypovolaemic shock from postoperative bleeding. The bleeding would most probably be the result of a slipped left gastric artery ligature. This is because the left gastric artery arising from the coeliac axis, is the largest branch, has a short course and hence most liable to have a slipped ligature. The patient needs to be resuscitated and taken to theatre.

The types of shock are:

- Hypovolaemic
- Septicaemic
- Cardiogenic
- Neurogenic
- Anaphylactic

The pathological outcome of shock is shown in **Figure 30.1**.

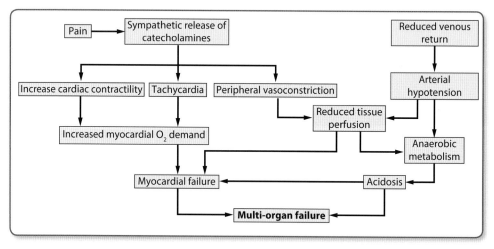

Figure 30.1 Pathological outcomes of shock, leading to multi-organ failure.

5. E Left ventricular aneurysm

This patient has a ventricular aneurysm, a delayed complication of left ventricular transmural myocardial infarct. It occurs in 10–15% of cases. A transmural infarct involves the full thickness of the ventricular wall while a subendocardial infarct involves one-third to half of the ventricular muscle. After thrombosis of the left circumflex and left anterior descending branches of the left coronary artery, the left ventricular muscle infarcts. The damaged area is later replaced by dense fibrosis, which then becomes solid, mature scar tissue. ECG shows persistent ST elevation. The scar tissue forms an aneurysm which can be true or false.

Chapter 31

Respiratory system

Questions

For each question, select the single best answer from the five options listed.

1. A 60-year-old man had a right hemicolectomy. On the first postoperative day he develops a temperature of 39°C, is very short of breath and looks slightly cyanosed; his oxygen saturation is 92%.

   What is the most likely diagnosis?

   A   Acute respiratory distress syndrome
   B   Aspiration pneumonia
   C   Atelectasis
   D   Lobar pneumonia
   E   Pulmonary embolus

2. A 28-year-old man, 1.93 m (6ft 4 in) tall, presents to the emergency department with sudden chest pain and rapid onset of breathlessness. A short time after admission, his pain improves although he continues to be breathless. Since childhood he has suffered from asthma for which he uses inhalers intermittently.

   What is the most likely diagnosis?

   A   Boerhaave's syndrome
   B   Cardiac tamponade
   C   Spontaneous pneumothorax
   D   Tension pneumothorax
   E   Tracheal rupture

3. A 55-year-old Caucasian man, who has been a smoker for 40 years, complains of recent haemoptysis. He has had a 'smoker's' cough for as long as he can remember. Recently, he has developed pain in his left shoulder and on examination has left Horner's syndrome.

   What is the most likely diagnosis?

   A   Carcinoma of the lung
   B   Mesothelioma
   C   Pulmonary metastasis
   D   Pulmonary tuberculosis
   E   Thoracic inlet (outlet) syndrome

4. A 45-year-old man, a non-smoker, complains of increasing shortness of breath for 5 days. He is orthopnoeic. During this period his neck, face and upper limbs have become swollen. The jugular veins are distended as are the veins on the front of his chest.

    What is the most likely diagnosis?

    A   Acute respiratory distress syndrome
    B   Chronic obstructive pulmonary disease
    C   Congestive cardiac failure
    D   Superior vena cava syndrome
    E   Surgical emphysema

5. A 55-year-old woman, a non-smoker, presents with haemoptysis and gradual shortness of breath for 2 months. Over the last 4 months she has developed a Cushingoid appearance. A chest X-ray shows a smooth shadow in the right lung with lower lobe collapse.

    What is the most likely diagnosis?

    A   Bronchiectasis
    B   Bronchial carcinoid tumour
    C   Pulmonary hamartoma
    D   Pulmonary secondary from an unknown primary
    E   Small cell lung carcinoma

6. A 62-year-old man presents with diffuse dull aching pain in the right side of his chest of 2 months' duration. The pain is exacerbated by deep breaths. Recently he has developed progressive shortness of breath which is quite disabling. He has night sweats, pyrexia and has lost 14 kg in weight during this period. A chest X-ray showed pleural effusion which on aspiration was blood-stained. Twenty years ago he worked in the asbestos industry and he has been a smoker all his life.

    What is the most likely diagnosis?

    A   Empyema
    B   Lymphoma
    C   Mesothelioma
    D   Pulmonary hypertension
    E   Tuberculosis

Answers

1. C Atelectasis

This patient has atelectasis. Examination will reveal poor basal air entry, bronchial breathing and dullness on percussion. Atelectasis is a collapse of lung tissue. This may affect part or all of one lung. The condition prevents normal oxygenation of tissues.

It is seen as a postoperative complication after major abdominal surgery. It results from mucus obstruction of a bronchus, the effect being exacerbated by reduced movement of the chest wall due to splinting of the respiratory muscles from pain. Postoperative atelectasis can be prevented and the risks reduced by: preoperative cessation of smoking for 6–8 weeks, physiotherapy and weight reduction, postoperative physiotherapy, adequate analgesia in the form of patient-controlled epidural to help coughing and deep breathing. The absence of surfactant will also lead to atelectasis.

Treatment is prompt and vigorous physiotherapy with humidified oxygen. If secondary infection supervenes, appropriate antibiotic treatment is instituted.

2. C Spontaneous pneumothorax

This young man has a spontaneous pneumothorax. It usually occurs in tall young men during exercise and in asthmatics. It presents with acute chest pain and shortness of breath. Pneumothorax is defined as air in the pleural cavity. It may be 'spontaneous' or 'tension', the latter being life-threatening. The cause of spontaneous pneumothorax is rupture of a pulmonary bulla produced by a defect in the connective tissue of the alveolar cells. There may also be underlying chronic obstructive pulmonary disease. It presents with shallow painful breathing, as the sensitive parietal pleura rubs on the lung surface. Small pneumothoraces may be left to resolve spontaneously. Larger ones may be aspirated. But if they reform or are causing respiratory distress a chest drain may be required. If they recur a pleurodesis may be required.

3. A Carcinoma of the lung

This patient, a long-term smoker with haemoptysis, has a primary lung cancer. His symptoms and signs suggest that the cancer is arising from the upper lobe. Horner's syndrome is due to involvement of the cervical sympathetic chain. Pain is from infiltration of the upper ribs and the lower cords of the brachial plexus. Involvement of the phrenic nerve can cause paralysis of the ipsilateral dome of the diaphragm (**Figure 4.3**); recurrent laryngeal nerve involvement will cause hoarseness of voice. A lung cancer that arises from the upper lobe is called a Pancoast tumour.

Carcinoma of the lung is the most common cause of cancer death worldwide. More than 85% of cases occur in cigarette smokers. There are two main types; non-small cell lung cancer (NSCLC) and small cell lung carcinoma (SCLC) which is also called oat cell carcinoma.

4. D Superior vena cava syndrome

This patient has superior vena cava syndrome. He is very short of breath with facial and neck swelling brought on by external compression and obstruction of the superior vena cava. As a result, he has distended jugular veins with collateral venous circulation on the chest wall. In advanced cases there may be brawny facial oedema of the upper arms, conjunctival oedema, visual disturbances, cyanosis and dysphagia – a symptom complex caused by gross mediastinal lymphadenopathy; in the younger age group this arises from primary malignancy of the lymph nodes such as a lymphoma. In the older age group it is more likely to be due to secondary metastases from a lung cancer.

In order to make a diagnosis an X-ray and CT of the chest may need to be followed by biopsy (CT guided or excision) of the enlarged lymph nodes. Treatment is radiotherapy and/or chemotherapy.

5. B Bronchial carcinoid tumour

This patient has bronchial carcinoid tumour. The unusual combination of pulmonary symptoms of haemoptysis and shortness of breath associated with the endocrine disturbance of a Cushingoid appearance gives the diagnosis. The chest X-ray shows a lung shadow with post-obstructive collapse from obstruction of the bronchus by the tumour. These features are typical of a bronchial carcinoid which account for up to 2% of primary lung cancers. These are neuroendocrine tumours that arise from neuroendocrine cells of the bronchial epithelium and not related to smoking. There are two types: a majority that have no endocrine manifestations and a group that has endocrine features such as Cushing syndrome where the tumour cells produce adrenocorticotrophic hormone. One-third of the tumours originate in the central bronchus, one-third is peripheral and one-third is in the middle of the lung. True carcinoid syndrome is manifested in only 1% of cases when there are liver metastases.

6. C Mesothelioma

This patient has all the clinical features of an underlying malignancy – weight loss, disabling dyspnoea, chronic chest pain and pyrexia. Past history of having worked in the asbestos industry gives a very strong indication of the diagnosis of a mesothelioma. This diagnosis should be very strongly suspected by the presence of a blood-stained pleural effusion which denotes underlying malignancy.

Macroscopically the tumour encases and compresses the lung extending into the fissures and interlobar septa, an appearance referred to as 'pleural rind'. Microscopically they show a biphasic pattern of epithelial and sarcomatous elements. When epithelial elements predominate, it may be difficult to differentiate from an adenocarcinoma. Immunohistochemistry differentiates a mesothelioma from an adenocarcinoma. Mesothelioma typically has absence of mucin and presence of hyaluronic acid with long slender microvilli on electron microscopy. Metastases can occur to lung parenchyma, mediastinal lymph nodes, liver, bones and peritoneum. It has a very poor prognosis.

Chapter 32

Gastrointestinal system

Questions

For each question, select the single best answer from the five options listed.

1. A 65-year-old woman complains of left iliac fossa pain associated with occasional passage of dark red blood per rectum. She is habitually constipated and takes regular laxatives for a satisfactory bowel action. She has had these symptoms for almost a year. She is overweight and is tender in the left iliac fossa.

   What is the most likely diagnosis?

   A   Colorectal carcinoma
   B   Crohn's disease
   C   Diverticular disease
   D   Ischaemic colitis
   E   Ulcerative colitis

2. A 70-year-old man complains of waking in the morning and having to rush to the lavatory to have a motion. He then finds that he only passes mucous, blood and watery stool. He has tenesmus and a continuous feeling of insufficient evacuation. This has been going on for the last 3 months during which time he has lost 10 kg in weight.

   What is the most likely diagnosis?

   A   Acute fissure-in-ano
   B   Fistula-in-ano
   C   Prolapse of rectum
   D   Rectal carcinoma
   E   Thrombosed piles

3. A 46-year-old man presents with a 6-month history of dyspeptic symptoms despite regular use of pantoprazole. On upper gastrointestinal endoscopy and biopsy and a rapid urease test, he is found to have a *Helicobacter pylori* infection.

   If left untreated over the long term, which one of the following conditions is most likely to develop?

   A   Acute gastric ulcer
   B   Acute duodenal ulcer
   C   Gastric lymphoma
   D   Hiatus hernia
   E   Oesophageal carcinoma

4. A 55-year-old man presents as an emergency with sudden onset of severe acute epigastric pain radiating to the back, of 4 hours' duration. He also complains of pain in the right shoulder tip, which he has had for a couple of hours. On examination, his pulse rate is 120 bpm and his blood pressure is 120/80 mmHg; his abdominal wall does not move with respiration and he has board-like rigidity. A chest X-ray shows free gas under the right dome of the diaphragm (**Figure 32.1**).

What is the most likely diagnosis?

A   Acute appendicitis
B   Acute pancreatitis
C   Intestinal obstruction from acute intussusception
D   Perforated duodenal ulcer
E   Ureteric colic

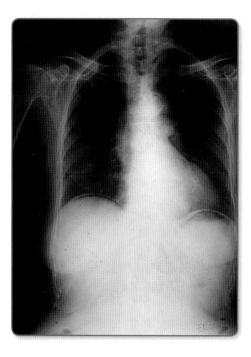

Figure 32.1 Gas under right dome of diaphragm.

5. A 19-year-old man is admitted with a 2-day history of right-sided abdominal pain, tenderness in the right iliac fossa and raised inflammatory markers. Following a clinical diagnosis of acute appendicitis, he is laparoscoped prior to his proposed appendicectomy. At laparoscopy, a 10 cm segment of the terminal ileum appears red, inflamed and thickened with free blood-stained fluid in the pelvis.

What is the most likely diagnosis?

A   Acute appendicitis
B   Acute intestinal ischaemia
C   Crohn's disease
D   Intussusception
E   Primary intestinal lymphoma

Answers

1. C Diverticular disease

An overweight woman who is constipated and has pain and tenderness in the left iliac fossa is most likely to be suffering from diverticular disease of the sigmoid colon (**Figure 32.2**). Diverticula are mucosal herniations that occur through the wall of the sigmoid colon at the point of maximum weakness which is the site of entry of the blood vessel. These are a consequence of a low-fibre diet, constipation, high intraluminal pressure, disordered motility and increased segmentation.

One-fifth of patients with diverticular disease are symptomatic – left iliac fossa cramps, bloating, pellet-like stools and the passage of mucus. Rupture of a peridiverticular submucosal blood vessel may result in sudden severe colonic haemorrhage. Inflammation results in acute diverticulitis. The inflamed segment may penetrate into adjacent structures causing a fistula – colo-vesical (**Figure 49.10**) colo-vaginal, colo-cutaneous, colo-enteric.

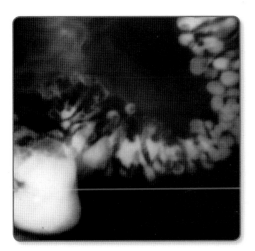

Figure 32.2 Barium enema showing diverticular disease of the sigmoid colon.

2. D Rectal carcinoma

The most likely diagnosis is a rectal carcinoma. Colorectal cancers are the second most common cause of cancer death in the United Kingdom, rectal cancers accounting for more than a third of them. The macroscopic types of rectal cancers are ulcerating (**Figure 48.9**), polypoid, tubular and annular (**Figure 48.10**), the latter two causing stenosing lesions. Polypoid cancers are more common in the right colon where the capacious lumen allows unimpeded growth; left colonic growths are more often annular or tubular. The vast majority are adenocarcinomas. A minority of them secrete mucin and hence are referred to as mucinous adenocarcinoma carrying a poorer prognosis. The degree of differentiation determines the prognosis, the greater the differentiation the better the prognosis.

They spread via the lymphatics to regional lymph nodes and by bloodstream to distant organs (34% liver, 22% lung). They are staged according to Dukes' classification (**Table 32.1**).

Table 32.1 Dukes' classification		
Stage	Description	5-year survival (%)
A	Beneath muscularis propria	90
B	Through muscularis propria	65
C	Spread to regional lymph nodes	35
D	Distant spread	10

3. D Gastric lymphoma

This patient might develop a gastric lymphoma if left untreated. Gastric mucosa-associated lymphoid tumour (MALToma) occurs in long-standing *Helicobacter pylori* chronic gastritis which provides the immunological stimulus for β cell proliferation. There are several causes of gastritis (**Figure 46.5**) of which *H. pylori* is one. Gastrointestinal lymphomas account for 10–15% of all primary lymphomas; stomach is the commonest site for a gastrointestinal lymphoma, and these make up 3–6% of all gastric malignancies. The tumour takes the form of a diffuse mucosal thickening, not unlike linitis plastica; ulceration may be present. The antrum and the pylorus are most commonly affected. Diagnosis is confirmed by deep biopsies on oesophagogastroduodenoscopy. The histology in the vast majority is a diffuse large non-Hodgkin's β-cell tumour. Lymphatic spread to the regional lymph nodes is late. The clinical presentation is similar to that of carcinoma – abdominal pain, anaemia, anorexia, asthenia and weight loss.

4. D Perforated duodenal ulcer

This patient has the hallmarks of a perforated intra-abdominal hollow viscus, the most common cause of which is a perforated duodenal ulcer. The sudden acute presentation with pain in the right shoulder tip (from referred pain due to diaphragmatic irritation as a result of peritonitis,) thoracic breathing and board-like abdominal rigidity are classical clinical features of a perforated duodenal ulcer. Within the first 4–6 hours of onset, the patient has chemical peritonitis; hence the patient is not shocked, with a normal pulse and blood pressure without pyrexia. After about 6 hours, if left untreated, bacterial peritonitis sets in and the patient will develop features of septic shock. The chronic complication of a duodenal ulcer is gastric outlet obstruction as a result of chronic cicatrisation of the pylorus with fibrosis. Treatment is operation and the perforation is closed with an omental patch.

5. C Crohn's disease

The most likely cause of this appearance is Crohn's disease, also called regional enteritis. The condition is a chronic transmural inflammatory disease that can affect any part of the gastrointestinal tract. The ileocaecal region is affected in about 40% of patients, small bowel disease in 30%, while in 20% the disease is confined to the large bowel with the right side more often affected than the left. Only 5% of patients have the disease limited to the anal or perianal region.

A characteristic feature of the disease is the patchy distribution of inflammation, with diseased segments interspersed between normal bowel called 'skip lesions'. Typically, all the layers of the bowel wall are involved giving rise to a strictured lumen. Macroscopically, the bowel lumen exhibits oedema with shallow, discrete aphthoid ulcers, serpiginous fissures, the mucosa showing a cobblestone appearance (**Figure 49.5**).

Chapter 33

Genitourinary system

Questions

For each question, select the single best answer from the five options listed.

1. A 52-year-old man complains of haematuria, discomfort in his right loin and irregular fever for the about a week. The haematuria is in the form of clots shaped like a worm. On examination, there is some fullness in the right loin with a suggestion of a mass that moves with respiration and it is bimanually palpable.

   What is the most probable clinical diagnosis?

   A Carcinoma of the kidney
   B Horseshoe kidney
   C Hydronephrosis
   D Pyelonephritis
   E Renal calculus

2. A 45-year-old woman presents with a first episode of right renal colic. On CT scan she is found to have a 3 mm calculus in her distal right ureter with no hydronephrosis. She is comfortable following analgesia; her renal function is normal and there is no sign of infection.

   What is the most appropriate treatment option?

   A Conservative management
   B Cystoscopy
   C Open ureterolithotomy
   D Percutaneous nephrolithotomy
   E Shockwave lithotripsy

3. A 73-year-old man presents to the urology department with a 2-week history of visible haematuria. He is investigated with a flexible cystoscope and CT urogram. The cystoscopy reveals a 1 cm papillary growth on the posterior wall of the bladder, which is excised.

   In the Western world, what is the most likely histological subtype of this bladder tumour?

   A Adenocarcinoma
   B Melanoma
   C Sarcoma
   D Squamous cell carcinoma
   E Transitional cell carcinoma

4. A 66-year-old man attends the urology outpatient clinic with progressive voiding lower urinary tract symptoms (hesitancy, poor flow and incomplete emptying). As part of his clinical examination he has a digital rectal examination, which reveals an enlarged, smooth and non-tender prostate, consistent with benign prostatic hyperplasia.

    In which zone of the prostate does benign prostatic hyperplasia largely develop?

    A   Peripheral zone
    B   Fibromuscular stroma
    C   Anterior zone
    D   Central zone
    E   Transitional zone

5. A 64-year-old man has had a transurethral resection of the prostate (TURP). Immediately following his surgery, he has stress incontinence which does not resolve with conservative measures. On subsequent cystoscopy, his verumontanum cannot be visualised.

    Which structure is most likely to have been damaged during this patient's TURP?

    A   Internal urethral sphincter
    B   Pelvic floor muscles
    C   External urethral sphincter
    D   Ureteric orifices
    E   Penile urethra

6. A 65-year-old man presents to his GP with fever, sweats, frequency of micturition, suprapubic pain and dysuria. On further questioning the man has had voiding lower urinary tract symptoms of poor urinary stream, hesitancy, and incomplete emptying for several months.

    What is the most likely underlying cause of this patient's urinary tract infection?

    A   Benign prostatic hyperplasia
    B   Bladder cancer
    C   Renal stone
    D   Colovesical fistula
    E   Ureteric reflux

7. A 40-year-old man presents with a 3-week history of left testicular swelling. He
    has no systemic upset and no history of trauma. He does have a history of bilateral
    orchidopexy when aged 2 years. On examination, he has a hard, craggy mass
    arising from his left testicular parenchyma and ultrasound confirms this as a likely
    testicular tumour. Tumour markers are given below.

Tumour marker	Result	Reference range
α-Fetoprotein	4 kU/L	<7.5 kU/L
Human chorionic gonadotrophin	2 IU/L	<9 IU/L
Lactate dehydrogenase	250 U/L	208–460 U/L

What is the most likely diagnosis?

A   Leydig cell tumour
B   Non-seminomatous germ cell tumour
C   Rhabdomyosarcoma
D   Seminoma
E   Sertoli tumour

Answers

1. A Carcinoma of kidney

This patient has the classical triad of haematuria, pain and mass in the loin indicating a renal cell carcinoma (RCC), unless otherwise proven. The patient should have a contrast CT scan to confirm and stage the disease and assess the vascularity which would help in surgical management as some of these tumours are extremely vascular (and may require preoperative embolisation of the renal artery).

Macroscopically the tumour arises from the proximal tubular epithelial cells. Typically, yellowish-orange in colour it is solid and cystic spaces with areas of necrosis and haemorrhage (**Figure 45.1**). The tumour contains an abundance of lipids and glycogen, which accounts for the clear cell cytoplasm. The tumour typically metastasises through the blood steam.

One in four patients with RCC present with their secondaries as an initial symptom, such as haemoptysis from lung secondaries, convulsion from brain metastasis, or a pathological fracture from a secondary in a long bone. Long bone secondaries are well known to present as a pulsating, hot tumour because of its vascularity. Renal cell carcinoma is known as a 'great mimic' because of the production of ectopic hormones that cause 'pyrexia of unknown origin' and paraneoplastic syndromes producing polycythaemia from excessive erythropoietin production and hypertension from renin production.

2. A Conservative management

In the absence of ureteric obstruction, renal impairment and infection, it is safe to adopt a conservative approach to small ureteric calculi, if pain can be controlled easily with simple analgesics (**Figures 33.1** and **33.2**). Stones <5 mm in size have approximately 90% spontaneous passage rate and this can be improved with the

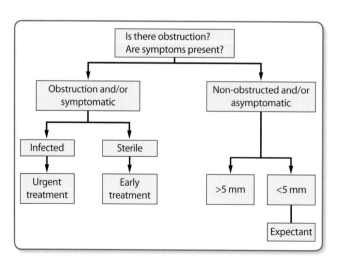

Figure 33.1
Management of ureteric stones depending on whether symptoms are present.

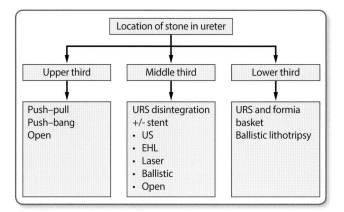

Figure 33.2
Management of ureteric stone depending on the location of the stone. URS, ureteroscopy; US, ultrasound; EHL, electrohydraulic lithotripsy.

addition of medical expulsion therapy, such as an alpha-blocker (e.g. tamsulosin). This relaxes the distal ureter and aids stone passage, and reduces analgesic requirements. Stones 5–9 mm in size have an approximate 50% spontaneous passage rate, while those >10 mm have <10% spontaneous passage rate.

3. E Transitional cell carcinoma

90% of bladder tumours in the Western world are transitional cell cancer. Squamous cell cancers are common (75%) where schistosomiasis is endemic (e.g. Egypt), it is caused by the ova of *Schistosoma haematobium*. Squamous cell cancers are also caused by chronic inflammatory states such as long-term catheterisation. Adenocarcinoma is rare; one third will originate in the urachus. Sarcoma and melanoma both occur very rarely in the bladder.

4. E Transitional zone

Benign prostatic hyperplasia develops in the transitional zone of the prostate. This makes possible resection of a benign enlarged prostate transurethrally. However, 75% of prostatic cancer occurs in the peripheral zone where it can easily be palpated by digital rectal exam.

5. C External urethral sphincter

Continence in men is mainly controlled by the external urethral sphincter. The internal sphincter does not add much to the control of urine. During a transurethral resection of the prostate (TURP) the internal sphincter is resected together with the prostatic urethra and the prostate adenoma. The position of the external urethral sphincter is approximately marked by the verumontanum where the ejaculatory ducts enter the prostatic urethra. As such, during a TURP the operator must be aware at all times where the verumontanum is situated in relation to the resection loop. If the verumontanum is damaged the external urethral sphincter may be damaged or resected completely. Pelvic floor muscle training may help some return to continence but if not further evaluation is required and surgery in the form of an artificial urinary sphincter or a male urethral sling may be necessary for cure.

6. A Benign prostatic hyperplasia

Benign prostatic hyperplasia (BPH) causes a range of symptoms in men as they grow older. There are two main classes of symptoms: voiding symptoms (hesitancy, poor flow, abdominal straining and incomplete emptying) and storage symptoms (frequency, nocturia and incontinence). In this case, the patient has voiding symptoms due to bladder outlet obstruction, most likely due to BPH. He will retain urine and have the feeling of incomplete emptying of urine. The urine will stagnate and be prone to urinary tract infection.

7. D Seminoma

Non-seminoma germ cell tumour (NSGCT) and seminoma (germ cell tumours) are the most common forms of testicular tumours; the others are rare. Cryptorchidism is a significant risk factor for both. NSGCT are more common in those aged 20–35 years, while seminoma is more common in those aged 35–45 years. Both α-fetoprotein and human chorionic gonadotrophin are more likely to be raised in NSGCT. Lactate dehydrogenase levels are raised in 10–20% of seminomas and can indicate the extent of disease but the test is not specific.

Chapter 34

Endocrine system

Questions

For each question, select the single best answer from the five options listed.

1. A 50-year-old man complains of early morning headache associated with occasional projectile vomiting of 2 months' duration. Recently, he has noticed that he has double vision and has difficulty seeing objects in the peripheral part of his vision. He finds that he is regularly bumping into doorways and people.

   What is the most likely diagnosis?

   A Anterior communicating artery aneurysm
   B Cavernous sinus thrombosis
   C Meningioma
   D Optic neuritis
   E Pituitary adenoma

2. A 70-year-old woman presents with severe explosive diarrhoea with colicky abdominal pain of 3 months' duration. She has an enlarged nodular liver, raised jugular venous pressure and features of pulmonary stenosis and tricuspid regurgitation. Eight years ago, she underwent a right hemicolectomy for a tumour arising from the terminal ileum.

   What is the most likely diagnosis?

   A Carcinoid syndrome
   B Cor pulmonale
   C Inflammatory bowel disease
   D Irritable bowel syndrome
   E Recurrent small bowel tumour

3. A 45-year-old woman complains of a central neck lump, present for 8 months, which moves upward with deglutition. Four months later, she developed more lumps on the left side of her neck.

   What is the most likely diagnosis?

   A Anaplastic carcinoma of the thyroid
   B Follicular carcinoma of the thyroid
   C Lymphoma of the thyroid
   D Multinodular goitre
   E Papillary carcinoma of the thyroid

4. A 35-year-old woman complains of episodic attacks of visual disturbances in
    the form of double and blurred vision associated with sweating, tremor, nausea,
    palpitations. On a couple of occasions she has lost consciousness. People brought
    her round by feeding her sugar cubes.

    What is the most likely diagnosis?

    A   Gastrinoma
    B   Glucagonoma
    C   Insulinoma
    D   Somatostatinoma
    E   VIPoma

5. A 35-year-old-woman has put on a considerable amount of weight mostly around
    her trunk for 4 months. During this period she has been found to be a diabetic
    with a blood pressure of 160/90 mmHg and noticed hair on her upper lip. She has
    amenorrhoea.

    What is the most likely diagnosis?

    A   Conn's syndrome
    B   Cushing's syndrome
    C   Incidentaloma
    D   Phaeochromocytoma
    E   Secondary metastasis in the adrenal

6. A 55-year-old man complains of increasing thirst, polyuria, abdominal pain and
    occasional vomiting for 3 months. He has felt unduly tired with malaise for which
    he saw his GP. The only abnormality on routine blood tests showed a serum
    calcium of 3.1 mmol/L.

    What is the most likely diagnosis?

    A   Diabetes mellitus
    B   Disseminated malignant disease
    C   Multiple endocrine neoplasia type 1
    D   Primary hyperparathyroidism
    E   Sarcoidosis

Answers

1. E Pituitary adenoma

This patient suffers from a pituitary adenoma. He has symptoms of raised intracranial pressure – early morning headache, projectile vomiting and visual disturbances. The latter symptom specifically is bitemporal hemianopia caused by the space-occupying lesion of the pituitary pressing upon the optic chiasma. Macroadenomas, as they enlarge produce pressure symptoms and may invade the cavernous sinus causing paralysis of the 3rd, 4th and 6th cranial nerves. Microadenomas more often cause endocrine disturbances. This depends upon the hormone secreted: galactorrhoea, amenorrhoea, impotence in a prolactinoma; Cushing's disease in an adrenocorticotrophic hormone producing tumour; acromegaly and gigantism in a growth-hormone secreting tumour. Rarely, pituitary adenomas are a part of multiple endocrine neoplasia syndrome type 1.

Depending upon how the cells stained by haematoxylin and eosin, they were classified as acidophil adenomas associated with overproduction of growth hormone, basophil adenomas producing excess adrenocorticotrophic hormone and chromophobe adenomas which are non-secretory.

2. A Carcinoid syndrome

This patient has carcinoid syndrome. This is due to the effects of excess circulating serotonin (5-hydroxytryptamine). She has an enlarged nodular liver, typical of hepatic secondaries from a carcinoid tumour from the ileum that was removed by right hemicolectomy in the past. Ileal carcinoids are often multiple and more aggressive. These tumours are neuroendocrine tumours that arise from the enterochromaffin cells also called APUD (amine precursor uptake and decarboxylation) cells. They constitute 10% of all small intestine tumours. Carcinoid syndrome occurs as a result of liver secondaries elaborating the enzyme 5-HT. This occurs in 5% of patients with carcinoid tumours.

Macroscopically, the tumour is yellowish-white in colour and arises as a submucous nodule; large tumours may be polypoid or annular with surface ulceration. Microscopically, there are nests, cords and rosettes of small, round cells. The classical presentation is explosive diarrhoea, episodic flushing, bronchospasm and pellagra-like skin lesions on the legs.

3. E Papillary carcinoma of the thyroid

This woman has typical papillary carcinoma of the thyroid (PCT), which has a predilection for women in this age group. She has a thyroid nodule with a mass of cervical lymph nodes on the side of the original lesion (**Figure 34.1**). This is the most common type (seen in 60–70% of all thyroid cancers). The diagnosis is confirmed by fine-needle aspiration cytology. In more than 75% of patients, PCT is multicentric

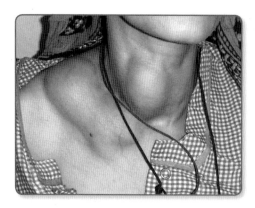

Figure 34.1 Papillary carcinoma of the thyroid.

in origin. This feature may represent multifocal origin of the tumour or lymphatic spread within the gland from a solitary tumour. Sometimes the condition may present as a mass of cervical lymphadenopathy without a clinically obvious thyroid lesion. The diagnosis is then made after a biopsy or fine-needle aspiration cytology of the lymph node which shows features of papillary carcinoma. To assess the aggressiveness of the tumour, various scoring systems are available.

4. C Insulinoma

This patient has an insulinoma (β-cell tumour), the commonest pancreatic endocrine tumour. She has the classical clinical symptoms of hypoglycaemia (diplopia and blurred vision) associated with the clinical features of catecholamine release (nausea, tremor, palpitations and sweating); these symptoms may progress to confusion, lethargy and loss of consciousness. This patient's symptoms are referred to as Whipple's triad: the three features are first, typical hypoglycaemic symptoms after fasting or exercise; second, blood glucose levels of <2.8 mmol/L and third, recovery after oral or intravenous glucose. In the vast majority of cases the diagnosis is strongly suspected by the biochemical demonstration of hypoglycaemia with inappropriate and excessive insulin secretion. This tumour occurs sporadically but may be a part of multiple endocrine neoplasia 1 syndrome. Histologically, the tumour cells resemble normal β-cells seen as nests in trabecular or solid patterns. Tumours showing a high mitotic rate denote malignancy.

5. B Cushing's syndrome

This woman has the classical features of Cushing's syndrome: recent onset of central obesity, diabetes, hirsutism, pigmentation of skin and menstrual irregularity (**Figure 34.2**). 85% of cases of this syndrome are ACTH-dependent (adrenocorticotrophic hormone dependent). Patients with this sub-group of Cushing's syndrome, caused by excessive secretion of ACTH from a pituitary adenoma, are labelled as having Cushing's disease. However, 15% of cases of Cushing's syndrome are actually caused by an adrenocortical adenoma or by ectopic ACTH production, as may occur in paraneoplastic syndrome from a small

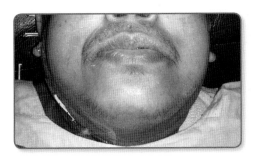

Figure 34.2 Cushing's syndrome. postoperative. Courtesy of Dr Nissanka Jayawardhana.

cell lung cancer. Adrenocortical carcinoma is very rare. In Cushing's disease, an excessive amount of ACTH is secreted, whereas in Cushing's syndrome the level of ACTH is low. Pathologically, the adenoma is encapsulated, firm, yellow and lobulated and about 5 cm in diameter. Adrenalectomy is the treatment of choice and gives good results.

6. D Primary hyperparathyroidism

This man has the features of primary hyperparathyroidism, the commonest cause of which is a parathyroid adenoma (80–90%). In a small minority, the cause is parathyroid hyperplasia (10–15%) while parathyroid carcinoma as a cause of hypercalcaemia is even rarer (1–5%). Secondary hyperparathyroidism occurs in chronic renal failure, in vitamin D deficiency and intestinal malabsorption; this is due to compensatory parathormone hypersecretion where all the glands are hyperplastic. Rarely, in these situations one of the glands may become an autonomous adenoma, when the condition is called tertiary hyperparathyroidism. In 20% an adenoma may occur as a part of multiple endocrine neoplasia syndrome type 1.

A parathyroid adenoma is a discrete, reddish brown tumour about 3 cm in diameter. Haemorrhagic and cystic areas are seen; histologically, sheets of chief cells are seen within a rich capillary network. They have a capsule which distinguishes it from parathyroid hyperplasia.

Chapter 35

Breast disorders

Questions

For each question, select the single best answer from the five options listed.

1. A 19-year-old woman presents to the one-stop clinic with a lump in her left breast. On examination there is a firm, 3 cm diameter, well circumscribed, mobile lump with no evidence of tethering. What is the most likely diagnosis in this patient?

   A   Breast abscess
   B   Breast cyst
   C   Fibroadenoma
   D   Galactocele
   E   Phylloides tumour

2. A 56-year-old woman complains of a painless lump in her in her left breast of 10 days' duration. She noticed it following a road traffic accident when the steering wheel hit her breast at the site of the lump. On examination, there is a hard lump deep to the nipple with an overlying bruise.

   What is the possible diagnosis?

   A   Carcinoma
   B   Fat necrosis
   C   Fibroadenosis
   D   Galactocele
   E   Phylloides tumour

3. A 48-year-old woman who had a silicone implant in her right breast complains of recent heaviness of her breast. On examination, there is an irregular lump deep to the scar of the breast augmentation procedure carried out almost 15 years ago.

   What imaging technique should be the procedure of choice as a part of a triple assessment?

   A   Digital mammography
   B   Magnetic resonance imaging
   C   Mammography
   D   Thermography
   E   Ultrasound

4. A 62-year-old woman complains of discharge from her left nipple of 6 weeks' duration. The discharge is greenish turbid in colour. On examination, there is some thickening in the subareolar area.

    What is the most probable clinical diagnosis?

    A Aberration of normal development and involution (ANDI)
    B Duct ectasia
    C Fibroadenosis
    D Galactocele
    E Paget's disease

5. A 54-year-old woman complains of a lump deep to her nipple of 6 weeks' duration. There is serous and blood-stained discharge from part of the areola of the nipple (**Figure 35.1**).

    What is the probable clinical diagnosis?

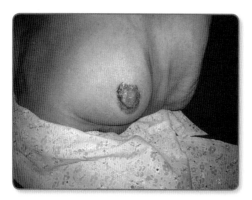

Figure 35.1 Paget's disease of nipple. Courtesy of Dr Nissanka Jayawardhaha.

    A Breast abscess
    B Granulomatous mastitis
    C Lobular carcinoma in situ
    D Paget's disease of nipple
    E Serocystic disease of Brodie

6. A 28-year-old woman who is 13 weeks pregnant complains of a painful lump in her left breast of 4 weeks' duration. On examination the breast is red, hot, tender and larger than the other side with an irregular lump.

    What is the probable diagnosis?

    A Acute mastitis
    B Breast abscess
    C Fibromatosis
    D Galactocele
    E Inflammatory carcinoma

Answers

1. C Fibroadenoma

This patient's breast lump is a fibroadenoma. Fibroadenoma is the most common type of benign tumour, which occurs mainly in young women. It arises from the breast lobule, both the loose connective tissue stroma and glands. Fibroadenomas undergo some of the same hormonally induced changes as the surrounding breast. They are well circumscribed with a lobulated appearance and is not tethered to the surrounding breast tissue.

It is considered to be an aberration of normal development and involution (ANDI). Clinically, it is typically very mobile and well defined from the surrounding breast tissue; hence it is often referred to as a 'breast mouse'. Very occasionally they may be large (>5 cm in diameter) and are called giant fibroadenoma.

Ideally it is removed by enucleation through a radial cosmetic incision. Microscopically there are two types: pericanalicular or hard, and intracanalicular or soft.

2. B Fat necrosis

The history of trauma should alert one to the diagnosis of traumatic fat necrosis. However, a history of trauma does not necessarily mean that this is a benign condition. Fat necrosis has all the clinical characteristics of a carcinoma – hard lump which may have underlying fixity and overlying skin tethering and nipple retraction. Bruising does not necessarily mean the condition is fat necrosis: the patient may have had a latent, malignant lump she was unaware of.

At the age of 65 she should undergo a triple assessment of clinical examination, imaging of mammography followed by fine-needle aspiration cytology and core biopsy to exclude carcinoma. If there is no evidence of malignancy, she should be observed on a regular basis until the lump has disappeared.

3. B Magnetic resonance imaging

All patients with a breast lump should undergo a triple assessment which consists of clinical examination, imaging and histopathological examination. There are two methods which are usually used in breast imaging: ultrasound and mammography are the most common, but in this particular scenario magnetic resonance imaging (MRI) is the best option. This is also regarded as the best imaging method for women with implants and high risk women.

It is particularly useful to distinguish scar tissue from recurrence in women who have had breast conservation surgery for cancer. However, in those within nine months of radiotherapy, MRI is less accurate as an imaging technique because of abnormal enhancement. MRI guided biopsy is technically complicated. Hence a repeat ultrasound-guided biopsy is better carried out.

4. B Duct ectasia

Greenish turbid discharge from the nipple is the result of duct ectasia. There may be nipple retraction with hyperproliferative ductal tissue which is inflamed. Initially there is dilatation of the lactiferous duct/s where there is stagnation of brownish-green stained discharge, which stains the undergarment. This stagnant fluid causes irritation leading to periductal mastitis from inspissated material; in extreme cases it may result in abscess and fistula formation. Rarely, an indurated mass may mimic a carcinoma, the suspicion being enhanced by nipple retraction. The typical scenario is one of nipple discharge, subareolar mass, abscess or duct fistula with nipple retraction. Breast cancer is excluded by triple assessment.

The cause of the condition is periductal inflammation with anaerobic bacterial infection; smoking can be an aetiology. Treatment consists of wide excision of all ducts under antibiotic cover (co-amoxiclav, metronidazole, flucloxacillin). Recurrence is common; giving up smoking helps in preventing recurrence.

5. D Paget's disease of nipple

Paget's disease is associated with an underlying invasive ductal carcinoma in situ (DCIS) causing nipple erosion. It constitutes 1–4% of all breast cancers. The cancer presents as erythema or an eczema-like change to the nipple and areola, with about 50% having a palpable mass. It needs to be differentiated from eczema which involves the areola first and the nipple second, whereas Paget's disease involves the nipple first. Eczema is usually bilateral.

Microscopically, glandular epithelial malignant cells are seen within the epidermis which contains clusters of ductal-type carcinoma cells that are large, ovoid with abundant, clear, pale cytoplasm containing mucin globules.

The diagnosis is reached by a triple assessment in a one-stop breast clinic. Management is discussed in a multidisciplinary team (MDT) and appropriate treatment instituted.

6. E Inflammatory carcinoma

This patient has inflammatory breast carcinoma. It should not be mistaken for a breast abscess. Triple assessment should be carried out with clinical assessment, imaging with ultrasound (mammography is best avoided as the patient is pregnant) followed by core biopsy.

This particular patient poses the greatest challenge in communication. Many conditions are to be taken into consideration – the age of the patient, whether she has a child already and her future family plans. It will be quite a challenge for the MDT to decide upon the best management which will be a combination of all three forms of cancer treatment – chemotherapy, radiotherapy and surgery.

This is a very aggressive form of breast carcinoma with the clinical hallmarks of advanced cancer: peau d'orange due to blockage of the dermal lymphatics; nipple retraction due to infiltration of the lactiferous ducts and skin dimpling from involvement of the ligaments of Cooper.

Chapter 36

Musculoskeletal system

Questions

For each question, select the single best answer from the five options listed.

1. A 35-year-old woman presents with a history of symmetrical polyarthropathy affecting the small joints of both hands and both feet. Examination reveals swan neck and boutonniere deformities in the fingers of both hands. Radiographs of the affected joints demonstrate varying degrees of joint space narrowing and bony erosions.

    Which finding would suggest Felty's syndrome?

    A Anaemia
    B Dry eyes and mouth
    C Neutropenia
    D Raised inflammatory markers (erythrocyte sedimentation rate, C-reactive protein)
    E Rheumatoid factor positive

2. A 63-year-old man presents with a painful left arm with no history of preceding trauma. Examination reveals pain over the proximal aspect of the left humerus and subsequent radiographs are consistent with a pathological fracture. A subsequent bone scan reveals further pathological lesions of the femur and spine.

    Which primary malignancy is the most probable cause of the secondary bony metastases?

    A Colonic carcinoma
    B Gastric carcinoma
    C Hepatoma
    D Pancreatic carcinoma
    E Renal cell carcinoma

3. A 42-year-old man presents with a one week history of sudden onset of increasing pain, swelling and redness to his left great toe. On examination there is tenderness, swelling and erythema over the metatarsophalangeal joint of the left hallux with an associated cellulitis. Tophi are also present. Subsequent blood tests demonstrate an elevated uric acid level and a diagnosis of gout was made.

   Which one of the following is a recognised risk factor for gout?

   A   Liver disease
   B   Raynaud's syndrome
   C   Renal impairment
   D   Smoking
   E   Steroids

4. A 69-year-old woman presents with history of increasing pain in both hips. Examination reveals an antalgic gait and a restriction of movement in both hips. Pelvic radiographs are suggestive of osteoarthritis.

   Which one of the following is a recognised characteristic of osteoarthritis on plain radiographs?

   A   Brodie's abscess
   B   Joint space widening
   C   Osteophytes
   D   Sequestrum
   E   Subchondral collapse

5. A 25-year-old old man presents with significant pain and swelling to the left forearm that has developed after the past 2 hours after being kicked by an opponent during a football match. On examination, there is significant swelling throughout the volar compartment with significant pain on passive stretch of the left wrist but with no sensory or motor abnormalities noted. Radiographs of the forearm reveal no bony injury. Despite adequate analgesia, 2 hours later the patient has persisting pain and continuous intracompartmental pressure monitoring of the forearm is compatible with compartment syndrome.

   What is the most appropriate treatment for this patient?

   A   Administer intravenous fluids to increase diastolic pressure
   B   Elevate arm and continue close observation
   C   Fasciotomy of the left forearm on the next available trauma list
   D   Increase analgesia
   E   Urgent fasciotomy of the left forearm

6. A 38-year-old man presents with a painful left wrist following a fall from his bicycle. On examination, he has a tender anatomical snuff box. Radiographs reveal a minimally displaced fracture through the waist of the left scaphoid. Following 6 months of treatment with immobilisation and subsequent mobilisation, the patient still has pain at the fracture site and check radiographs reveal no bone growth at the fracture site with no cortex bridging.

What is the most likely diagnosis?

A   Atrophic non-union
B   Delayed union
C   Hypertrophic non-union
D   Infected non-union
E   Union

7. A 3-year-old boy presents with a limp but no history of preceding trauma. Examination reveals a decreased range of movement with severe pain in the left hip. The patient is pyrexial with raised inflammatory markers and subsequent imaging reveals a significant effusion that was aspirated. On microbiological analysis using chocolate agar Gram-negative, rod-shaped organisms were identified.

What is the most likely causative organism?

A   *Haemophilus influenzae*
B   *Neisseria gonorrhoea*
C   *Staphylococcus aureus*
D   *Staphylococcus epidermidis*
E   Streptococci

8. A 14-year-old boy presents with pain, tenderness and localised swelling to the mid-shaft region of his right femur. Radiographs reveal a lytic lesion with a classic 'onion skin' periosteal reaction.

What is the most likely diagnosis?

A   Chondrosarcoma
B   Ewing's sarcoma
C   Fibrosarcoma
D   Osteochondroma
E   Osteosarcoma

Answers

1. C Neutropenia

Felty's syndrome is characterised by rheumatoid arthritis, splenomegaly and neutropenia. The most common form of inflammatory arthropathy is rheumatoid arthritis with peak incidence between 30–50 years old. The female:male ratio is approximately 3:1. Pathogenesis is not conclusively known but is thought to be associated with an unidentified trigger in genetically susceptible individuals (HLA-DR4 and DR1). This leads to activation of an immune and inflammatory process with lymphocytes, plasma cells and macrophages causing chronic joint and tissue inflammation.

Clinical features include an exacerbating remitting symmetrical polyarthropathy, with stiffness and swelling predominantly affecting the small joints of the hands and feet, although any joint can be involved. Hand deformities include:

- Swan neck deformity
- Ulnar and volar deviation of the fingers
- Boutonnière deformity
- Prominent ulnar styloid

Known extra-articular and systemic features include vasculitis, rheumatoid nodules, Sjögren's syndrome, pericarditis, pulmonary fibrosis, lung nodules, normochromic normocytic anaemia, thrombocytosis and amyloidosis. Routine blood tests demonstrate raised inflammatory markers, with immunological tests including Rheumatoid factor positive, anti-cyclic citrullinated protein antibody positive, and antinuclear antigen positive. X-ray findings include bony erosion, periarticular osteoporosis, and joint space narrowing. Treatment is with disease-modifying agents, steroids, non-steroidal anti-inflammatory drugs, biologicals, joint injections and arthroplasty.

2. E Renal cell carcinoma

Secondary bone tumours often metastasise from:

- Prostate (sclerotic lesions)
- Breast (lytic lesions)
- Kidney (lytic lesions)
- Lung (lytic lesions)
- Thyroid (lytic lesions)

Patients with bony metastasis may present with symptoms from their primary lesion and/or with symptoms and signs of their secondary lesion(s) including bone pain, pathological fracture or spinal cord compression. Pathological fractures are characterised by fracture following a low energy injury, through a region of bone with a pre-existing abnormality due to destruction of the bone architecture. Investigation includes radiographs, blood tests (calcium and alkaline phosphatase), bone scan and bone biopsy. The Mirels scoring system is used to guide treatment of pathological lesions (prophylactic fixation $\geq$ 8) and is based on four categories each scored 1–3:

- Pain (mild, moderate, mechanical)
- Tumour location (upper limb, lower limb, peritrochanteric/proximal femur)
- Lesion type (blastic, mixed, lytic)
- Lesion size (<1/3, 1/3–2/3, >2/3 of cortex involved)

Treatment includes analgesia, bisphosphonates, radiotherapy, chemotherapy and surgery to stabilise actual or impending pathological fractures.

3. C Renal impairment

Gout is characterised by hyperuricaemia (increased production or decreased excretion of uric acid) leading to the deposit of crystals within the joints and soft tissues, resulting in an inflammatory arthropathy. It predominantly affects men (8:1) and the peak age incidence is 20–40 years. Factors associated with increased production of uric acid include genetics (Lesch–Nyhan syndrome) and concomitant diseases (myeloproliferative and lymphoproliferative disorders). Factors associated with decreased excretion include renal impairment, thiazide diuretics and excess alcohol intake.

Investigations include blood tests (leucocytosis, raised C-reactive protein and erythrocyte sedimentation rate, abnormal urea and electrolytes, raised urate), imaging (bony erosions, loss of joint space, osteosclerosis) and joint aspiration (polymorphs, urate crystals, no organisms). Management for an acute attack requires rest, analgesia (e.g. non-steroidal anti-inflammatory drugs), colchicine and/or joint injections with steroid. Risk reduction strategies include lifestyle changes (alcohol reduction, avoiding purine rich foods, weight loss) and medications (e.g. allopurinol, probenecid).

Pseudogout is a predominantly large joint inflammatory arthropathy characterised by calcium pyrophosphate crystals deposition within joints and is associated with osteoarthritis. Less commonly associated diseases include endocrine disorders (e.g. diabetes mellitus, hyperparathyroidism, hypothyroidism, and acromegaly) and liver disorders (e.g. haemochromatosis, Wilson's disease). It predominantly affects women and the peak age incidence is 60–80 years.

Investigations include blood tests (leucocytosis, raised C-reactive protein and erythrocyte sedimentation rate, raised calcium), imaging (chondrocalcinosis) and joint aspiration (polymorphs, rhomboid shaped CPP (calcium pyrophosphate) crystals, no organisms).

4. C Osteophytes

Osteoarthritis is characterised by joint cartilage damage with joint space narrowing, osteophytes, subchondral sclerosis and subchondral cysts found on radiographs of the affected joint(s). Subchondral collapse is characteristic of avascular necrosis, whereas sequestrem and a Brodie's abscess are associated with osteomyelitis.

Risk factors for osteoarthritis include obesity, manual occupation, previous trauma or septic arthritis, developmental dysplasia of the hip (DDH), hypermobility syndrome, Perthes disease and Paget's disease. The hips, knees, spine and hands are most commonly involved and presentation with pain, swelling (osteophytes, e.g. Bouchard's and Heberden's nodes in the hands) and stiffness of the affected joint(s) that is exacerbated by weight bearing and movement. Blood tests and joint aspirations are usually unremarkable.

Management includes lifestyle modification (weight loss, physiotherapy), analgesia (e.g. non-steroidal anti-inflammatory drugs), intra-articular steroid injections and surgery (arthroplasty).

5. E Urgent fasciotomy of the left forearm

Acute compartment syndrome is a surgical emergency. It occurs when the contents of an inelastic walled compartment of the body swell and raise the pressure within that compartment. In this case the muscles have swollen up within the fascia. Once the pressure reaches a critical level the capillaries then the veins draining the compartment (which are thin walled) collapse under the external pressure. Arterial blood continues to enter but venous drainage is blocked. Pressure will then rapidly rise to mean arterial pressure when circulation in the compartment ceases and ischaemia starts. The muscles most commonly affected are those in the lower leg, and forearm. Less commonly affected are the intrinsic muscles of the hand and foot.

There does not need to be a fracture for a compartment syndrome to develop. Crushing injuries and severe bruising are potent causes. Indeed, open fractures are unlikely to cause this problem because the fascia is also likely to be breached. The diagnosis is a clinical one (intercompartmental pressure measurements are unreliable), but an intercompartmental pressure within 30 mmHg of diastolic pressure is claimed to be diagnostic. If there is severe pain especially on passively stretching the affected muscles then a compartment syndrome is likely and a fasciotomy should be performed whatever the intercompartmental pressures are found to be. The warm ischaemic time for limbs is not normally more than 3–6 hours so fasciotomy must be performed urgently if it is to succeed. Fasciotomy after 24–48 hours is likely to do more harm than good as a reperfusion syndrome will result leading to myoglobinuria and renal failure.

When a fasciotomy is performed all the compartments which might be involved (four in the lower leg) must be fully decompressed along their whole length. The wounds should be left open and no attempt made to close them until the swelling has gone down. Regular inspections are needed to identify and remove dead tissue.

6. A Atrophic non-union

Fractures of the proximal pole or waist of the scaphoid are a known risk factor for delayed or non-union of the scaphoid. Radiological union is frequently defined as the bridging of three out of the four cortices at the fracture site. Delayed union is defined as a persistent absence of clinical and radiological signs of fracture union, with the fracture taking longer than expected to unite. The time before a delayed union is defined as a non-union is fracture dependent. In a scaphoid fracture, this is often defined as the absence of trabeculae bridging the fracture site at 16 weeks. Non-union may be atrophic with no callus formed and thinning of the fractures ends. The cause is likely to be loss of blood supply. Excessive movement at the fracture site leads to hypertrophic non-union which is seen on radiographs as expansion of the bone ends and excessive callus formation but no bridging of the fracture site. Risk factors for delayed or non-union are shown in **Table 36.1**.

Table 36.1 Risk factors for delayed or union categorised according to patient, injury and treatment characteristics		
Patient factors	**Injury factors**	**Treatment factors**
Age	Open fracture	Prolonged immobilisation
Smoking	Extensive soft tissue trauma	Poor fracture reduction
Diabetes mellitus	Infection	Poor fracture fixation
Medications, e.g. non-steroidal anti-inflammatory drugs	Neurovascular injury Site of fracture (diaphysis/metaphysis) Degree of bone loss Polytrauma, e.g. head injury Pathological fracture	

7. A *Haemophilus influenzae*

Bacterial infection of a native or prosthetic joint is an orthopaedic emergency. In the native joint it can lead to joint destruction and in all patients can lead to severe sepsis. Risk factors include co-existing joint diseases, e.g. rheumatoid arthritis, previous joint arthroplasty, extremes of age, immunosuppression, diabetes and social deprivation. Common infecting organisms include *Staphylococcus aureus*, *Streptococcus*, *Neisseria gonorrhoeae*, *Haemophilus influenzae* and *Staphylococcus epidermidis*. *Staphylococcus* and *Streptococcus* are gram-positive organisms. *N. gonorrhoeae* infection is commonly seen in sexually active young adults and is

Table 36.2 Risk factors for delayed or union categorised according to patient, injury and treatment characteristics (adapted from Miller MD, Thompson SR and Hart J. Review of Orthopaedics, 6th ed. Philadelphia: Elsevier; 2012)	
Age	**Common organisms**
<12 months	*Staphylococcus* Group B *Streptococcus*
6 months – 5 years	*Staphylococcus* *Haemophilus influenzae*
5–12 years	*Staphylococcus aureus*
12–18 years	*Staphylococcus* *Neisseria gonorrhoea*

associated with polyarthralgia, tenosynovitis, urogenital symptoms and a pustular rash. *Staphylococcus epidermidis* is the common causative organism following joint arthroplasty. The common affecting organisms in children are shown in **Table 36.2**.

8. B Ewing's sarcoma

Ewing's sarcoma is a particularly malignant very rare small round cell tumour of the bone that frequently affects male teenagers. A genetic translocation is associated with the tumour (t 11;22). Localisation is often in the diaphysis of long and tubular bones, e.g. femur, pelvis ribs, humerus or spine. Radiographs demonstrate bone destruction and soft tissue swelling with a characteristic 'onion-skin' periosteal reaction.

Osteochondroma is a common cartilage tumour of cartilage that predominantly affects the metaphyses of long-bones in children and adolescents. The majority of tumours are asymptomatic. They have a 'mushroom type' appearance on imaging. Chondrosarcoma is a rare malignant bone tumour that is predominantly seen in older people (peak incidence is around 45 years) rather than children. The majority are found within the medulla of the proximal femur, pelvis, proximal humerus, ribs and spine. Endosteal scalloping is seen on imaging. Osteosarcoma is the most common malignant bone tumour of both children and adults (excluding myeloma). Risk factors include male gender, Paget's disease, retinoblastoma and radiation exposure. The tumours are destruction in nature and are often localised to the metaphyseal ends of the long bones, e.g. distal femur. Skip lesions are common. Metastases to the lung can occur. Radiographs demonstrate sclerosis, bony destruction, Codman's triangle and sunray spicules.

Chapter 37

Lymphoreticular system and liver

Questions

For each question, select the single best answer from the five options listed.

1. A 30-year-old woman, a recent immigrant from Africa, complains of an ulcer on the right side of her neck, which appeared 4 weeks ago. It was preceded by a matted lump, which first appeared 6 months ago. She has regular episodes of fever in the evenings.

   What is the most likely diagnosis?

   A   Branchial fistula
   B   Hodgkin's lymphoma
   C   Infected sebaceous cyst
   D   Secondary cervical metastasis
   E   Tuberculous sinus from tuberculous cervical lymphadenitis

2. A 38-year-old man presents with a painless, solid, firm, mass on the right side of his neck, which has been slowly growing in size over the last 8 months. He has hepatosplenomegaly; he complains of malaise, evening pyrexia with night sweats, pruritus and has recently lost some weight.

   What is the most likely diagnosis?

   A   Branchial cyst
   B   Carotid body tumour
   C   Hodgkin's lymphoma
   D   Secondary cervical metastasis
   E   Tuberculous lymphadenitis

3. A 40-year-old woman complains of malaise, tiredness and itching all over her body for almost 1 year. Her daughter noticed that for the last few months, she has a yellowish tinge to her conjunctiva. She has smooth hepatomegaly. Her serum bilirubin is 37 µmol/L and alkaline phosphatase is 720 units/L.

   What is the most likely diagnosis?

   A   Common bile duct stones
   B   Portal hypertension
   C   Primary biliary cirrhosis
   D   Primary sclerosing cholangitis
   E   Secondary metastases in liver

4. A 25-year-old man complains of recurrent intermittent jaundice for 2 years. He has episodes when he feels lethargic and unduly tired. He looks slightly jaundiced and has an enlarged spleen. On one occasion he had fever, abdominal pain, nausea and vomiting when he looked very anaemic. He has developed a 3 cm superficial ulcer on his leg.

   What is the most likely diagnosis?

   A   Chronic leukaemia
   B   Hereditary spherocytosis
   C   Idiopathic thrombocytopenic purpura
   D   Myelofibrosis
   E   Splenic infarction

5. A 72-year-old man complains of yellowish discoloration of his skin and sclera of 3 weeks' duration. This has been associated with malaise and right upper quadrant pain. On examination, he is jaundiced with an enlarged hard nodular liver and a long well-healed midline scar from an extended right hemicolectomy carried out 3 years ago for a carcinoma of the hepatic flexure. His blood results show:

   Haemoglobin 9 g/L
   C-reactive protein 92 mg/L
   Bilirubin 82 µmol/L
   Serum albumin 33 g/L
   Alkaline phosphatase 210 units/L
   Aspartate aminotransferase 84 units/L
   Alanine aminotransferase 110 units/L
   α-Fetoprotein 135 units/mL

   What is the most likely diagnosis?

   A   Biliary cirrhosis
   B   Cholangiocarcinoma
   C   Hepatoma
   D   Portal hypertension
   E   Secondary metastases

Answers

1. E Tuberculous sinus from tuberculous cervical lymphadenitis

This woman from Africa has the typical features of tuberculous cervical lymphadenitis. This has resulted in cervical lymph node swelling preceding the formation of a sinus. The nodes are matted. She also has the classical feature of evening pyrexia. The bacillus enters through the tonsil. Humans can be infected by both the bovine and the human form. A primary pulmonary focus should be excluded.

The node caseates, breaks down and forms a cold abscess (**Figure 37.1**), so called because it is not warm or tender. The pus, initially confined by the deep cervical fascia, tracks through the fascia superficially to form a biloculated abscess called a 'collar-stud' abscess resembling a dumb-bell. Left untreated, it bursts forming a sinus (**Figure 37.2**) which typically has an overhanging edge. The diagnosis is confirmed by biopsy. This shows caseating necrosis in which the dead tissue lacks any structure.

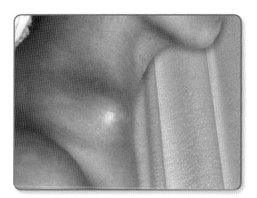

Figure 37.1 Cold abscess. Courtesy of Professor Ahmad Fahal.

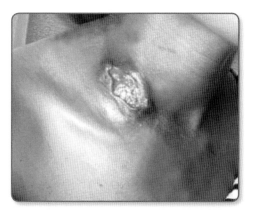

Figure 37.2 Tuberculous sinus with overhanging edge. Courtesy of Professor Ahmad Fahal.

2. C Hodgkin's lymphoma

This man has a neck lump typical of Hodgkin's disease – he has a mass of firm lymph nodes (**Figure 37.3**), slowly growing in size of several months' duration and enlarged liver and spleen. He has constitutional symptoms, referred to as 'B' symptoms, such as fatigue, pruritus, and cyclical temperature (Pel–Ebstein fever). The diagnosis is confirmed by lymph node biopsy. The extent of the disease is evaluated by haematological and biochemical investigations, imaging by chest X-ray, CT scan of the neck, chest and abdomen and bone marrow biopsy. This is a generalised disease of the reticuloendothelial system. Prior to definitive treatment the condition should be staged according to the Ann Arbor system devised in 1971. Pathologically, four different types of Hodgkin's lymphoma are recognised: nodular sclerosis, mixed-cellularity, lymphocyte-rich and lymphocyte-depleted. Microscopically lymphocytes, eosinophils, macrophages, neutrophils, plasma cells and. fibroblasts are present.

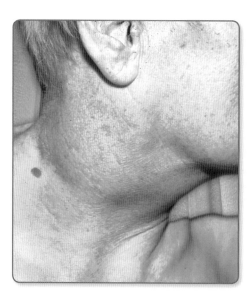

Figure 37.3 Lump on right side of neck: Hodgkin's lymphoma.

3. C Primary biliary cirrhosis

This patient has primary biliary cirrhosis. By far the vast majority of sufferers are women who present with gradual onset of fatigue and pruritus over a long period, jaundice being apparent later on. Hepatomegaly with scratch marks from pruritus is clinically apparent. Raised serum bilirubin and alkaline phosphatase should alert one to the diagnosis. This is confirmed by the presence of antimitochondrial antibodies, raised serum immunoglobulin (IgM). 85% of patients with primary biliary cirrhosis have at least one other autoimmune disease such as chronic thyroiditis, rheumatoid arthritis, scleroderma, Sjögren's syndrome or systemic lupus erythematosus. Liver ultrasound shows altered architecture.

Ultimate confirmation is by liver biopsy. The condition is a chronic progressive cholestatic liver disease causing destruction of intrahepatic bile ducts. Three stages are recognised: ductal lesion, scarring and cirrhosis. In stage 3, the end-stage, cirrhosis results with the liver becoming dark green in colour due to bile stasis.

4. B Hereditary spherocytosis

This young man with splenomegaly, intermittent jaundice and a leg ulcer suffers from hereditary spherocytosis. It is also called acholuric jaundice as there is no bile pigment in the urine in the presence of jaundice. This is because, the jaundice is from unconjugated bilirubin that is not water soluble and hence is not excreted by the kidney. Absence of pruritus is also a feature of unconjugated hyperbilirubinaemia. The acute clinical episode in the patient of fever, abdominal pain, nausea and vomiting and extreme anaemia is caused by a haemolytic crisis. These patients have a high chance of developing pigment gallstones which might be silent.

In this condition, there is a premature destruction of red cells caused by the monocyte/macrophage system in the spleen. The fundamental defect is an autosomal dominant hereditary disorder typified by a spherical red blood cell as opposed to the normal biconcave shape.

5. E Secondary metastases

This patient had a right hemicolectomy for cancer 3 years ago and now has hepatomegaly with deranged liver function tests with raised CEA. This is typical of liver secondaries. He should be thoroughly investigated and referred to the hepatobiliary surgeon for further treatment. As it is 3 years since his original resection, consideration should be given to the possibility of resection. As a general rule the longer the recurrence free interval, the better are the chances of success after resection of secondary. The patient is then discussed in a multidisciplinary team meeting. Some patients may be suitable for downstaging with various therapies followed by resection. Therefore, the following staging procedures should be carried out to assess for resectability:

- Colonoscopy and review previous histology to make sure that the original tumour has not recurred
- US, CT, PET-CT +/– MRI of abdomen and pelvis with contrast
- Chest CT
- Staging patient's comorbid status

Chapter 38

Orthopaedic pathology

Questions

For each question, select the single best answer from the five options listed.

1. A 5-year-old boy is brought to the clinic by his mother, who complains that the child has been crying with pain around the lower part of his right thigh since the previous evening. The boy refuses to move the limb and appears lethargic. Examination reveals that the child is febrile, and that his right distal thigh is swollen, warm and tender. The mother mentions that he recently recovered from an upper respiratory tract infection.

   Which region of the bone does the disease described in the above scenario commonly affect?

   A   Diaphysis
   B   Epiphysis
   C   Metaphysis
   D   No definite region affected
   E   The entire bone is generally affected diffusely

2. A 35-year-old man presents to the orthopaedic clinic complaining of discharge from a sinus over his left shin, with mild pain. He had sustained a fracture of his left tibia a year ago, for which a nailing of the tibia was performed. He recalls the problem starting within a few weeks postoperatively. The pain and discharge subside with antibiotics from the GP only to recur after a short period of relief. He can walk, however, bearing full weight on the affected limb. The attending orthopaedic surgeon orders radiographs of the affected leg.

   What would you expect to find on the X-rays?

   A   Brodie's abscess
   B   Mal-positioned tibial nail
   C   Mal-union of the tibial fracture
   D   Non-union of the tibial fracture
   E   Sequestrum, involucrum and periosteal reaction

3. A 48-year-old man presents with excruciating pain over his left, big toe, which came on suddenly the previous night. He says that the pain is so severe it wouldn't allow him to wear socks. He had five pints of beer last night. His toe is swollen, red and tender at the metatarsophalangeal joint.

What abnormality do you expect to find on his blood tests?

A   High calcium levels
B   High serum uric acid levels
C   Low potassium levels
D   Markedly high white cell count
E   Reversal of albumin/globulin ratio

4. A 24-year-old man sustained a humeral shaft fracture and injury to his radial nerve 4 months ago, with follow-up at regular intervals in the orthopaedic clinic. His clinical records document a progressing Tinel's sign with gradual improvement of motor function, noted first in the wrist extensors and then in the finger extensors.

What type of nerve injury is he most likely to have sustained?

A   Axonotmesis
B   Damage to the motor end plate
C   Neurapraxia
D   Neurotmesis
E   None of the above

5. A 22-year-old man presents to the orthopaedic clinic with low back pain for the past few months. He complains of stiffness in the back, which is worse in the mornings, and when he gets up from his chair in the evening. The surgeon notes limitation of flexion of the lumbar spine, and maximum chest expansion being 2 cm. He orders a radiograph of the pelvis.

What diagnosis is the clinician likely to make from the radiograph in this case?

A   Bilateral sacro-iliitis
B   Congenital vertebral anomaly
C   Old wedge compression fracture of L1
D   Reduced disc spaces in the lumbar spine
E   Secondaries in the lumbar spine from carcinoma of the lung

6. A 40-year-old woman presents to the orthopaedic clinic with pain involving multiple joints for several months, which has increased in severity for the past few weeks. The pain involves the small joints of both hands and she complains that her hands feel stiff for about an hour after waking up in the morning.

Which statement best describes the pathological findings seen in a joint affected by the symptoms above?

A   Cartilage metaplasia of the synovium
B   Deposition of calcium pyrophosphate
C   Erosion of articular cartilage by an inflammatory pannus
D   Granulomatous inflammation with caseous necrosis
E   Presence of negatively birefringent crystals in the joint

7.   A 45-year-old man presents with a lump around his left knee (**Figure 38.1**), which he noticed a few months ago. He undergoes radiographic evaluation of his knee, which reveals a lesion in the distal femur showing a soap-bubble appearance (**Figure 38.2**). This is followed by a biopsy from the lesion, which reveals numerous multinucleated giant cells.

What is the likely diagnosis?

A   Chondrosarcoma
B   Ewing's tumour
C   Giant cell tumour
D   Osteoma
E   Osteosarcoma

8.   A 37-year-old woman presents with pain extending from her neck down her left arm and to the end of her ring fingers. She also complains of frequent numbness affecting these fingers. On examination, there appears to be wasting of the intrinsic muscles of the hand. The physician notes that when he abducts and externally rotates the affected arm, the patient's symptoms are markedly exacerbated.

X-rays of the cervical spine are requested. What bony abnormality would you expect to find?

A   Cervical rib
B   Increased prevertebral shadow`
C   Multiple syndesmophytes
D   Occult vertebral fracture
E   Reduced disc spaces affecting C3, C4 and C5 disc spaces

9.   A 13-year-old boy presents after noticing a hard lump on the side of his knee while taking a shower. It does not cause him any pain or any restriction of his knee movements. On examination a hard, non-tender lump is felt on the medial aspect of his distal femur. X-rays reveal a pedunculated bony outgrowth from the metaphysis.

What is the most likely diagnosis?

A   Chondromyxoid fibroma
B   Ewing's sarcoma
C   Non-ossifying fibroma
D   Osteochondroma
E   Osteoid osteoma

Answers

1. C Metaphysis

The disease described in the question is acute pyogenic osteomyelitis, which affects children aged between 2 and 7 years. The source of the infection is usually a tooth with caries, an upper respiratory infection (as in this case), or an infected wound. The most common bacterial species implicated in acute osteomyelitis is *Staphylococcus aureus*. The infection spreads through the bloodstream to enter the bone, and establishes at the metaphyseal region. The reason for this metaphyseal predilection is the arrangement of blood vessels in the form of hair-pin loops, which causes stasis of blood in this region, creating a favourable environment for bacteria to proliferate. The metaphysis is also relatively poor in the number of reticulo-endothelial cells as compared to the diaphysis, which may be another reason for infection establishing at the metaphysis.

Treatment involves drainage of pus through drill holes in the affected region of bone, and appropriate antibiotics for about 6 weeks.

2. E Sequestrum, involucrum and periosteal reaction

This patient is suffering from chronic osteomyelitis which can result after an open fracture or from acquiring an infection during surgery (usually involving implants), i.e. postoperative osteomyelitis.

Thickening and irregularity of the involved bone, along with fixity of the sinus to the bone, is unequivocal evidence of chronic osteomyelitis (**Figure 38.1**).

Pathologically, dead infected bone is surrounded by infected granulation tissue, and is the focus of persisting infection. This is known as the sequestrum. The surrounding bone tries to wall off this infected focus, forming new sclerotic bone around the sequestrum – known as the involucrum. Radiologically, the sequestrum appears as a dense region, lined by a thin lytic zone representing the granulation tissue (**Figure 38.2**). This is surrounded by dense sclerotic new bone representing the involucrum. The most useful investigation is a sinogram, where a radio-opaque dye is injected via the sinus to identify the source of persisting infection.

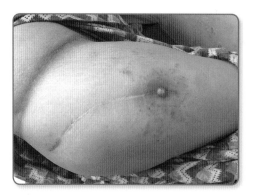

Figure 38.1 A sinus discharging pus 6 months after hip surgery using implants. A tell-tale sign of chronic osteomyelitis.

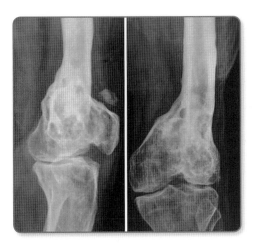

Figure 38.2 Radiographic appearance of an osteomyelitic distal femur.

3. B High serum uric acid levels

This man is suffering from an attack of acute gout, which is usually seen in obese and hypertensive middle-aged men.

The acute attack manifests as sudden of onset severe pain, usually involving the first metatarsophalangeal joint. The joint is red, hot and exquisitely tender. The cause is the precipitation of uric acid crystals in the joint space, which occurs when uric acid levels exceed their threshold of solubility in the plasma. Although usually clinically obvious, the diagnosis is confirmed by the presence of uric acid crystals in the joint space. These are typically negatively birefringent when viewed under a polarising microscope. Treatment of the acute attack involves administration of an NSAID and colchicine, which is now less favoured due to side-effects.

Urate lowering drugs should not be administered during an acute attack of gout, because they result in mobilisation of uric acid stores and worsening of the attack.

4. A Axonotmesis

Axonotmesis involves anatomical damage to the nerve fibres or axons. However, the endoneurial sheath surrounding the axons remains intact. The axon distal to the point of injury undergoes degeneration and fragmentation – Wallerian degeneration. As the axon regenerates, the muscles supplied proximally recover first, followed by those supplied distally. Similarly, tapping the skin over the point of the regenerating axon produces a tingling sensation along the course of the nerve (Tinel's sign) which signifies an attempt at nerve regeneration. As the regeneration progresses distally, so does the point at which Tinel's sign is elicited, signifying progressing regeneration.

According to Seddon's classification the other types of nerve injuries are:

- Neurapraxia, which is a physiological block of the nerve akin to concussion
- Neurotmesis, where the nerve is completely severed

5. A Bilateral sacro-iliitis

This patient is suffering from ankylosing spondylitis (AS), of which a typical finding is inflammation of the sacro-iliac joints. The cause of AS has been linked to the presence of the genetic marker HLA-B27.

Restriction of lumbar flexion noted by the Schober's test suggests AS. Further evidence can be obtained from the limitation of chest expansion, which is usually 5–7 cm in a healthy young male. While standing against a wall, the back of the hips, shoulders and occiput should normally simultaneously touch the wall, which does not happen in a patient with spinal deformity due to AS.

The earliest radiological feature is presence of inflammation in both sacro-iliac joints, which is evident as haziness of the joint space and sclerosis of the joint margins. Later, the entire spine is fused due to the presence of bridging syndesmophytes, giving the typical appearance of 'bamboo spine.'

6. C Erosion of articular cartilage by an inflammatory pannus

The diagnosis is rheumatoid arthritis (RA). Important features of the disease are:

- the involvement of small joints of the hands and feet
- a bilaterally symmetrical involvement
- presence of morning stiffness which lasts more than 30 minutes
- presence of RA factor and anti-CCP in serum
- presence of rheumatoid nodules which occur mainly over the extensor surfaces (back of forearms, elbows etc.)
- symptoms lasting more than 6 weeks

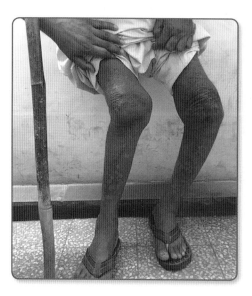

Figure 38.3 Knee deformity in advanced untreated rheumatoid arthritis.

Pathologically, the disease begins as proliferative synovitis, the synovium being infiltrated by inflammatory cells. Persistent inflammation results in the release of proteolytic enzymes, which destroy the articular cartilage of the joint. Also, a layer of granulation tissue arising from the inflamed and congested synovium invades the articular cartilage directly, and this is known as the pannus. Left untreated, the inflammatory process destroys the joint surfaces and results in permanent crippling deformities (**Figure 38.3**).

7. C Giant cell tumour

This patient is suffering from a giant cell tumour (GCT), also known as osteoclastoma. Although mostly benign, some GCTs show aggressive behaviour, and about 5% metastasise. The tumour is known to have a high rate of local recurrence after curettage (**Figure 38.4**).

Pathologically, the tumour is composed of numerous multinucleated giant cells in a background of stromal cells. The pathological appearance of the tumour has little value in identifying those that demonstrate an aggressive behaviour.

Radiologically, GCT displays the three Es: **E**ccentrically situated, **E**piphyseal, **E**xpansile lesion that abuts the articular cartilage (**Figure 38.5**). Further imaging (CT/MRI) is necessary to ensure that the tumour has not breached the joint margin or the cortex of the involved bone.

Treatment is surgical and involves extended curettage of the lesion. Wide excision with reconstruction is employed only in cases of recurrent tumours or those with significant extraosseous extension.

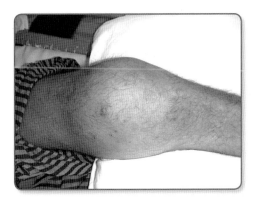

Figure 38.4 Clinical appearance of a giant cell tumour involving the distal femur.

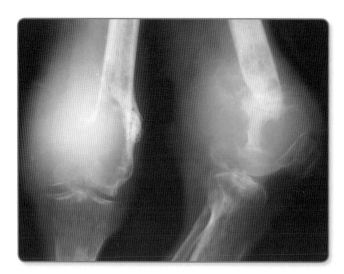

Figure 38.5 The radiological appearance of a giant cell tumour.

8. A Cervical rib

This patient has thoracic inlet/outlet syndrome. The first rib, with the scalenus anterior and scalenus medius, forms a triangle, through which pass the subclavian vessels and the lower trunk of the brachial plexus (formed by C8 and T1). Compression of these structures as they pass through this triangle, produces vascular and neurological symptoms. The causes of such compression are:

- a true cervical rib articulating with C7 vertebra
- an enlarged transverse process of C7
- a fibrous band that extends from the transverse process of C7

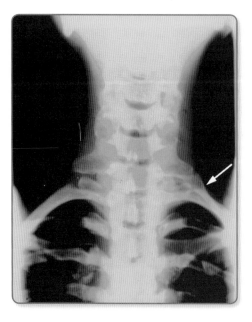

Figure 38.6 Radiograph showing the presence of cervical ribs (arrow).

Adson's test, where the patient's neck is extended and turned towards the affected side, aggravates this compression and causes loss of the radial pulse, or reproduces the patient's neurological symptoms, suggesting thoracic outlet syndrome.

X-rays will show a cervical rib (**Figure 38.6**) although a true cervical rib may often be an incidental finding.

Nerve entrapment syndromes are discussed in Chapter 56.

9. D Osteochondroma

The given clinical scenario and imaging findings clinch the diagnosis of an osteochondroma. An osteochondroma, also known as an exostosis, is a benign, aberrant bony outgrowth from the growth plate, which grows towards the diaphysis of the involved bone (**Figure 38.7**). It is generally noticed in growing children before fusion of the physis. It may be pedunculated or sessile, and its end bears a cartilage cap. It ceases to grow after the physis fuses. Very rarely, the cartilaginous cap may undergo a malignant change and transform into a chondrosarcoma or osteosarcoma.

Pain may occur if the stalk of the lesion fractures, or if the outgrowth impinges against a tendon or causes inflammation of a bursa. It may also impinge on the surrounding neurovascular structures causing symptoms.

If symptomatic, the osteochondroma should be excised only after the completion of skeletal growth, because of the high possibility of recurrence.

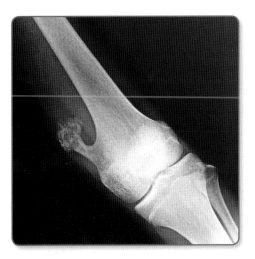

Figure 38.7 Pedunculated osteochondroma.

Principles of surgery in general

Chapter 39

Perioperative care

Questions

Theme: American Society of Anaesthesiologists classification

Options for Questions 1–4:

A	I-E		**D**	IV-E
B	II-E		**E**	V-E
C	III-E		**F**	VI-E

For each of the following cases, select the single most appropriate ASA class. Each option may be used once, more than once or not at all.

1. A 28-year-old man who is normally fit and well, has been declared brain dead following a head injury sustained during an alleged assault. He has no other injuries and is awaiting organ harvesting.

2. A 78-year-old man with a history of hypertension presents to the emergency department with abdominal pain and signs of hypovolaemic shock. He is not responding to fluid resuscitation. He has just arrived in theatre for emergency abdominal aortic aneurysm repair.

3. A 36-year-old woman requires laparoscopic cholecystectomy for acute cholecystitis. She has a goitre but is euthyroid on treatment with levothyroxine.

4. A 58-year-old woman is admitted as an emergency with a perforated sigmoid diverticulum for a Hartmann's procedure. She has a history of chronic obstructive pulmonary disease (COPD), presents dyspnoea on minimal exertion and requires treatment for exacerbations of COPD several times a year.

Theme: Nerve injury during anaesthesia

Options for Questions 5–7:

A	Common peroneal nerve	E	Radial nerve
B	Facial nerve	F	Supraorbital nerve
C	Femoral nerve	G	Tibial nerve
D	Median nerve	H	Ulnar nerve

For each of the following cases, select the single most likely nerve injury. Each option may be used once, more than once or not at all.

5. A 62-year-old man in the prone position for lumbar discectomy complains of loss of sensation to the anterior half of his scalp.

6. A 64-year-old man complains of sensory loss in the medial one-and-a-half digits of her hand following laparoscopic cholecystectomy.

7. A 52-year-old man complains of sensory loss over the lateral dorsal aspect of the hand and a wrist drop following open fasciectomy for an ipsilateral Dupuytren's contracture.

Theme: Monitoring of the anaesthetised patient

Options for Questions 8–10:

A	Airway pressure monitor	H	Intra-arterial blood pressure monitor
B	Bispectral analysis	I	Nasopharyngeal temperature probe
C	Electrocardiograph – lead II		
D	Electrocardiograph – lead V5	J	Noninvasive blood pressure monitor
E	End-tidal carbon dioxide analyser		
F	End-tidal anaesthetic agent analyser	K	Peripheral nerve stimulator
G	Inspired oxygen analyser	L	Pulse oximeter

For each of the following cases, select the single most useful monitor. Each option may be used once, more than once or not at all.

8. A 49-year-old man undergoing lumbar discectomy, to assess adequacy of ventilation.

9. A 27-year-old woman at the end of a laparoscopic cholecystectomy, to assess whether reversal of muscle relaxation is required.

10. A 74-year-old man undergoing femoral endarterectomy under spinal anaesthesia. He has had a recent myocardial infarction to monitor myocardial ischaemia.

Answers

1. F VI-E

This patient has been declared brain dead and is waiting for organ harvest for the purpose of organ donation. He is therefore ASA VI. The E denotes the fact that it is an emergency not a planned procedure. The patient was normally fit and well prior to the assault but he is now no longer regarded, as ASA I. ASA classification is not a very sensitive predictor of anaesthetic mortality but it does offer a reasonable estimate of overall outcome. It does not require calculation of a complex scoring system. The predicted mortality following surgery by ASA class is shown in **Table 39.1**.

Table 39.1 Predicted mortality following surgery by American Society of Anaesthesiologists class	
ASA class	**Predicted mortality (%)**
I	0.05
II	0.4
III	4.5
IV	25
V	50
VI	100
ASA, American Society of Anaesthesiologists	

2. E V-E

This patient has haemorrhagic shock secondary to a ruptured abdominal aortic aneurysm. His haemodynamic status is not improving with fluid resuscitation and he is moribund so the only chance of survival is with operative management hence his ASA V status. The patient has a history of hypertension so before his aneurysm rupture, he would have been considered ASA II but this is no longer the case.

3. B II-E

This patient would be categorised as having mild systemic thyroid disease, i.e. an ASA II patient. This patient has a goitre so the anaesthetist will undertake careful preoperative assessment of the airway as the goitre may make management of the airway more challenging, e.g. by tracheal compression if it extends retrosternally. Ideally, hypothyroid patients should be rendered euthyroid before surgery to avoid the potential effects of hypothyroidism including myocardial depression, decreased ventilatory drive, abnormal baroreceptor function, reduced plasma volume, anaemia and altered hepatic drug metabolism. The perioperative risk is probably greater in hyperthyroidism especially in view of the cardiovascular effects, which include atrial fibrillation, congestive cardiac failure and ischaemic heart disease. Thyroid storm is a serious complication of hyperthyroidism where a life-threatening hypermetabolic crisis develops.

4. C III-E

This patient would be considered to have systemic disease which is severe but which is not a constant threat to life, i.e. ASA III. Her dyspnoea does not occur at rest, which would put her into an ASA IV category. It can be difficult to decide which class patients are assigned to because the American Society of Anaesthesiologists does not provide specific guidance but various groups of experts have suggested some consensus guidelines to help with this, e.g. the National Institute for Health and Care Excellence preoperative investigation guidelines.

5. F Supraorbital nerve

The supraorbital nerve is a terminal branch of the frontal nerve. It exits the skull via the supraorbital foramen after which it can be compressed by suboptimal head position during prone positioning. The areas to which it provides sensory supply include the conjunctiva of the eye and the skin from the forehead as far back as the vertex. Adequate padding of the bony prominences can prevent compression injury.

6. H Ulnar nerve

The ulnar nerve originates from the medial cord of the brachial plexus (C8–T1) and descends on the posteromedial aspect of the humerus. At the elbow it passes posteriorly to the medial epicondyle of the distal humerus and is vulnerable to injury at this point.

During laparoscopic cholecystectomy, the arms are often placed by the patient's side to provide optimal surgical access to the abdomen. Devices used to secure the arms in this position can compress the ulnar nerve against the medial epicondyle of the humerus if they are not positioned appropriately. Damage to the ulnar nerve can produce a clawed hand and sensory loss in the little finger and medial half of the ring finger.

Whilst the ulnar nerve is derived from the brachial plexus, the signs and symptoms suggest damage at a specific point distal to the brachial plexus.

7. E Radial nerve

The radial nerve originates from the posterior cord of the brachial plexus (C5–T1). During open fasciectomy for Dupuytren's contracture, a tourniquet is applied to the upper arm to minimise blood loss and provide optimal surgical conditions. If this tourniquet is not adequately padded or if the tourniquet pressure is excessively high (leading to damage from mechanical compression and ischaemia) or too low (resulting in passive congestion of the arm). Nerve tissue is more vulnerable to compression injury whereas muscle is more susceptible to ischaemia. Care should be taken to ensure that the minimum tourniquet pressure required to obtain bloodless field is used at all times and that the recommended time for tourniquet inflation is never exceeded. The highest risk of nerve damage is seen in patients who are cachectic, have flaccid skin or conical shaped arms.

8. E End-tidal carbon dioxide analyser

The end-tidal carbon dioxide analyser or capnography is one of the basic requirements for monitoring during anaesthesia according to the Association of Anaesthetists of Great Britain and Ireland. It is used to assess adequacy of ventilation, i.e. the clearance of CO_2 from the body. It does not provide any information about oxygenation. End-tidal CO_2 is a good proxy for alveolar CO_2 in normal anaesthetised patients with a difference of only 0.4–0.7 kPa. If end-tidal CO_2 is above the normal range, consideration should be given to increasing minute ventilation in patients who are receiving positive pressure ventilation. The capnograph trace rapidly drops or falls to zero with a decrease in cardiac output or after cardiac arrest. It is also useful in the detection of oesophageal rather than tracheal intubation and blockage or disconnection of the breathing system.

9. K Peripheral nerve stimulator

The degree of neuromuscular blockade can be assessed by applying a supramaximal stimulus to a peripheral nerve with a peripheral nerve stimulator, and then assessing the associated muscular response. It is important to assess neuromuscular function prior to waking the patient up and attempting tracheal extubation because complications such as residual airway obstruction, regurgitation and aspiration, weakness and respiratory failure may result from residual paralysis. Clinical assessment is also important and may include assessment of the tidal volume or ability to cough or achieve a sustained head lift. If required, non-depolarising muscle relaxants such as atracurium can be reversed by administering the anticholinesterase neostigmine. There is a relatively new drug called sugammadex which can be used to reverse a particular class of non-depolarising muscle relaxant which includes rocuronium by encapsulating rocuronium molecules and preventing their action at the neuromuscular junction.

10. D Electrocardiograph – lead V5

For real time perioperative monitoring, a continuous electrocardiograph trace is displayed on the monitoring screen. Most patients require only a 3-lead ECG with the electrodes being placed on the right arm, left leg and left arm. This allows recording of leads I, II and III with lead II being most commonly displayed on the monitor because it allows the best identification and interpretation of arrhythmias.

In patients who are at increased risk of myocardial ischaemia, a 5-lead ECG can be used to generate a V5-lead which will demonstrate 90% of detectable myocardial ischaemic changes and also provide arrhythmia monitoring.

Electrocardiograph monitoring during surgery can be difficult as lead placement may be suboptimal to allow better surgical access and interference from diathermy is common despite an electromagnetic filter being used to try and reduce this.

Chapter 40

Postoperative management and critical care

Questions

Theme: Hypoxaemia in surgical patients

Options for Questions 1–4:

A	Acute lung injury	E	Opioid induced respiratory
B	Acute respiratory distress		depression
	syndrome	F	Pulmonary embolism
C	Atelectasis	G	Pneumonia
D	Fat embolism		

For each of the following cases, select the single most likely diagnosis. Each option may be used once, more than once or not at all.

1. A 25-year-old man attends the emergency department following a road traffic accident. A femoral shaft fracture is seen on X-ray and femoral nailing is carried out the following morning. Six hours postoperatively, he develops pyrexia, confusion and petechial rash on the anterior chest wall.

2. A 42-year-old woman is admitted to the surgical ward with acute pancreatitis, and is receiving 10 litres per minute of oxygen via a non-rebreathe mask (estimated FiO_2 0.80). Her PaO_2 is 8 kPa. Bilateral infiltrates are visible on a chest X-ray taken that morning.

3. A 34-year-old woman is in the recovery room following an elective laparoscopic cholecystectomy for biliary colic. She complains of being in severe abdominal pain. She is obese (BMI = 33 kg/m^2) and smokes 20 cigarettes a day but is otherwise well. Respiratory rate is 16 breaths per minute, heart rate is 103 beats per minute and blood pressure is 142/84 mmHg. She requires 6 L/min of oxygen to maintain SpO_2 94%.

4. A 67-year-old man is in the surgical high dependency unit 72 hours following anterior resection for bowel cancer. He complains of breathlessness at rest and some right-sided pleuritic chest pain but denies other cardiorespiratory symptoms. He does not appear to be sedated or in pain and is receiving analgesia via a patient-controlled morphine pump (PCA). He is haemodynamically stable but is hypoxic and tachypnoeic. His chest sounds clear. An arterial blood gas has shown PaO_2 of 6.8 kPa and $PaCO_2$ of 3.6 kPa on 5 L/min of oxygen.

Theme: Electrolyte disturbances

Options for Questions 5–6:

A	Hypercalcaemia	F	Hypocalcaemia
B	Hyperchloraemia	G	Hypochloraemia
C	Hyperkalaemia	H	Hypokalaemia
D	Hypermagnesaemia	I	Hypomagnesaemia
E	Hypernatraemia	J	Hyponatraemia

For each of the following cases, select the single most likely electrolyte disturbance. Each option may be used once, more than once or not at all.

5. A 38-year-old woman is an inpatient in the surgical unit following total thyroidectomy 12 hours ago. She previously had difficulty breathing and circumoral paraesthesia.

6. A 45-year-old man is reviewed at the pre-assessment clinic prior to a inguinal hernia repair and noted to be in atrial fibrillation. He has a history of significant alcohol excess. Serum potassium is 4.5 mmol/L.

Theme: Cardiovascular complications following surgery

Options for Questions 7–10:

A	Broad QRS complexes, tented T waves	E	P waves unrelated to QRS complexes
B	Disorganised waveform, broad QRS complexes	F	Regularly irregular rhythm P waves present
C	Irregularly irregular rhythm, absent P waves	G	Sinus tachycardia, low-voltage QRS complexes
D	Lead I: prominent S wave, lead III: Q wave, inverted T wave	H	ST elevation in the anterior leads

For each of the following cases, select the single most likely ECG finding. Each option may be used once, more than once or not at all.

7. A 68-year-old man is in the high dependency unit 48 hours following an oesophagogastrectomy for cancer. There is concern regarding anastamotic breakdown.

8. A 55-year-old man in the high dependency unit 72 hours following an elective abdominal aortic aneurysm repair. He gets an episode of severe chest pain which is not relieved by glyceryl trinitrate spray.

9. A 32-year-old woman presents to the emergency department. She was trapped in a car for several hours following a road traffic accident with extensive soft tissue injuries to both legs. She is tachycardic and her creatine kinase is 6300 mmol/L.

10. A 65-year-old woman is in the orthopaedic ward 48 hours after left total hip arthroplasty. She complains of shortness of breath and pleuritic chest pain. Her chest is clear. A recent blood gas shows hypoxaemia and a recent chest X-ray detected no abnormality.

Answers

1. D Fat embolism

Fat emboli can be a found in lung parenchyma and peripheral circulation after long bone fracture or other trauma. Non-traumatic causes of fat embolism include pancreatitis, diabetes mellitus and steroid treatment are less common.

This case describes the classic triad of symptoms seen in fat embolism in the context of a high risk injury. This triad generally presents 24–72 hours postinjury:

- Respiratory compromise: 50% of patients develop severe hypoxaemia and may require intubation.
- Neurological dysfunction: caused by cerebral emboli, which can cause an acute delirium or focal neurological deficit, which are generally transient.
- Petechial rash: this occurs last and only in 60% cases. May appear on the chest wall, conjunctiva and oral mucous membranes etc.

The management of fat embolism is supportive so efforts should be made to prevent it occurring by limiting intraosseous pressure and avoiding cement and reaming when possible. Overall mortality remains between 5 and 15%.

2. B Acute respiratory distress syndrome

Acute pancreatitis can be complicated by multiple organ dysfunction. The respiratory complications can be severe and often herald a poor outcome.

There are a number of causes of hypoxaemia in acute pancreatitis:

- Acute respiratory distress syndrome (ARDS)
- Pneumonia
- Pleural effusion
- Atelectasis
- V/Q mismatch with no radiological abnormality

The diagnostic criteria for ARDS are:

- Acute onset
- Bilateral infiltrates on chest X-ray
- No evidence of left atrial hypertension, with pulmonary artery occlusion pressure of ≤ 18 mmHg if measured
- PaO_2/FiO_2 ratio ≤ 27 kPa

ARDS is associated with diffuse damage to the alveoli and endothelial leakage and injury. The early phase lasting from days 1–5 is characterised as being 'exudative' with leakage of protein rich fluid into the interstitium and air spaces. The later phase is typically 'fibroproliferative' in nature with architectural changes including emphysema and pulmonary fibrosis developing.

The treatment of ARDS is supportive. Patients generally require intubation and ventilation in the intensive care unit to optimise oxygenation and to manage other failing organ systems.

3. C Atelectasis

Atelectasis describes the absence of gas from part of, or the entire, lung. It is caused by obstruction of aeration of the alveoli. The gas trapped within the alveoli is eventually absorbed leaving nothing to splint open the alveoli so they collapse. Gas exchange and oxygenation are then markedly decreased. This occurs in the dependent region of normal lungs during anaesthesia. Other causes include endobronchial intubation. In this patient, smoking will make the sputum thick and sticky putting her at risk of sputum retention. Her uncontrolled pain will reduce chest movement and subsequently aeration of that area of lung postoperatively the failure to reinflate the lung produces atelectasis.

There is already supplemental oxygen therapy in situ. The priorities should now be:

- getting the patient to sit up to improve respiratory mechanics and increase functional residual capacity
- optimising analgesia so the patient can freely cough and take a deep breath and
- arranging chest physiotherapy to ensure that the collapsed areas of lung are reinflated to avoid chest sepsis postoperatively

4. F Pulmonary embolism

Pulmonary embolism is mechanical obstruction of a pulmonary artery or arteriole with thrombus which is often derived from a deep vein thrombosis in the legs or pelvis. It may present with pleuritic chest pain, tachypnoea, tachycardia and cyanosis unless the PE is massive in which case hypotension or cardiac arrest may occur.

This patient has a number of risk factors for pulmonary embolism including malignancy, major abdominal/pelvic surgery and immobility. He should have been given venous thromboembolism prophylaxis including an anticoagulant, e.g. low molecular weight heparin and mechanical prophylaxis, i.e. graduated compression stockings.

Confirmation of the diagnosis using either CT pulmonary angiography or ventilation-perfusion scanning should occur followed by treatment with low molecular weight heparin or unfractionated heparin if concerns about postoperative bleeding persist.

5. F Hypocalcaemia

Hypocalcaemia following thyroid surgery is caused by damage to the parathyroid glands which produce parathyroid hormone (PTH), which is integral to the regulation of serum calcium.

Deficiency in PTH leads to hypocalcaemia which in the post-thyroidectomy setting may be permanent (0.4–13.8% of patients) due to direct trauma, (inadvertent) surgical removal or compromise of blood supply; or it may be transient (2–53% of patients) due to reversible ischemia or hypothermia.

Most patients are asymptomatic. Classic symptoms include: circumoral paraesthesiae, tetany, carpopedal spasm, laryngospasm, seizures, prolonged QT interval on ECG, and cardiac arrest.

Routine postoperative check of PTH and calcium will identify patients at risk of hypocalcaemia following thyroidectomy. In patients symptomatic of hypocalcaemia, replacement should be by the intravenous route titrated to symptoms and blood levels. Oral calcium supplementation should then be commenced alongside replacement of vitamin D.

6. J Hypomagnesaemia

Patients with a history of alcohol excess have a number of reasons for developing atrial fibrillation one of which is electrolyte imbalance. Other causes of hypomagnesaemia are listed below:

- Reduced intake
- Increased gastrointestinal loss
- Increased renal loss

The clinical features can be divided into:

- Neuromuscular: tetany, muscle weakness, seizures, nystagmus
- Cardiovascular: ST depression, T wave inversion, prolonged QT interval, arrhythmias, e.g. atrial fibrillation, ventricular fibrillation

Atrial fibrillation needs to be controlled prior to surgery so this should prompt further assessment of the patient.

Magnesium replacement can be either intravenous or oral. Severe symptomatic hypomagnesaemia should be treated intravenously. The efficacy of this treatment is limited by the magnesium reabsorption in the loop of Henle and up to 50% of this dose may be excreted. Oral magnesium supplementation should be used in asymptomatic patients. With both intravenous and oral replacement, it is important to monitor patients for signs and symptoms of hypermagnesaemia.

7. C Irregularly irregular ventricular rhythm, absent P waves

This description is suggestive of atrial fibrillation (AF). AF is a supraventricular tachycardia where there is uncoordinated atrial contraction. If atrioventricular conduction remains intact, the ventricular response is rapid and irregular. Causes of atrial fibrillation can be divided into cardiac causes which include: postmyocardial infarction, hypertension, valvular heart disease, congenital heart disease.

Other causes which include: alcohol excess, pulmonary embolism, lower respiratory tract infection and hyperthyroidism

In postoperative patients, AF can be a sign of surgical sepsis. In a patient who has recently undergone oesophagectomy, priorities are management of the arrhythmia and looking for an underlying cause which may be anastamotic breakdown or pneumonia.

Management of the arrhythmia should focus on controlling the ventricular rate and if possible, restoration of sinus rhythm. The method of choice is dependent on haemodynamic status; the main options are either chemical or electrical cardioversion. Once haemodynamic stability has been achieved, consideration should be given to preventing recurrence of atrial fibrillation and preventing thrombotic complications.

8. H ST elevation in the anterior leads

This description is suggestive of anterior myocardial infarction. The perioperative period can be associated with large and unpredictable changes in atherosclerotic plaque biology with an increased risk of plaque rupture. It also can lead to a mismatch of myocardial oxygen supply and demand with significant variation in heart rate, blood pressure, anaemia and hypoxaemia.

Perioperative ischaemia is a significant predictor of mortality and morbidity from non-cardiac surgery. Perioperative ischaemia can be silent and very difficult to treat due to the increased risk of bleeding with anticoagulants, antiplatelet agents and thrombolysis.

A more effective strategy may be to identify high risk patient preoperatively and investigate them. Optimisation of pharmacological treatment and revascularisation options can then be considered. This will not avoid all risk as unpredictable plaque rupture may still occur.

9. A Broad QRS complexes, tented T waves

This description is suggestive of hyperkalaemia. This is a clinical emergency and treatment should be instituted immediately with calcium gluconate as a slow bolus to stabilise the myocardium with continuous ECG monitoring, then treatments such as insulin/dextrose infusion to drive potassium intracellularly.

In this scenario, it is related to the development of rhabdomyolysis. Rhabdomyloysis may be:

- Traumatic: following crush injury, excessive muscle activity, electrocution
- Nontraumatic: infective causes, electrolyte disturbances, metabolic and immune mediated disorders

Irrespective of the aetiology, the final common pathway is release of myocyte components into the systemic circulation which causes hyperkalaemia, acidosis and acute renal failure.

Creatine kinase should be checked and if this is greater than 5000 mmol/L, acute renal failure should be expected in approximately 50% of cases. The urine may be dark and test positively for blood on urinalysis. Urinalysis cannot differentiate between myoglobin and haemoglobin.

Prompt crystalloid fluid resuscitation should be commenced and consideration given to alkalinisation of the urine with sodium bicarbonate to increase the solubility of myoglobin and reduce the severity of renal dysfunction. Renal replacement therapy may be required.

10. D Lead I: prominent S wave, lead III: Q wave, inverted T wave

The description 'Lead I: Prominent S wave, lead III: Q wave, inverted T wave' is consistent with suspected pulmonary embolism (PE). The most common ECG finding in PE is a sinus tachycardia. The classical 'S1Q3T3' ECG changes shown in **Figure 40.1** are not as commonly seen in clinical practice. Right heart strain patterns, e.g. right axis deviation, right bundle branch block and T wave inversion in leads V1–V4 may also occur. ECG is of limited diagnostic value in PE but can be helpful in ruling out obvious myocardial ischaemia from the differential diagnosis.

Hip arthroplasty is major surgery and the incidence of postoperative deep vein thrombosis diagnosed on venography is 70% with <1% fatal PE, if no prophylaxis is given. This rate significantly decreases with prophylaxis.

Clinical features depend on the severity of PE with pleuritic chest pain, dyspnoea and haemoptysis in milder cases and hypotension, cyanosis and raised jugular venous pressure in more significant PEs. Smaller PEs have less haemodynamic effects but infarction of an area of lung tissue may occur. Multiple PEs can cause pulmonary hypertension.

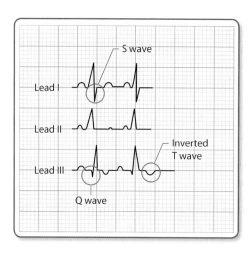

Figure 40.1 S1Q3T3 ECG pattern.

Chapter 41

Surgical technique and technology

Questions

Theme: Types of suture material used with needles

Options for Questions 1–3:

A	Chromic catgut 4/0	E	Polydioxanone 5/0
B	Metal clips	F	Polygalactin 2/0
C	Plain catgut 3/0	G	Polypropylene 5/0
D	Polyamide 4/0	H	Silk 1/0

For each of the following scenarios, select the single most appropriate suture material. Each option may be used once, more than once or not at all.

1. A 35-year-old man undergoes an open suprapubic cystolithotomy for removal of a large bladder calculus. The bladder is repaired in two layers.

2. A 19-year-old man falls from height and is brought to the emergency department with a scalp laceration. The laceration is closed.

3. A 56-year-old man undergoes a reversed saphenous vein femoropopliteal bypass for occlusive disease of the superficial femoral artery. An arterial anastomosis is carried out.

Theme: Surgical wound closure and anastomotic technique

Options for Questions 4–6:

A	Continuous suture	E	Single layer interrupted serosub-mucosal (extramucosal) suture
B	Horizontal mattress		
C	Interrupted suture	F	Subcuticular suture
D	Laparostomy and use of Bogota bag	G	Tension suture
		H	Vertical mattress suture

For each of the following scenarios, select the single most appropriate suturing technique. Each option may be used once, more than once or not at all.

4. A 65-year-old man is undergoing colorectal anastomosis after anterior resection. A hand-sewn anastomosis is performed.

5. A 70-year-old woman on the 6th postoperative day following a mid-line laparotomy for a perforated duodenal ulcer has developed a wound dehiscence. The patient is on steroids and is taken to theatre for resuture of the abdomen.

6. A 56-year-old man is known to suffer from chronic obstructive airways disease and presents with perforated appendicitis. After laparotomy, appendicectomy and peritoneal lavage, it is difficult to approximate the abdominal wall with conventional suturing technique due to gross abdominal distension.

Theme: Sterilisation techniques

Options for Questions 7–9:

A	Autoclaving	D	Ethylene oxide gas
B	Cetrimide and chlorhexidine solution	E	Formaldehyde
		F	Povidone iodine solution
C	Chlorine dioxide solution	G	Ultraviolet rays

For each of the following implements used at surgery, select the single most appropriate method of sterilisation. Each option may be used once, more than once or not at all.

7. Abdominal drain.

8. Deaver's retractor.

9. Gastroscope.

Theme: Energy sources

Options for Questions 10–12:

A	Argon beam coagulator	E	Monopolar coagulation current
B	Bipolar current	F	Monopolar cutting current
C	Chemical cautery	G	Thermal cautery
D	Cryotherapy	H	Ultrasonic shears

For each of the following scenarios, select the single most likely energy source. Each option may be used once, more than once or not at all.

10. A 25-year-old man presents to the emergency department with a crush injury to his hand. His wound is being explored under tourniquet and Bier's block. Haemostasis needs to be achieved.

11. A 40-year-old woman is due to have a right hemicolectomy for carcinoma of the caecum. The operation is due to be carried out by the usual open procedure.

12. A 70-year-old woman with a pacemaker and left-sided hemiarthroplasty of her hip has to undergo laparotomy for suspected colonic perforation from carcinoma. Haemostasis needs to be achieved by special technique in view of the presence of a prosthesis and a pacemaker.

Answers

1. F Polygalactin 2/0

Polygalactin is a synthetic multifilament absorbable suture material. Absorbable sutures are preferred for bladder closure so that no foreign material stays in the bladder wall avoiding a nidus for any subsequent stone formation. Bladder closure is usually done in two layers and is water tight with 2/0 or 1/0 suture.

2. H Silk 1/0

Scalp is a tough layer of the skin and is closed with a nonabsorbable suture like silk. Silk is easier to knot and does not slip. This quality is a great help in the presence of profuse bleeding. Due to the strength of the skin of the scalp and to avoid suture breakage during knotting a thicker suture like 1/0 or 2/0 is to be used.

3. G Polypropylene 5/0

Fine monofilament polypropylene suture is used for vascular anastomosis. Size of the suture varies from a finer 4/0 or 5/0 in femoral or popliteal arteries to heavier sutures like 2/0 or 3/0 for the abdominal aorta.

4. E Single layer interrupted serosubmucosal (extramucosal) anastomosis suture

In colorectal surgery this method of anastomosis is now regarded as the method of choice. Interrupted nonabsorbable sutures taking bites of the serosa and submucosa but excluding the mucosa are taken. This will preserve the blood supply and not narrow the lumen after the anastomosis. This technique would ensure a water-tight anastomosis that heals well in spite of the inherent tenuous blood supply of the colon.

5. G Tension suture

For resuture of a wound dehiscence tension sutures are used. The term 'tension suture' is a misnomer because they are never tied under tension. They are so called because they are tied in such a way that they should relieve abdominal tension. Strictly speaking they should be called 'through-and-throughs' as they go through all the layers of the abdominal wall including skin. The suture is taken at least 2 cm from the wound edge and the knot tied over a fine rubber tube so that the nylon suture does not dig into the abdominal skin. The sutures are left in place for 2 weeks. Sometimes such sutures are used prophylactically in patients such as the immunocompromised, the jaundiced, those with chronic renal failure and patients on steroids, who are vulnerable to developing burst abdomen.

6. D Laparostomy and use of Bogota bag

Any attempt to close the abdomen forcibly under tension causes increased pressure in the abdominal cavity risking the possibility of abdominal compartment syndrome. This condition leads to reduced venous return (from pressure on inferior vena cava) and severely affects respiration (from diaphragmatic splinting) resulting in type 2 respiratory failure. In such cases, the abdominal wall is left open (laparostomy) and the exposed bowel can be covered with a soft plastic bag (Bogota bag) cut into a size to fit the defect and sutured to the rectus sheath all around. This was devised from a sterilised urology fluid bag in 1984 by Dr Oswaldo Borraez, a trauma surgeon, while he was a resident in Bogota. Once the acute stage of oedema and infection has settled, it is usually possible to approximate the abdominal wall or leave it for closure by secondary intention.

7. D Ethylene oxide gas

Ethylene oxide gas is used for disposable material such as plastic tube drains and catheters made of polyvinylchloride, latex or rubber. This highly penetrative gas requires 12 hours to be effective which includes the time for aeration to rid the article of the residual toxic gas. It is also used for instruments that cannot withstand temperatures above 60°C.

8. A Autoclaving

Autoclaving is steam under pressure used for metallic instruments except for sharp objects such as scissors which would become blunt by this method. Used at 134°C at 30 per square inch (psi) for 3 minutes or 121°C at 15 psi for 15 minutes, this technique is one of the most reliable and efficient methods of sterilisation.

9. C Chlorine dioxide solution

Chlorine dioxide solution is used to disinfect gastroscopes. This is an oxidising and germicidal agent a clear colourless and odourless solution used to disinfect fibreoptic endoscopes. In the past 2% glutaraldehyde was used for this purpose. A 20 minute immersion would get rid of most micro-organisms but not spores. It was extremely irritant and toxic to the skin; hence it has been replaced with chlorine dioxide.

10. B Bipolar current

Bipolar current is a safe current as the path of the current is limited between the two poles and no stray current passes to the patient's tissues. It is used where the blood vessel is an end artery particularly in fingers and toes. There is no patient electrode. The active and return electrodes are at the operation site – the two blades of the forceps perform both functions. It is ideally used in a patient with a pacemaker and for delicate surgical procedures.

11. E Monopolar coagulation current

Monopolar coagulation current is the one most commonly used in conventional open surgery. The active electrode is at the surgical site; the return electrode is usually on patient's thigh. The pad is 70 cm^2; before it is applied the hair at the site is shaved. Other precautions to be taken are: there should be no fluid in the vicinity; the patient should not touch any metal objects; and in a patient with prosthesis, the patient electrode should be as far away as possible from the prosthesis.

12. H Ultrasonic shears

Ultrasonic shears achieve haemostasis using vibration at ultrasonic frequency. There is no passage of electrical current through the patient's tissues. Hence, it is safe in patients who have implanted pacemakers or metallic prostheses.

Chapter 42

Management of legal issues in surgery

Questions

Theme: Communication skills

Options for Questions 1–2:

A	Acknowledge good work	G	Make sure that you know everyone's names and their responsibilities
B	Acknowledge that there is a problem as soon as possible		
C	Get the facts first	H	Remain calm, delegate duties
D	Give the people involved a severe ticking off	I	Set some ground rules for discussion
E	Make sure that everyone who needs to know is informed	J	Take copious notes
F	Make sure that you have a quiet room where you will not be disturbed		

For each of the following situations, select the single most appropriate initial action, which is most likely to achieve a successful outcome. Each option may be used once, more than once, or not at all.

1. There is a dispute between two members of staff over duties on the ward. Both have given their side of the story. A meeting is called to try to resolve the issue.

2. Four ambulances arrive simultaneously at the emergency department with four seriously injured patients from a car crash. They have not given any notice of their arrival.

Theme: Breaking bad news

Options for Questions 3–5:

A   The environment was not appropriate

B   A check should have been made as to whether the patient wanted someone with them

C   The interviewer should have found out how much the patient wanted to know before starting

D   Adequate time should have been left to complete the task

E   Simpler language could have been used

F   This was handled correctly

For each of the following scenarios, select the single most appropriate critique. Each option may be used once, more than once or not at all.

3.   A 60-year-old retired man has smoked all his life. He developed a cough and an X-ray shows a suspicious shadow. Tracheal cytology confirms the presence of an adenocarcinoma. On scanning, there is evidence of metastases in the brain and in the vertebrae. An interview is arranged with the patient and his wife. It is explained that there is a cancer in his lungs and that it has spread throughout his body, such that only palliative treatment would be appropriate. He is shown both the scans and it is explained where metastases can be seen. The patient and his wife seem shocked, but have no questions. But the wife does mention that she had not wanted her husband told just at this moment since he was being treated for depression.

4.   A 30-year-old married woman has had a breast lump removed. At clinic 1 week later she is told that the lump was an aggressive form of cancer and that she needs a mastectomy and radiotherapy. She is very upset by the news and needs a great deal of support and reassurance. The clinic nurse phones her husband to arrange for her children to be collected from school and to ask him to come and collect her from the clinic as she feels too upset to drive.

5.   A 30-year-old man has a phaeochromocytoma. It is explained that surges in hormones released by the tumour are leading to instability in the blood pressure homeostasis mechanisms and that these fluctuations are responsible for his symptoms. The doctor then goes on to explain how difficult the tumour can be to find and that there may be rebound side-effects after it has been successfully removed. The patient seems a little dissociated from the interview but has no questions.

Theme: Evidence-based surgical practice

Options for Questions 6–8:

A Enter keywords into an internet search engine

B Perform a literature review for the Cochrane collaboration

C Perform an audit

D Perform a randomised controlled trial (RCT)

E Give a presentation based on the patients seen

F Search for NICE or SIGN guidelines

For each of the following situations, select the single most appropriate action, which is most likely to give a clinically useful answer. Each option may be used once, more than once, or not at all.

6. A consultant has designed a new method for ligating perforating varicose veins, using a small metal coil which he has had designed and had made for him by a local company. He is now going to start implanting these.

7. There are two different knee replacements used in the hospital, and it has been agreed that the unit should only use one. But it cannot be decided which is the one which should be used.

8. There appear to be too many cases of wound infection on the ward. This may be a result of there being no hand-gel available at the end of each patient's bed.

Theme: Ethics and medical negligence

Options for Questions 9–11:

A There was a breach of duty of care

B On the balance of probabilities there is negligence

C The patient has come to harm, but so far no more than this can be said

D There is no legal issue here

E There is no negligence as there is no breach of care

For each of the following situations, select the single most likely conclusion that will be drawn when legal advice is sought. Each option may be used once, more than once, or not at all.

9. A 30-year old woman has a swab left in her abdomen following a laparotomy, but she is otherwise well.

10. A 10-year old boy is given penicillin. It was not thought that the patient was allergic to penicillin. He comes out in a rash, which settles within hours.

11. A 70-year old man has a total hip replacement. On rounds the following morning it is noticed that he has a foot drop. This subsequently turns out to be permanent.

Theme: Handling a complaint

Options for Questions 12–14:

A	Acknowledge as soon as possible before you know the facts	**E**	Gather the facts together before calling a meeting
B	Arrange a meeting and explain what has happened	**F**	Keep the complaint on a 'need to know' basis so that morale in the unit is maintained
C	Apologise first even before you have the facts	**G**	Promise to learn from what has happened
D	Bring the case up first at a clinical governance meeting on a 'no-name' basis	**H**	Write immediately that 'You are sorry that you feel this way'

For each of the following situations, select the single most appropriate action. Each option may be used once, more than once, or not at all.

12. A 70-year-old man had a total hip replacement 2 weeks ago. He has now been told that the joint is infected and that it will need to be changed. His wife complains about this and says that lots of the patients treated by this service have become infected. This is checked with the consultant and the infection control officer. A recent audit of the unit shows that the unit has had three infections in the 150 hip replacement operations performed in the last year. The national infection rate is reported as being between 1 and 3%. All measures which should be taken to prevent infection have been taken.

13. A 90-year-old woman falls out of bed when slightly confused. This occurred because the cot sides were down at the time of the accident. There are instructions in the nursing notes that the sides should be kept up at all times. The sides were apparently down because the nurses were all busy with another patient who had collapsed.

14. A 60-year-old man complains because he has to return to theatre after a ligature has slipped on a large vessel. The ligature had not been double tied. The doctor proposes to see the patient and apologise personally for what has happened.

Answers

1. I Set some ground rules for discussion

When setting up a meeting for 'conflict resolution' there need to be clear ground rules. These must be agreed before negotiation starts as otherwise the situation can be made worse not better. Examples might be:

- There is to be no abusive language
- Either side can call 'time-out' if they feel that the meeting is going out of control

2. H Remain calm, delegate duties

This is another example where the ability of the department to respond is at risk of being overwhelmed by the medical need. You may well need to triage the casualties and you will certainly need to calmly allocate your staff to where they can do the most good for the maximum number.

3. C The interviewer should have found out how much the patient wanted to know before starting

Breaking bad news is not simple. It is important to find out how much the patient wants to know before proceeding. It may be that they want to take information in smaller pieces separated by time so that they can digest the change in their life. The wife's wishes that her husband should not be told at that time do not take priority over his wishes, but they need to be taken into account.

4. B A check should have been made as to whether the patient wanted someone with them

Most people would like to have someone they trust and respect with them when coping with bad news. In this case, it might have been better for this patient to have her husband with her while given the news.

5. E Simpler language could have been used

Language which may be simple to you, may be completely incomprehensible to the patient. Conversely, highly educated patients, especially doctors, may find layman's language patronising. It is therefore important to check regularly that you are using language appropriate to the patient's needs.

6. E Give a presentation based on the patients seen

There will be nothing in the literature. So, the first thing is to review the results which this technique has achieved. Presentation of these results and comparison with those achieved by other units using other techniques has no scientific validity, but is useful because it will show what questions need to answered by a properly set-up prospective trial.

7. D Perform a randomised controlled trial (RCT)

This issue could be resolved by choosing the cheapest implant, but it would be much better if a check was made first on whether there was any difference in outcome attributable to the implant, not the surgeon or any other confounding factor. Large numbers will be needed to achieve study validity so a multi-centre trial may need to be organised.

8. C Perform an audit

This is a clear example of where an audit is needed. First find out what exactly is your infection rate, and how this compares with other units. Then, if your rate is high, try an intervention (such as putting hand gel at the bedside) and review to see if your rate has now fallen. This process of identifying a problem, implementing a solution and then checking the results is called closing the audit loop.

9. A There was a breach of duty of care

It falls below an acceptable standard of care for a swab to have been left in after surgery, causing a 'breach of care'. This is the first 'hurdle' that has to be crossed by the plaintiff if medical negligence is to be proven. We do not know from this scenario whether the other preconditions of negligence have been met.

10. C The patient has come to harm, but so far no more than this can be said

The patient has come to harm as a result of the penicillin being given. It is not yet proven that there is a breach of care (perhaps the patient did not admit to being allergic to penicillin despite being asked). Nor is it clear that the patient has 'consequences' as a result of this harm, e.g. he has had to take time off school. 'Coming to harm' is a second condition for medical negligence which needs to be proven in British law for a case to succeed.

11. D There is no legal issue here

Here, there are consequences of the surgery: the patient is going to be left with a permanent foot drop. 'Consequences' is the third condition required if medical negligence is to be proved, but the scenario does not tell us whether the other conditions ('breach of care' and 'harm') have occurred, as we do not know why the patient has a foot drop. It is likely that the sciatic nerve was damaged at surgery, but other possibilities need to be excluded.

12. B Arrange a meeting and explain what has happened

You know the facts. This appears to have been an 'act of God'. All reasonable precautions were taken, and there is no need for an apology. Your figures for infection are in the middle of the national average. However, a meeting is needed to explain the situation to the patient and wife. This should help everyone come to terms with what has happened. If the patient's wife continues to blame the service for events, you should not say 'I am sorry that you feel this way' (option H). That is not an apology, it is a rather irritating way of saying that you disagree with their view.

13. C Apologise first even before you have the facts

This patient should not have fallen out of bed. It is important to apologise for this mistake. An apology does not lay you open to litigation. The evidence is that frequently a full and heartfelt apology satisfies the patient and prevents litigation. It would be good to explain that measures are to be taken to ensure that this does not happen again, and to bring the subject up at the next clinical governance meeting to remind everyone to check cot sides all the time.

14. G Promise to learn from what has happened

You will meet with the patient and apologise because an error has been made. Now ensure that the patient feels happier about things and, if possible, litigation is avoided. This is to explain that every possible measure is to be taken to ensure this 'never happens again'. One way in which this can be done is to hold a clinical governance meeting to explore what happened in a 'no blame' environment and explore what extra measures could be introduced to prevent a recurrence.

Chapter 43

Clinical microbiology

Questions

Theme: Pathogen likely to be isolated

Options for Questions 1–3:

A β-haemolytic *Streptococcus*
B *Candida albicans*
C *Clostridium welchii*
D *Escherichia coli*
E *Staphylococcus aureus*
F *Staphylococcus epidermidis*
G *Streptococcus pyogenes*

For each of the following cases, select the single most likely organism to be cultured. Each option may be used once, more than once or not at all.

1. A 70-year-old woman has a routine hip replacement. All goes well initially but over the next few months, she complains of increasing pain in the hip. Her C-reactive protein is raised at 50 mg/L and she is apyrexial. A needle aspiration of the hip joint is performed.

2. A 70-year-old man has a repair of a recurrent inguinal hernia. Within 48 hours the wound is red and swollen and the patient is pyrexial. Blood cultures are sent for.

3. A 70-year-old woman has been receiving chemotherapy for carcinoma of the breast. She is put on a broad spectrum antibiotics for a chest infection which takes 10 days to clear. On day 8, while she is still on antibiotics, she complains of a red and sore mouth with white plaques on the tongue and cheeks. A swab is taken from one of these plaques.

Theme: Appropriate treatment of infections

Options for Questions 4–6:

A Amoxicillin	F Nitrofurantoin
B Cefuroxime	G Oral penicillin
C Clotrimoxazole	H Penicillin V
D Flucloxacillin	I Vancomycin
E Gentamycin	

For each of the following cases, select the single most appropriate therapy. Each option may be used once, more than once or not at all.

4. A 65-year-old man is scheduled for a total hip replacement which needs to be covered by a prophylactic antibiotic.

5. A 70-year-old woman has had a mastectomy develops a purulent discharge from the wound. Two other patients on the ward have also developed wound infections.

6. An 18-year-old man has cut his hand on a tin that he was opening. The wound has been closed, but cellulitis is spreading in pink streaks up the arm from the wound.

Theme: Preventing cross-infection

Options for Questions 7–9:

A Autoclaving	E Universal precautions or standard
B Disposable instruments	precautions (health care)
C Peritoneal washout	F Washing instruments before
D Skin cleaning with povidone	autoclaving
iodine	

For each of the following cases, select the single most appropriate technique for the prevention of cross-infection. Each option may be used once, more than once or not at all.

7. A 70-year-old man undergoes an emergency Hartmann's resection for perforated diverticulitis with faecal peritonitis.

8. A 25-year-old healthy man sustains a needle stick injury while clearing up a trolley following a lumbar puncture. The patient on whom the lumbar puncture was performed is known to be hepatitis B-positive.

9. A 20-year-old man attends the emergency department with a laceration to his forehead involving the eyebrow. This needs to be sutured.

Theme: Side effects of antibiotics

Options for Questions 10–11:

A	Aplastic anaemia	D	Staining of teeth
B	Hearing loss	E	Skin rash
C	Pseudo-membranous colitis		

For each of the following cases, select the single most likely side-effect. Each option may be used once, more than once or not at all.

10. An 80-year-old woman is being treated with gentamycin for a *Pseudomonas* infection of a leg ulcer. Routine blood results show a raised blood level of the antibiotic.

11. A 5-year-old girl with tonsillitis is given tetracycline in case there is a bacterial component to the infection.

Theme: Management in accidental contamination

Options for Questions 12–14:

A	Conference of all ward staff immediately	E	Post exposure prophylaxis and cessation of treatment, if subsequently risk is found to be low
B	Incise the wound at point of injury to make it bleed freely		
C	Post exposure prophylaxis treatment started immediately	F	Wash the area and report the incident
D	Suck the wound followed by post exposure prophylaxis		

For each of the following cases, select the single most appropriate management option. Each option may be used once, more than once or not at all.

12. A 30-year-old woman, a ward auxilliary receives a needle stick injury from a discarded needle while emptying a rubbish bag in the main treatment room. There are no known 'high risk' patients on the ward.

13. A 22-year-old student nurse is clearing away a trolley just used to take a bone marrow sample from a patient who is known to be HIV-positive. She receives a needle stick injury but is worried it was her fault and does not report it for 4 hours.

14. A 25-year-old nurse is taking down an intravenous infusion from a patient, who is not known to be carrying HIV, or any form of hepatitis, but is a patient with a potentially high-risk lifestyle. She receives a deep needle stick injury from the intravenous cannula, which is covered in the patient's blood. There is no information in the notes to suggest that the patient has an HIV infection, and there is nothing to suggest that they are high-risk.

Answers

1. F *Staphylococcus epidermidis*

Total joint replacements are performed under super-sterile conditions, but it is impossible to remove all skin commensals from the operating field. The one most likely to contaminate the wound and infect the implant is *Staphylococcus epidermidis*, which normally is not a pathogen.

2. E *Staphylococcus aureus*

Staphylococcus aureus is the organism most likely to infect a wound in hospital. In some cases, this will be methicillin-resistant *Staphylococcus aureus* (MRSA) an organism of low virulence but high infectivity which spreads from patient-to-patient in hospitals and nursing homes where patients have low resistance to infection.

3. B *Candida albicans*

Antibiotic treatment may destroy the body's natural bacterial flora and leave the patient open to attack by fungi such a thrush (oral candidiasis). The mucous membranes will be red and sore with plaques of white material.

4. B Cefuroxime

When giving prophylactic antibiotics it is important to cover the most likely infecting organism as well as less likely culprits. Therefore, a broad-spectrum antibiotic such as cefuroxime may be better, rather than a narrow spectrum one such as flucloxacillin which will cover *Staphylococcus* (the most likely infective organism) but may not be of value against gram-negative organisms.

5. I Vancomycin

A hospital-acquired infection is likely to be resistant to first line antibiotics and so an antibiotic such as vancomycin needs to be considered, as it is more likely to be effective. The sensitivity of the organism will need to be checked by taking cultures, preferably when the patient is not on any antibiotic.

6. G Oral penicillin

The organism is likely to be *Streptococcus pyogenes* which is very sensitive to penicillin. It would be quite reasonable to give the penicillin orally.

7. C Peritoneal washout

The surgeon would be working in a field contaminated with *Escherichia coli*. Washing out the peritoneal cavity with several litres of warm normal saline will reduce the contamination load, and give the body a better chance of combating the effects of faecal peritonitis and further effects of sepsis.

8. E Universal precautions or standard precautions (health care)

Universal precautions or standard precautions (healthcare) consist of a system of behaviour geared towards preventing staff and patients from being cross infected. They are valuable for avoiding needle stick injuries, which are a potent cause of hepatitis infection.

9. B Disposable instruments

Prions are not reliably destroyed by conventional sterilisation techniques such as autoclaving or ionising radiation. The only way to be certain of not transmitting prions between surgical cases is to have disposable instruments.

10. B Hearing loss

Gentamycin has a very narrow therapeutic range: too low a concentration and it is ineffective, too high and it causes deafness. It is excreted by the kidneys and so the dose needs to be very carefully titrated in patients with renal insufficiency.

11. D Staining of teeth

Tetracycline is taken up by growing bone and teeth, and can be used in histological studies of both. However, in children it has the side-effect of staining teeth yellow and so should be avoided.

12. F Wash the area and report the incident

Any contamination from a patient should be treated with copious washing with soap and water. There is no place for sucking the wound or vigorous scrubbing (B). The guidelines for post exposure prophylaxis (PEP) should then help to decide the chances of contamination containing HIV and the chance of this being transmitted. If there is no broken skin and mucous membranes are not involved then the risk is so low that the complication risk of PEP outweigh the benefits. Again if the source of contamination is a low risk patient, then again PEP should not be given as the risks outweigh the benefits. It will be valuable to have a clinical governance meeting on this case and use the problems raised to heighten awareness. The staff member will need support and counselling.

13. E Post exposure prophylaxis and cessation of treatment, if subsequently risk is found to be low

This is a high risk injury (penetrating injury from a positive patient). Therefore, PEP should be given, starting as soon as possible. PEP is thought to be effective if given within 72 hours of exposure, so this patient is within the time limits, but will require counselling.

14. E Post exposure prophylaxis and cessation of treatment, if subsequently risk is found to be low

The risk here is uncertain but might be 'high' risk as the patient comes from a high-risk group (intravenous drug user, homosexual contact, those living in parts of the world where HIV is common). Therefore, consent should be obtained from the patient to test for HIV. However, post exposure prophylaxis should be started right away. If the HIV test result on the patient comes back negative then PEP can be stopped.

Chapter 44

Emergency medicine and trauma management

Questions

Theme: Pathophysiology of trauma

Options for Questions 1–2:

A	Acute respiratory distress syndrome	F	Class III hypovolaemic shock
B	Anaphylactic shock	G	Class IV hypovolaemic shock
C	Cardiogenic shock	H	Fat embolism syndrome
D	Class I hypovolaemic shock	I	Neurogenic shock
E	Class II hypovolaemic shock	J	Septic shock
		K	Tension pneumothorax

For each of the following cases, select the single most appropriate diagnosis. Each option may be used once, more than once or not at all.

1. A 22-year-old man presents with multiple injuries following a fall from his motorcycle at high speed. Injuries identified include a significant head injury, splenic rupture and an open right tibial diaphyseal fracture. He undergoes urgent splenectomy, with wound debridement and intramedullary nailing of his tibial fracture. He returns to the intensive therapy unit intubated and ventilated on inotropic support. On day 2 postoperatively his oxygen and ventilator requirements increase and chest radiographs reveal diffuse fluffy pulmonary infiltrates with a $PaO_2/FiO_2 < 200$ mmHg.

2. A 74-year-old man presents with a sudden onset of abdominal pain radiating to the flanks. In the emergency department, he has a palpable abdominal mass, a tachycardia of 125 beats per minute, a blood pressure of 80/40 mmHg, a urine output of less than 5 mL/h, a respiratory rate of 35 breaths per minute, and is confused.

Theme: Trunk and neurological trauma

Options for Questions 3–6:

A	Anterior cord syndrome	F	Intracerebral haemorrhage
B	Brown-Séquard syndrome	G	Pneumothorax
C	Central cord syndrome	H	Subarachnoid haemorrhage
D	Cardiac tamponade	I	Subdural haemorrhage
E	Extradural haemorrhage	J	Tension pneumothorax

For each of the following cases, select the single most appropriate diagnosis. Each option may be used once, more than once or not at all.

3. A 48-year-old man with a background of alcohol excess presents following a fall whilst intoxicated. On examination, he is found to have substantial abrasions around the right side of his head, but with no other injuries found and is lucid with a Glasgow Coma Score of 14 (eye opening 4, verbal response 4, motor response 6). Following 2 hours in the emergency department, his score falls with an associated bradycardia and hypertension, and is found to have a fixed and dilated pupil on the right-hand side.

4. A 32-year-old woman presents complaining of thoracic pain following a fall from a horse whilst out riding. On examination, she is tender in the region of T6–T8 with evidence of swelling and bruising in this region. Imaging reveals compression fractures of T6 and T7 with impingement of the fragments on the vertebral canal. On detailed neurological assessment, she is found to have loss of power below the level of the fracture, with an associated loss of power and temperature sensation. Proprioception and touch remain intact.

5. A 24-year-old man presents following a penetrating wound to his anterior chest wall following an altercation. On examination, he is found to have 2 cm penetrating wound on the anterior chest wall in the region of the 5th intercostal space mid-clavicular line. He has tachycardia with a pulse of 132 beats per minute, a blood pressure of 76/42 mmHg, with a raised jugular venous pressure and muffled heart sounds.

6. A 28-year-old woman presenting following a fall from a height of approximately 30 ft. On primary surgery she is found to have high oxygen requirements and cardiovascular instability with a raised jugular venous pressure, tracheal deviation to the right and diminished breath sounds on the left hand side of the chest. Radiological findings include multiple left sided rib fractures, a pelvic fracture, an open long bone fracture and a significant head injury.

Theme: Orthopaedic trauma

Options for Questions 7–9:

A	Cannulated screw fixation	H	Total hip replacement
B	Dynamic hip screw fixation	I	Traction
C	External fixation	J	Wound debridement and washout
D	Hip hemi-arthroplasty	K	Wound debridement and washout
E	Intramedullary fixation		with fracture fixation
F	Nonoperative treatment	L	Wound debridement, washout
G	Open reduction internal fixation		and closure with fracture fixation

For each of the following cases, select the single most appropriate management. Each option may be used once, more than once or not at all.

7. A 31-year-old man presents with an open fracture of his right tibia following a direct blow from a horse to his right leg. On examination, there is 5 cm wound over the anteromedial aspect of his right leg with evidence of contamination. No distal neurovascular deficit is found.

8. A 48-year-old woman presents following a simple twisting injury to her left ankle. She has no past medical history of note and it is an isolated injury. On examination, it is a closed injury and she is neurovascularly intact. Anteroposterior and lateral radiographs of the left ankle reveal an undisplaced lateral malleolus fracture at the level of the syndesmosis, with no disruption of the ankle mortice.

9. A 78-year-old woman presents following a simple mechanical fall whilst out doing her shopping and is complaining of right sided hip pain and an inability to weight bear. She has a past medical history of osteoarthritis, hypertension, hypothyroidism and hyperlipidaemia. It is an isolated injury. On examination, her right lower limb is shortened and externally rotated. Radiographs demonstrate evidence of a right intertrochanteric neck of femur fracture with moderate to severe arthritic changes in the ipsilateral hip.

Answers

1. A Acute respiratory distress syndrome

Acute respiratory distress syndrome is the acute onset of severe refractory hypoxaemia following either direct or indirect injury to the lungs in the absence of cardiac failure. Two phases of injury include an acute inflammatory exudative phase (complement activation), followed by abnormalities in lung mechanics leading to decreased lung compliance. Potential causes include:

- Direct lung contusion, fat embolus, aspiration, inhalation injury, near drowning
- Indirect trauma, sepsis, burns, massive blood transfusion, pancreatitis, cardiac bypass

Defined criteria for diagnosis include:

- Identified precipitating factor
- Acute onset of symptoms
- Refractory hypoxaemia
  - $PaO_2/FiO_2 < 200$ mmHg
  - $PaO_2/FiO_2 < 300$ mmHg = acute lung injury
- Absence of cardiac failure
  - Pulmonary artery wedge pressure <18 mmHg
- Bilateral diffuse 'fluffy' pulmonary infiltrates on chest radiograph

Management is supportive including ventilation with high positive end-expiratory pressure and steroids, with treatment of the underlying cause. The mortality rate is 50–60%.

2. F Class III hypovolaemic shock

Shock is an acute circulatory failure leading to inadequate tissue perfusion pressure, thus resulting in the inability to meet the metabolic requirements for aerobic cellular respiration. Types of shock include:

- Hypovolaemic
- Cardiogenic
- Neurogenic
- Septic
- Anaphylactic

For trauma patients, hypovolaemic shock is most common. Hypovolaemic shock is classified in **Table 44.1**.

Table 44.1 Classification of hypovolaemic shock				
	I	II	III	IV
Blood loss (mL)	< 750	750–1500	1500–2000	2000+
% blood volume (70 kg adult)	15	15–30	30–40	40+
Pulse rate (beats per minute)	< 100	> 100	> 120	140+
Blood pressure	↔	↔	↓	↓
Pulse pressure	↔	↓	↓	↓
Respiratory rate (breaths per minute)	14–20	20–30	30–40	> 40
Urine output (mL/h)	> 30	20–30	5–15	Anuric
Central nervous system	Restless	Anxious	Anxious and confused	Confused and lethargic
Fluid required	Crystalloid	Crystalloid and colloid	Colloid and blood	Colloid and blood

↔ Normotensive or hypertensive, i.e. the parameter may be normal or higher than expected but not lower

3. E Extradural haemorrhage

Patients who sustain significant head injuries may suffer from intracranial bleeding. This can be categorised into:

- Extracerebral (extradural, subdural, subarachnoid; **Table 44.2)**
- Intracerebral

Table 44.2 The contrasting presentations of extracerebral haemorrhages		
Type	**Cause**	**Clinical presentation**
Extradural	Bleed between skull and dura matter. Low energy trauma possible. Associated with fracture and subsequent injury to artery or dural venous sinus, e.g. middle meningeal artery injury secondary to temporal fracture	Boggy swelling, e.g. in temporal region
Concussion followed by lucid interval
Rapid decline (↓Glasgow Coma Score, bradycardia, blood pressure)
Dilated ipsilateral pupil
Contralateral hemiparesis
CT appearance is a biconvex lens
Subdural	Bleed between dura matter and arachnoid. Associated with shearing injury to bridging veins. Chronic presentation in elderly patients after minor trauma, with better prognosis	Initial injury
Rapidly worsening headache and ↓ Glasgow Coma Score
CT appearance is a crescent shape

4. A Anterior cord syndrome

Injuries to the spinal cord can be classified as shown in **Table 44.3**.

Table 44.3 Classification of spinal cord injuries		
Category	**Cause**	**Clinical presentation**
Complete cord	Complete transection of spinal cord	Total irreversible paralysis and loss of sensory distal to level
Anterior cord	Involvement of the corticospinal and spinothalamic tracts with preservation of the dorsal columns Associated with anterior spinal artery occlusion, anterior dislocations, disc herniation, vertebral compression fractures	Loss of motor function below level (corticospinal tract) Loss of pain and temperature below level (spinothalamic tract) Touch and proprioception remain intact (dorsal columns)
Posterior cord	Involvement of the dorsal columns only Hyperextension injuries, posterior vertebral fractures, posterior spinal artery occlusion	Loss of touch and proprioception with ataxia Pain, power and temperature intact below level
Central cord	Spinothalamic and corticospinal involvement Associated with trauma in young patients, elderly patients with cervical spondylosis, syringomyelia, spinal tumours	Loss of pain and temperature below level Loss of upper limb power Some preservation lower limb sensation and power Touch and proprioception remain intact (late involvement only)
Brown–Séquard	Lateral cord hemisection or mass with ipsilateral pyramidal tract and dorsal column involvement Associated with penetrating injuries, tumours affecting one side, infection, multiple sclerosis	Loss of power and proprioception below lesion on ipsilateral side Loss of pain and temperature below level on contralateral side

5. D Cardiac tamponade

Cardiac tamponade (pericardial tamponade) is a trauma emergency and occurs when there is a rapid accumulation of fluid within the fibrous pericardial sac, leading ultimately to obstructive shock. The most common cause is a penetrating injury to the chest, with the left and right ventricle frequently injured. Clinical findings include:

- Tachycardia, tachypnoea, declining Glasgow Coma Score
- Beck's triad: hypotension (↓ stroke volume), raised jugular venous pressure (impaired venous return), muffled heart sounds (blood in pericardial sac)
- Pulsus paradoxus: ≥10 mmHg in blood pressure on inspiration
- Kussmaul's sign: raised jugular venous pressure on inspiration
- ECG: small amplitude QRS complexes, ST segment change
- ECHO: small or collapsed ventricle, distended pericardium

Without urgent treatment with pericardiocentesis, pulseless electrical activity arrest will result.

6. J Tension pneumothorax

A pneumothorax occurs when there is air within the pleural cavity. A tension pneumothorax occurs when there is a 'one way valve' at the site of air entry into the pleural cavity, where air is entering the pleural cavity on inspiration (valve open), but with no expulsion of air on expiration (valve closed).

Clinical findings include:

- Tachycardia, raised jugular venous pressure, hypotension, tachypnoea, hypoxia,
- Ipsilateral signs: diminished breath sounds, hyper-resonance, expanded, decreased movement
- Chest X-ray: lung collapse, trachea deviated away from side of injury

Without urgent needle decompression, pulseless electrical activity arrest will result. Decompression involves insertion of a large bore cannula in the second intercostal space (mid-clavicular line) on the affected side, followed by chest drain insertion.

7. K Wound debridement and washout with fracture fixation

The Gustilo–Anderson classification of open fractures is:

- I: wound < 1 cm, clean, minimal soft tissue damage, no periosteal stripping
- II: wound > 1 cm, moderate soft tissue damage, no periosteal stripping
- IIIA: extensive soft tissue damage, periosteal stripping, but adequate coverage no flap needed
- IIIB: extensive soft tissue damage, periosteal stripping, inadequate coverage and flap needed, massive contamination
- IIIC: open fracture associated with arterial injury requiring repair

Irrespective of the size of the wound or soft tissue damage, some injuries are classified as a grade III, e.g. high-energy, segmental fracture, traumatic amputation, heavy contamination (e.g. farm injuries, gunshot wounds).

8. F Nonoperative treatment

The ankle joint is a hinge type mortice joint with an articulation between the body of the talus and the distal aspects of the tibia (tibial plafond and medial malleolus) and fibula (lateral malleolus). Injuries commonly occur following a twisting mechanism. Integrity of the skin may be compromised and urgent reduction should be carried out if found. Assessment of neurovascular status is essential.

Classification of ankle fractures is with the AO–Weber classification using anteroposterior and lateral radiographs of the ankle joint. The classification is:

- Weber A: Horizontal avulsion fracture of lateral malleolus below the level of the syndesmosis

- Weber B: Fracture of the lateral malleolus at the level of the syndesmosis
- Weber C: Fracture of the lateral malleolus above the level of the syndesmosis

Isolated Weber A fractures are stable injuries and can be treated nonoperatively. Isolated stable Weber B fractures, with no evidence of medial ligament disruption (undisplaced ankle mortice on radiographs), can be treated nonoperatively. Unstable Weber B and Weber C fractures or best treated with open reduction and internal fixation.

9. B Dynamic hip screw fixation

A proximal femoral fracture frequently occurs as the result of a low energy fall. In elderly osteoporotic women, the mean age at the time of injury is approximately 80 years and almost a third of patients die within the first year following fracture. Fractures of the hip can be classified according to disruption of the capsular blood supply to the femoral head:

- Intracapsular or subcapital
- Extracapsular
  - Intertrochanteric
  - Subtrochanteric

Intracapsular neck of femur fractures are commonly classified according to the Garden classification:

- Garden I: incomplete or valgus impacted fracture
- Garden II: complete undisplaced fracture
- Garden III: complete fracture with partial displacement but contact between fracture fragments
- Garden IV: complete fracture with total displacement

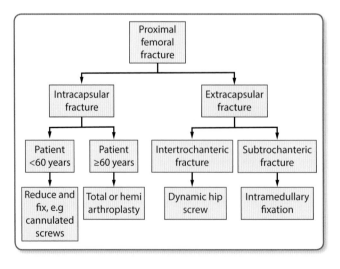

Figure 44.1 Management of proximal femoral fractures.

Treatment of proximal femoral fractures is described in **Figure 44.1**. Undisplaced intracapsular hip fractures are routinely managed with fixation. Consideration of co-morbidities including osteoporosis and alcohol excess in patients less than 60 years of age with displaced intracapsular hip fractures is needed as some may be better managed with a hip arthroplasty.

Chapter 45

Principles of surgical oncology

Questions

Theme: Aetiology of malignant tumours

Options for Questions 1–3:

- A Chemical carcinogens
- B Genetic inheritance
- C Infections
- D Metaplasia
- E Physical carcinogens

For each of the following situations, select the single most likely aetiology. Each option may be used once, more than once or not at all.

1. A 58-year-old man suffered from gastro-oesophageal reflux disease (GORD) with heartburn, acid regurgitation and repeated attacks of chest infection for many years. He has been on regular upper gastrointestinal endoscopic surveillance (OGD) and medical treatment. Of late he has been having some dysphagia with food sticking in the lower retro-sternal region.

2. A 55-year-old man has been referred to the one-stop haematuria clinic with periodic, profuse and painless haematuria for the past 2 months. On examination, there are no physical findings except for slight anaemia.

3. A 50-year-old man complains of anorexia, weight loss, upper abdominal pain and occasional vomiting. On oesophagogastroduodenoscopy he has a fungating mass in the pylorus from which biopsies have been taken.

Theme: Pathological types of malignant tumours

Options for Questions 4–6:

- A Adenocarcinoma
- B Basal cell carcinoma
- C Malignant melanoma
- D Osteosarcoma
- E Soft tissue sarcoma
- F Squamous cell carcinoma
- G Teratoma
- H Transitional cell carcinoma

For each of the following situations, select the single most likely pathological diagnosis. Each option may be used once, more than once or not at all.

4. A 35-year-old woman complains of a mole over her left shoulder region. She noticed that recently it has become itchy and has started bleeding. She would like it removed because of blood-staining of her clothes.

5. A 48-year-old man complains of colicky left-sided abdominal pain associated with intermittent constipation of 6 weeks' duration. He started taking laxatives for a satisfactory bowel action without much benefit. A CT colonography showed an 'apple core deformity' in the splenic flexure. This was followed by a colonoscopy which showed an ulcerative tumour in the upper descending colon.

6. A 56-year-old man complains of intermittent, profuse, progressive, painless, haematuria for the last 4 weeks. He has no other symptoms except for shortness of breath which is due to a haemoglobin of 80 g/L. He was seen in the one-stop haematuria clinic where on flexible cystoscopy he was found to have a papilliferous growth in the left side of the bladder.

Theme: Tumour markers

Options for Questions 7–9:

A   α-Fetoprotein
B   β-Human chorionic
   gonadotrophin
C   Calcitonin

D   Cancer antigen 125
E   Carcinoembryonic antigen
F   Erythropoietin
G   Prostate specific antigen

For each of the following situations, select the single most suitable tumour marker. Each option may be used once, more than once or not at all.

7. A 25-year-old man complains of a hard lump in his right testicle, which he found as he felt a sense of heaviness in his scrotum. Ultrasound of the testis showed a solid lump and in the abdomen a solid firm mass was felt in the umbilical region.

8. A 62-year-old man complains of increasing constipation. A barium enema showed a shouldered deformity in his upper descending colon. Colonoscopic biopsy showed a well-differentiated adenocarcinoma and the liver was free of secondaries. He is due to undergo a radical left hemicolectomy.

9. A 42-year-old woman underwent a total thyroidectomy for a carcinoma which was a part of MEN2 syndrome. Histology showed stromal amyloid with areas of focal calcification. It also contained mucin, melanin and polypeptide hormones detected by immunohistochemistry. Metastatic cervical lymph nodes also contained amyloid.

Theme: Systemic effects of cancer

Options for Questions 10–12:

A   Amyloidosis
B   Cachexia
C   Haematologic syndromes (anaemia, eryhthrocytosis)
D   Hypercoagulable state (venous thrombosis)

E   Neurologic and neuromuscular syndromes
F   Paraneoplastic syndromes
G   Pyrexia

For each of the following situations, select the single most suitable type of systemic effect. Each option may be used once, more than once or not at all.

10. A 51-year old man complains of pain and swelling of his entire right lower limb for a couple of weeks. He has also had anorexia and epigastric pain for about a month. On examination, he has a swollen right lower limb with a mass in the epigastrium.

11. A 58-year-old man complains of gradual weight loss over 4 months. He has anorexia with epigastric dull ache radiating to the back. He gets some relief from his pain by leaning forwards whilst sitting up in bed. On examination, there is nothing to find except evidence of weight loss in the form of ill-fitting loose clothes.

12. A 50-year-old man, a heavy smoker of many years, complains of cough with streaks of blood in his sputum for 4 months. He also complains of pain in the right side of his chest. A chest X-ray shows a large shadow in the mid-zone of his right lung. His family has noticed that he has become obese, particularly swollen facial features. His doctor found that recently he has become a type 2 diabetic.

Theme: Palliation in malignant disease

Options for Questions 13–15:

A   Adjuvant therapy
B   Chemotherapy
C   Drugs and medical treatment
D   Interventional radiology

E   Radiotherapy
F   Stenting
G   Surgery

For each of the following situations, select the single most suitable palliative procedure. Each option may be used once, more than once or not at all.

13. A 75-year-old man has had a channel transurethral resection of the prostate for cancer prostate with bladder outflow obstruction. At the time of diagnosis he was found to have sclerotic bone secondaries in his lumbar vertebrae and pelvis. He has disabling backache. His prostate-specific antigen is raised.

14. A 60-year-old woman presents with quite severe features of carcinoid syndrome in the form of flushing, explosive watery diarrhoea, colicky abdominal pain and episodic sudden attacks of shortness of breath. She has a much raised urinary

5-hydroxyindoleacetic acid and liver ultrasound shows multiple solid tumours. Almost 6 years ago she underwent a right hemicolectomy for an ileal carcinoid tumour.

15. An 80-year-old man complains of intense pruritus. His family noticed that he is extremely icteric and his urine very dark yellow. On abdominal examination, he has a smooth, globular mass in the right hypochondrium and an enlarged liver.

Theme: Cancer screening

Options for Questions 16–18:

A	Barium enema	E	Oesophagogastroduodenoscpy
B	Colonoscopy	F	Smear test
C	Faecal occult blood testing	G	Tumour markers
D	Genetic screening		

For each of the following situations, select the single most suitable cancer screening modality. Each option may be used once, more than once or not at all.

16. A 30-year-old woman, who is completely asymptomatic has an elder brother who underwent an extended right hemicolectomy for Dukes stage B transverse colon carcinoma. Their father died from liver secondaries at the age of 68 years after an anterior resection at the age of 65 years.

17. A 35-year-old woman is concerned about her family history of breast cancer. Her mother died of secondaries from breast cancer at the age of 62 years. She has a sister who had breast cancer diagnosed and treated at the age of 42 years.

18. A 50-year-old woman has suffered from ulcerative colitis for 10 years during which time she has been on medical treatment with mesalazine, intermittent steroids and azathioprine. At present she has two to three bowel actions a day with some blood and mucus, a clinical situation which is no different over the last year or so.

Answers

1. D Metaplasia

Patients with long-standing GORD are susceptible to developing metaplastic changes in the lower one-third of the oesophagus. Metaplasia is an adaptive response to chronic persistent injury. In this case, it is the reflux of acid from the stomach into the lower oesophagus due to the loss of competence of the lower oesophageal sphincter (LOS). As a result, the squamous epithelium of the oesophagus is replaced by gastric columnar epithelium: this change is referred to as Barrett's oesophagus. The squamo-columnar junction moves up and strictures can occur at the new squamo-columnar junction. There is a 25 times greater chance of developing adenocarcinoma following this metaplastic change. Barrett's oesophagus may be diagnosed if there is any intestinal metaplasia in the lower oesophagus although previously it used to be diagnosed if there was at least 3 cm of columnar epithelium. The risk of cancer increases with the increased length of the abnormal mucosa.

2. A Chemical carcinogens

This patient has urinary bladder cancer unless otherwise proven. The aetiology is a chemical carcinogen, aromatic amines and azo dyes. Workers in the aniline dye, leather, rubber, paint and organic chemical industries are highly susceptible to urinary bladder cancer. Polycyclic hydrocarbons from cigarette smoke are an important risk factor of urinary bladder carcinoma as is β-naphthylamine to which dye industry workers are exposed. The aromatic amines and azo dyes are metabolised in the liver to form hydroxylamino derivative; these are then detoxified by conjugation with glucuronic acid. In the bladder, hydrolysis of glucuronide releases hydroxylamine causing DNA damage to the urothelial cell and cancer.

3. D Infections

This patient has a carcinoma of the stomach, the cause of which in the vast majority is *Helicobacter pylori* infection. In gastric cancer patients, there is a high incidence of *H. pylori* infection found serologically many years before the onset of the disease. Patients who are seropositive for *H. pylori* are three times more likely to develop the condition. The organism affects almost 70% of the world's population. In some parts of the world almost 9 out of 10 in the population are infected. It is thought to cause atrophic gastritis, peptic ulceration, mucosa-associated lymphoid tissue tumours (MALTomas) and cancer. The stomach is the most common site of extra-nodal lymphoma. Most gastric lymphomas are B-cell tumours and have been known to regress after eradication of *H. pylori* infection.

4. C Malignant melanoma

This patient's history and the description of the lesion are typical of a malignant melanoma, which is a neoplasm arising from the melanocytes. Exposure to sun and persistent sunburn is associated with this condition; therefore, ultra-violet radiation is the responsible physical carcinogen. Malignant melanoma occurs mostly in white-skinned people. The skin of darker races is protected from the harmful effects of ultraviolet radiation by the greater amount of melanin.

The changes in the skin lesion that makes one suspect transformation into malignant melanoma can be summarised as ABCDE: geometrical **A**symmetry in two axes, irregular **B**order, lesion showing at least two different **C**olours, maximum **D**iameter > 6 mm and **E**levation of lesion. The types of malignant melanoma are:

*   Superficial spreading (70%)
*   Nodular melanoma (15%)
*   Lentigo maligna melanoma (5–10%)
*   Acral lentiginous melanoma (2–8% in white-skinned, more common in the dark-skinned)

5. A Adenocarcinoma

This is an adenocarcinoma of the colon. Most of these cancers arise in adenomatous polyps. Mutation in the APC (adenomatous polyposis coli) gene plays an important role in the development of most colorectal cancers. The risk factors in the development of adenocarcinoma of the large bowel are: genetic (HNPCC – hereditary non-polyposisis colic cancer), ulcerative colitis and Crohn's disease, consumption of red meat and animal fat and low residue diet. The degree of differentiation influences the prognosis with well-differentiated tumours carrying a better prognosis.

Macroscopically the tumours are ulcerative that present with bleeding and mucoid discharge, polypoid that may cause intussusception, annular and tubular that present with obstructive symptoms such as abdominal pain, constipation and as an emergency with intestinal obstruction. These tumours spread by direct extension and through lymphatics to regional lymph nodes and by the blood stream to the liver and lungs; rarely to bones and brain.

6. H Transitional cell carcinoma

This patient has a transitional cell carcinoma (TCC) which is the most common urothelial tumour. The vast majority of the cancers that arise from the renal pelvis down to the terminal urethra are TCC. Rarely, in the bladder, a squamous carcinoma may arise from long-standing irritation from a vesical calculus or Bilharzial infestation. Adenocarcinoma of the bladder may be a direct extension from a colorectal carcinoma.

The patient's cancer should be staged with a CT scan, intravenous urogram (IVU) (**Figure 45.1**), MRI and chest X-ray, EUA and bimanual examination, and then discussed in a MDT meeting to institute the most appropriate treatment. This may be surgery (endoscopic or open), radiotherapy or a combination of both.

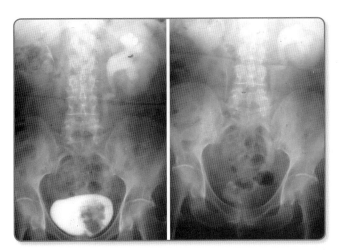

Figure 45.1 IVU showing carcinoma of left side of the bladder obstructing the left ureter.

7. A α-Fetoprotein

This young man has a solid mass in his testicle which is a testicular tumour. In view of his age, this is most likely a teratoma (non-seminomatous germ cell tumour). The tumour marker is α-fetoprotein (AFP). Blood should be sent to estimate this as soon as the diagnosis is suspected. The abdominal mass is a pre- and para-aortic group of lymph node secondaries. With such a clinical picture elevation of AFP is almost certain. The tumour marker level also helps in the staging of the tumour. T1M staging indicates that there are no secondaries but elevated marker level. Having done the tumour marker level preoperatively, it should be repeated shortly after orchidectomy. There is a protocol for follow-up at which this is repeated. If levels are elevated, secondaries should be sought on chest X-ray and CT of the abdomen and liver.

8. E Carcinoembryonic antigen

Carcinoembryonic antigen is the tumour marker that should be routinely carried out in colorectal carcinoma. It should be done as a baseline prior to surgery, in this radical left hemicolectomy. Thereafter, it is repeated at every follow-up. Elevated levels should alert one to the possibility of secondaries particularly in the liver or a recurrence or a metachronous carcinoma. Investigations should be carried out to look for recurrence and appropriate management instituted.

Carcinoembryonic antigen is also a tumour marker in medullary carcinoma of thyroid and mucinous adenocarcinoma of pancreas.

9. C Calcitonin

The histology of this patient's thyroid is typical of medullary carcinoma of the thyroid (MCT). Moreover, in this patient the MCT is part of MEN syndrome. The tumour marker is calcitonin. The tumour arises from the parafollicular C cells of the thyroid and produces calcitonin. This should be used prior to the patient's operation, as a baseline, and then to monitor the patient during follow-up.

Another use of calcitonin as a tumour marker in MCT is to diagnose the condition in family members. The blood test should be offered as a screening tool for the patient's first degree family members: children and siblings.

A tumour marker is a circulating biochemical substance that can be detected in the cells or in the body fluids indicative of a malignant neoplasm. A marker is most useful when it is specific, sensitive and proportional to the tumour load (**Table 45.1**).

Table 45.1 Use of tumour markers	
Type of tumour	**Use(s) of tumour marker**
Gastrointestinal	• Carcinoembryonic antigen in colorectal cancer
Hepatobiliary	• α-fetoprotein in hepatoma
Genitourinary	• Erythropoietin in Wilms' tumour • Prostate-specific antigen in prostate cancer In testicular tumours: • β-human chorionic gonadotropin • α-fetoprotein
Endocrine	• Calcitonin in medullary thyroid carcinoma • Other endocrine tumours
Gynaecology	• Ca-125 in ovarian cancer

10. D Hypercoagulable state

Armand Trousseau, a French Physician, described venous thromboembolism and thrombophlebitis in himself as he died from pancreatic cancer, although he thought he had gastric cancer. This patient has the features of a gastric cancer – anorexia, upper abdominal pain and epigastric mass. Venous thrombosis in the leg in gastric cancer is therefore referred to as Trousseau's sign. In pancreatic cancer, there is a 50 times greater incidence of venous thromboembolism. Cancers of the breast, prostate, ovary and gastrointestinal tract are particularly susceptible to this complication. In pancreatic cancer and in gastric mucinous adenocarcinoma a hypercoagulable state exists which commonly leads to venous thromboembolism in the deep veins of the leg, often a cause of death from pulmonary embolism.

11. B Cachexia

This patient has weight loss, anorexia and backache relieved by bending forward. This is very suggestive of a carcinoma of the body of the pancreas; by bending forward the patient tries to relieve pressure on the coeliac plexus by the growth. Cachexia is a classical presentation of pancreatic cancer probably brought on by their decreased caloric intake from anorexia and abnormalities of taste. The diminished food intake does not always explain the significant wasting. This is thought to be due to tumour necrosis factor α and cytokines (interferons, interleukin-6) producing a wasting syndrome often described as a part of a paraneoplastic syndrome.

12. F Paraneoplastic syndromes

This patient has all the features of a carcinoma of the right lung. The clinical features noticed by his family are suggestive of Cushing's syndrome, a diagnosis strengthened by the recent onset of diabetes. Small cell lung carcinoma, also known as 'oat cell' carcinoma, accounts for about one-fifth of all bronchogenic cancers. This is a highly malignant epithelial tumour often demonstrating paraneoplastic syndromes due to the ectopic secretion of adrenocorticotropic hormone, resulting in the cushingoid appearance with hypokalaemia, hyperglycaemia, hypertension and weakness. The other feature of paraneoplastic syndrome is hypercalcaemia which can occur in the absence of skeletal metastases due to the secretion of a parathormone-like peptide from a lung or breast cancer.

13. E Radiotherapy

This patient has pain from bony secondaries from his cancer prostate which is being palliated locally by channel transurethral resection of prostate. This is also corroborated by his raised prostate-specific antigen. He should be palliated by radiotherapy to his lumbar vertebrae and pelvis. Should that not relieve his pain or there is recurrent pain in future, bilateral subcapsular orchidectomy should be considered.

14. D Interventional radiology

This woman has classical carcinoid syndrome from multiple hepatic secondaries. The diagnosis is strongly supported by a raised urinary 5-hydroxyindoleacetic acid (5-HIAA) which confirms secondaries. The enzyme serotonin elaborated from the secondaries cause very distressing symptoms. The ideal palliative treatment is interventional radiology and hepatic artery embolisation. This renders the secondaries ischaemic, thereby making them non-functional. The patient's symptoms would be much relieved with a fall in the urinary 5-HIAA.

15. F Stenting

This elderly man is extremely bothered by pruritus as a result of obstructive jaundice from a carcinoma of the head of the pancreas. The patient has conjugated hyperbilirubinaemia. Normally, the icterus does not bother the patient as much as his family members. He is not suitable for resection. The ideal palliation is endoscopic retrograde insertion of a stent into his common bile duct. Rarely, if this is not possible for technical reasons, the second option would be to do a cholecystojejunostomy and a gastrojejunostomy to prevent gastric outlet obstruction in future.

16. B Colonoscopy

This 30-year-old woman should be offered regular colonoscopic surveillance (at least annually). She belongs to a family with hereditary non-polyposis colorectal cancer. This is an autosomal dominant inherited disease accounting for 3–5% of all large bowel cancers. The clinical features of these patients are: onset at a young age, colon proximal to splenic flexure mostly affected, may have synchronous cancers and may develop extracolonic cancers – of the endometrium, ovary, stomach, and hepatobiliary tract and transitional carcinoma of the upper urinary tract.

17. D Genetic screening

This woman has a strong family history of breast cancer with two first degree relatives suffering from the condition. This risk is enhanced if the relatives had the disease at a young age or had bilateral disease. *BRCA1* (breast cancer-1) and *BRCA2* are the two high-risk genes that account for 20–50% of these cancers. *BRCA1* and *BRCA2* are tumour suppressor genes that are important in repair of DNA and regulation of mitotic phases. Mutations in these genes create the instability in cells of the breast and ovary encouraging the formation of cancer. Hence this woman should be offered genetic screening. If the patient proves to be 'gene positive' she could be given the choice of bilateral prophylactic mastectomy.

18. B Colonoscopy

As this woman has suffered from ulcerative colitis for 10 years, she has an enhanced chance of developing colorectal cancer. She should be subjected to annual colonoscopic surveillance and biopsy. Those that have high grade dysplasia should have the colon removed to prevent cancer. This risk is higher when the disease starts at a young age, when there is a very severe first attack and if the entire colon is involved. Often there may be a synchronous colon cancer when it occurs in ulcerative colitis.

Chapter 46

The abdomen

Questions

Theme: Abdominal pain

Options for Questions 1–2:

A Abdominal aortic aneurysm	**D** Chronic cholecystitis
B Carcinoma of stomach	**E** Gastro-oesophageal reflux disease
C Carcinoma of body of pancreas	

For each of the following situations, select the single most likely diagnosis. Each option may be used once, more than once or not at all.

1. A 50-year-old woman complains of epigastric pain radiating to the back associated with heartburn of 4 months' duration. The pain does not have any regular pattern and not specifically related to food. She feels occasionally nauseous and is rarely sick. She has water brash and suffers from cough although she is not a smoker. On examination, she is overweight and has signs of basal crepitus in her lungs.

2. A 55-year-old man complains of constant epigastric pain radiating to the back of 3 months' duration. The pain is constant, dull and unrelated to food. It keeps him awake at night. The only relief he obtains is by sitting up and bending forwards. During this time, he has lost 10 kg in weight. There are no physical findings except for evidence of weight loss obvious by his very loose-fitting clothes.

Theme: Abdominal masses

Options for Questions 3–4:

A	Abdominal aortic aneurysm	D	Hydronephrosis
B	Carcinoma of the caecum	E	Mucocele of the gallbladder
C	Carcinoma of head of the pancreas		

For each of the following situations, select the single most likely diagnosis. Each option may be used once, more than once or not at all.

3. An 84-year-old woman complains of intense itching all over her body of 2 months' duration. This has been associated with gradual progressive jaundice and weight loss. On examination there are scratch marks all over her body and a smooth globular non-tender mass in the right upper quadrant which moves with respiration. There is also hepatomegaly (**Figure 46.1**).

4. A 65-year-old woman complains of recent shortness of breath whilst going about her daily routine activities for the last 2 months. On examination, she looks pale with a haemoglobin of 72 g/L. Abdominal examination reveals a mass in the right iliac fossa which is mobile and non-tender (**Figure 46.2**).

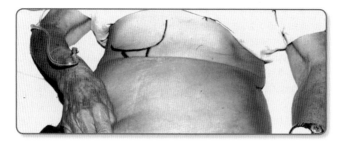

Figure 46.1 Jaundiced patient with hepatomegaly and enlarged gallbladder.

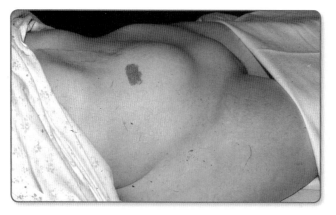

Figure 46.2 Lump in the right iliac fossa from carcinoma of caecum.

Theme: The acute abdomen

Options for Questions 5–6:

A Acute appendicitis

B Acute biliary colic

C Acute pancreatitis

D Leaking abdominal aortic aneurysm

E Ureteric colic

For each of the following situations, select the single most likely diagnosis. Each option may be used once, more than once or not at all.

5. A 70-year-old man complains of sudden onset of very severe abdominal pain radiating to the back and left side of the abdomen of 4 hours' duration. He has a distended abdomen with a blood pressure of 90/60 mmHg, pulse rate of 120 beats per minute is cold and clammy and looks pale. Abdominal examination shows a grossly distended abdomen more on the left side with tenderness and guarding.

6. A 26-year-old woman complains of severe dull pain in the right iliac fossa of 12 hours' duration. It started as a colicky pain around the umbilicus almost 24 hours ago before it moved to the right iliac fossa. She has been anorexic with nausea and vomited once. On examination she has a temperature of 100°C with tenderness, rigidity and rebound tenderness in the right iliac fossa.

Theme: Intestinal obstruction

Options for Questions 7–8:

A Gallstone ileus

B Incarcerated femoral hernia

C Large intestinal obstruction from left colonic carcinoma

D Upper small intestinal obstruction from adhesions

E Volvulus of the sigmoid colon

For each of the following situations, select the single most likely diagnosis. Each option may be used once, more than once or not at all.

7. A 78-year-old man from the geriatric medical ward has been referred with gradual abdominal distension, particularly on the left side of almost a week's duration. His last bowel movement was 5 days ago. He complains of generalised abdominal pain. On examination, he is short of breath from his distended abdomen. His blood pressure is 110/80 mmHg and pulse is 100 beats per minute. The abdomen is tympanitic; rectal examination reveals an empty ballooned rectum.

8. A 79-year-old woman has been admitted as an emergency with abdominal distension, faeculent vomiting, dull generalised abdominal pain and constipation of 4 days' duration. On examination she looks unwell with gross generalised abdominal distension, marked dehydration as evidenced by sunken eyes, dry tongue and loss of skin turgor. There are no masses palpable. A CT scan shows gas in the biliary tree with small bowel distension.

Theme: Peritonitis and abdominal abscess

Options for Questions 9–10:

A   Acute perforated appendicitis
B   Pelvic abscess
C   Pelvic inflammatory disease
D   Perforated diverticulitis
E   Subphrenic abscess

For each of the following situations, select the single most likely diagnosis. Each option may be used once, more than once or not at all.

9. A 70-year-old woman complains of sudden onset of severe lower abdominal pain spreading to the entire lower half of abdomen of 6 hours' duration. Prior to this acute episode she has been suffering from constipation for several months for which a barium enema was carried out shown in **Figure 46.3**. On examination, she has septic shock with tenderness, rigidity and rebound tenderness all over her lower abdomen.

10. A 50-year-old woman underwent a laparoscopic closure of a perforated duodenal ulcer one week ago. Immediately following the operation, she progressed satisfactorily for 4–5 days. After that she developed swinging pyrexia, complaining of pain in her right shoulder tip. She is breathless and tender in the right upper quadrant. A chest X-ray shows right pleural effusion.

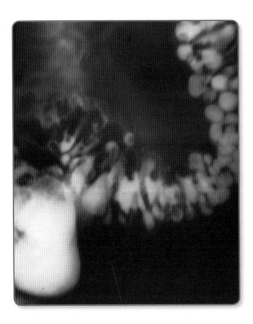

Figure 46.3 Barium enema showing severe diverticular disease of sigmoid colon.

Theme: Gastrointestinal haemorrhage

Options for Questions 11–12:

A   Aortoenteric fistula
B   Bleeding peptic ulcer
C   Leiomyoma of stomach
D   Mallory–Weiss syndrome
E   Oesophageal varices

For each of the following situations, select the single most likely diagnosis. Each option may be used once, more than once or not at all.

11. A 60-year-old man, a smoker, has been admitted as an emergency with sudden-onset severe acute haematemesis preceded by a few days of loose black stools. He has suffered on and off for years with indigestion for which he self-medicated. Recently, he took some nonsteroidal anti-inflammatory drugs for his arthritic knee. On examination he has features of hypovolaemic shock.

12. A 70-year-old man has been brought to the emergency department with sudden-onset severe acute haematemesis in the form of clots. He has hypovolaemic shock. On abdominal examination he has a well-healed mid-line scar extending from the xiphisternum to the pubic symphysis for an elective abdominal aortic aneurysm operation 6 years ago.

Theme: Hernia

Options for Questions 13–14:

A   Epigastric hernia
B   Femoral hernia
C   Incisional hernia
D   Inguinal hernia
E   Obturator hernia

For each of the following situations, select the single most likely diagnosis. Each option may be used once, more than once or not at all.

13. A 68-year-old man complains of discomfort in his lower abdomen of 8 months' duration. His discomfort dates back to the finding of a lump in his right groin which is slightly tender. On examination, he has a 3–4 cm lump at the medial end of his inguinal ligament. This lump is mobile, slightly tender, not reducible, situated below the inguinal ligament and lateral to the pubic tubercle.

14. A 65-year-old woman complains of pain in her left knee of about 6 months' duration. The pain starts in the groin and radiates down the inner side of the thigh and is made worse on coughing or any form of straining. On examination, she looks in some discomfort in her left groin and finds relief from the pain when she keeps her hip flexed, abducted and externally rotated. There is fullness under the pectineus muscle where a cough impulse can be felt.

Answers

1. E Gastro-oesophageal reflux disease

This 50-year-old woman has abdominal pain with heartburn, water brash and features of chest infection – tell-tale features of gastro-oesophageal reflux disease. Her chest infection is due to the aspiration of stomach contents from reflux. She needs an oesophagogastroduodenoscopy to assess the degree of reflux and oesophagitis and to look for any shortening of the oesophagus. A biopsy should be taken to look for dysplasia. There are various grades of oesophagitis, the most common being streaks of mucosal inflammation. Initially, she should be on medical treatment. This should be followed by regular endoscopies and a biopsy to make sure the condition is healing, and there is no metaplasia and dysplasia.

2. C Carcinoma of body of pancreas

This man has the typical symptoms of a patient with carcinoma arising from the body of the pancreas – abdominal pain that is unremitting radiating to the back due to the cancer pressing on the coeliac plexus. The pain is gnawing in nature and relieved by sitting and leaning forward which makes the enlarged pancreas fall away from the coeliac plexus of nerves. Weight loss is another prominent symptom partly brought on by anorexia. The condition usually presents late with most having metastasised at the time of presentation. 10% of patients present with migratory thrombophlebitis (Trousseau's sign). This sign may occasionally be the first clinical evidence of cancer of the body and/or tail of the pancreas. Diagnosis is confirmed by CT scan. Treatment is centred on palliation of intractable pain.

3. C Carcinoma of the head of the pancreas

This patient has typical obstructive jaundice causing her intense pruritus with scratch marks all over her body. The obstructive jaundice is the result of a carcinoma of the head of the pancreas causing obstruction to the lower end of the common bile duct. This results in a distended gallbladder. In any patient with a palpable non-tender gallbladder with obstructive jaundice, the cause of obstruction is unlikely to be gallstones because previous cholecystitis would have rendered the gall gallbladder to become thick and contracted; therefore, the underlying pathology would be something sinister such a cancer of the head of the pancreas as in this patient. This is referred to as Courvoisier's law or sign.

The diagnosis should be confirmed by an ultrasound and CT scan followed by staging. The majority are not suitable for resection. Palliation for pruritus is achieved by stenting of the common bile duct.

4. B Carcinoma of the caecum

This woman has a carcinoma of the caecum causing the mass in the right iliac fossa. She has typical symptoms of anaemia – undue shortness of breath from daily normal activities. On examination, she has a mass in the region of the caecum. Iron deficiency anaemia is a classically elective clinical presentation of caecal and right-sided colonic carcinoma. This is because of chronic bleeding. The patient would have low haemoglobin, with stools being positive for faecal occult blood. Confirmation of diagnosis is achieved by colonoscopy and biopsy. This is followed by a staging CT scan. Management is discussed in a MDT meeting followed by appropriate treatment, which would be a radical right hemicolectomy with adjuvant chemotherapy depending upon the staging outcome.

5. D Leaking abdominal aortic aneurysm

This 70-year-old man has had an acute abdominal catastrophic pain with features of hypovolaemic shock – pallor, hypotension, tachycardia and cold clammy skin. He has a distended abdomen, more marked on the left side with tenderness and rigidity. This man has a leaking abdominal aortic aneurysm. He needs immediate resuscitation with crystalloids using two wide-bore intravenous cannulae, an indwelling catheter and should be transferred to theatre for immediate surgery. Some vascular surgeons perform a CT on the way to the theatre but time should not be wasted if the diagnosis is obvious. The patient's blood pressure should not be raised to any more than 90 mmHg because this would be counter-productive.

6. A Acute appendicitis

This patient has the classical history of acute appendicitis. The pain commences around the umbilicus because the appendix is a structure of midgut origin. It later settles in the right iliac fossa when the parietal peritoneum becomes inflamed with all the typical physical findings of peritonitis – tenderness, rigidity and rebound tenderness, the latter elicited by pain on coughing or moving. About 50% of patients present with a typical history; atypical presentation is more common in the extremes of age. The position of the appendix can vary – 75% are retrocaecal and 20% are pelvic.

While various investigations can be carried out to confirm the diagnosis, there are scoring systems; unfortunately, none are absolutely accurate. It is essentially a clinical diagnosis. However, in women of child bearing age gynaecological conditions can confuse the issue. Under those circumstances, laparoscopy is the ideal method of confirmation. The treatment is emergency appendicectomy, either laparoscopic or open.

7   E Volvulus of the sigmoid colon

This elderly man has features of acute-on-chronic large bowel intestinal obstruction. His symptoms have been going on for almost a week. He has constipation and abdominal distension and some pain. He does not have features of strangulation such as hypotension, temperature or marked tachycardia. His abdominal distension is mainly on the left side. Pain is not a prominent feature as would happen in a patient who has a closed-loop large bowel obstruction from a left colonic carcinoma. This patient needs an intravenous line, indwelling urinary catheter, confirmation of the diagnosis by a plain abdominal X-ray which would show a massively dilated and twisted sigmoid colon; a Gastrografin enema can also be done. Initial management is by colonoscopic deflation. If conservative management is unsuccessful, operation will be necessary at which sigmoid colectomy is done as a Hartmann's type procedure.

8   A Gallstone ileus

This patient has the typical features of distal acute small bowel obstruction with abdominal pain, distension and faeculent vomiting which is a sign of distal ileal obstruction. Her symptoms have been going on for a few days, now reaching an acute stage with total obstruction of the distal ileum. This is evidenced by faeculent vomiting, which is a sinister sign. Although gallstone ileus is rarely a preoperative diagnosis, and is usually diagnosed in surgery, in this patient the diagnosis can be made preoperatively on the CT scan which shows gas in the biliary tree. The gas in the biliary tree is caused by a cholecystoduodenal fistula from a stone that has fistulated into the duodenum. Thereafter it travels down to the narrowest part of the small bowel, obstructing the terminal ileum, and resulting in gallstone ileus. The treatment is resuscitation with intravenous fluids and emergency laparotomy.

9   D Perforated diverticulitis

This woman has lower abdominal peritonitis with features of septic shock. Her history of constipation and her obesity should alert one to the possibility of diverticular disease. The previous barium enema (**Figure 46.3**) confirms that she has severe diverticular disease. Features of peritonitis in the presence of septic shock should suggest faecal peritonitis from perforated diverticulitis. The clinical presentation of acute diverticulitis is depicted in **Figure 46.4**. She should be resuscitated with analgesia, intravenous fluids, indwelling catheter, central venous pressure line and intravenous antibiotics. An erect chest X-ray may show gas under the right dome of the diaphragm. Once she is optimised she should be taken to the theatre for laparotomy.

At laparotomy she should undergo a Hartmann's operation and thorough peritoneal lavage. Septic complications of diverticulitis are classified according to the Hinchey system (**Figures 46.5** and **46.6**).

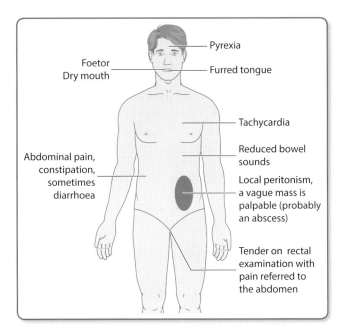

Figure 46.4 Clinical presentation of acute diverticulitis +/− paracolic abscess.

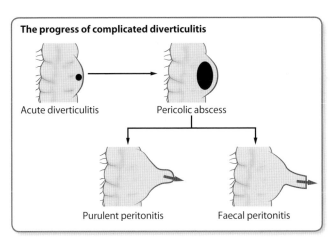

Figure 46.5 Hinchey classification of septic complications of acute diverticulitis.

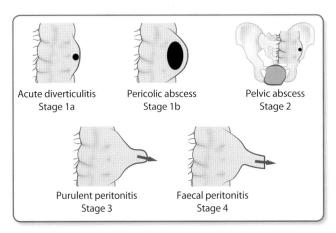

Figure 46.6 Modified Hinchey staging of acute diverticulitis.

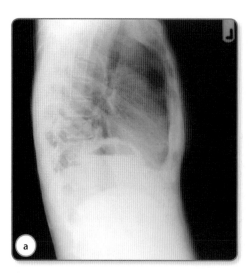
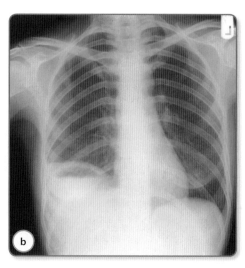

Figure 46.7 Two chest X-rays. Lateral (a) and anteroposterior (b) views showing raised right dome of diaphragm, under which there is a large air–fluid level.

10. E Subphrenic abscess

After laparoscopic closure of a perforated duodenal ulcer, this patient made a good recovery initially. However, a week later she has pyrexia with signs of intra-abdominal sepsis. She has pain in the right shoulder tip from diaphragmatic irritation and signs in the right upper quadrant with pleural effusion. She has a right subphrenic abscess. On chest X-ray she would have an elevated right dome of the diaphragm under which there would be a fluid level (**Figure 46.7**). She needs an ultrasound and/or CT scan of the subphrenic spaces to localise the abscess. This would most probably be in the right anterior subdiaphragmatic space or in the hepatorenal pouch (Morrison's pouch). She would require a CT-guided drainage of the abscess. This may need to be performed more than once as the abscess may be multi-loculated. Rarely, an abscess requires extraperitoneal drainage.

11. B Bleeding peptic ulcer

This 60-year-old man has features of long-standing peptic ulceration. He now has hypovolaemic shock with upper abdominal tenderness. He is bleeding from a peptic ulcer, almost certainly a duodenal ulcer.

He needs immediate resuscitation: two wide bore intravenous cannulae through which crystalloids are infused followed by blood transfusion, indwelling catheter to monitor urinary output, central venous pressure line and urgent oesophagogastroduodenoscopy. In the case of a bleeding duodenal ulcer, this would show an ulcer crater on the posterior wall of the first of the duodenum. Attempts may be made to stop the bleeding with minimal access surgical methods such as lasers, argon diathermy and injection methods. A bleeding gastric ulcer from the posterior wall penetrates into the splenic artery when a partial gastrectomy may be necessary **(Figure 46.8)**. The overall management of acute upper gastrointestinal haemorrhage is summarised in **Figure 46.9.**

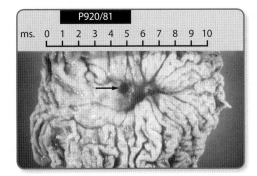

Figure 46.8 Partial gastrectomy specimen for bleeding posterior gastric ulcer. The arrow points to the bleeding point.

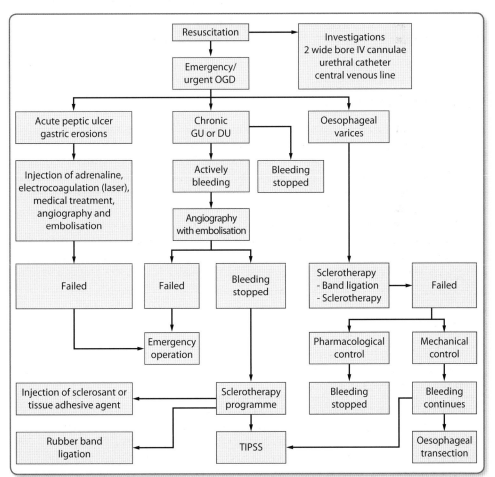

Figure 46.9 Management of acute upper gastrointestinal haemorrhage. OGD, oesophagogastroduodenoscopy; MAS, minimal access surgery; GU, gastric ulcer; DU, duodenal ulcer; TIPSS, transhepatic portosystemic stent shunt.

12. A Aortoenteric fistula

Any patient who has a vascular graft and a gastrointestinal bleed should be presumed to have an aortoenteric fistula unless otherwise proven. This man who had an operation for abdominal aortic aneurysm in the past has now an acute haematemesis. This patient requires urgent resuscitation on the same lines as the preceding patient to be followed by oesophagogastroduodenoscopy. The latter may be difficult because of severe bleeding from the duodenum. If the bleeding has stopped, the experienced endoscopist may see the site of fistula between the duodenum and the aortic graft. This patient needs an immediate operation by an expert vascular surgeon. At operation the fistula has to be disconnected, the aortic graft removed, the duodenal hole closed, the ends of the aorta closed off followed by an axillobifemoral extra-anatomic bypass graft.

13. B Femoral hernia

This patient has an irreducible tender lump at the medial end of his right groin. This lump is below the inguinal ligament and lateral to the pubic tubercle, the site of the femoral canal. He therefore has a femoral hernia which probably contains irreducible omentum that is the cause of his lower abdominal discomfort. He needs an operation. Whilst there are several approaches, the simplest elective procedure is to do a low approach. An oblique incision is made along the medial half and 2 cm below the inguinal ligament, the hernial sac is isolated, opened, the contents reduced and the sac transfixed, ligated and removed. The femoral ring is obliterated by approximating the medial part of the inguinal ligament to the pectineal ligament. Femoral hernia is more common in the female, although inguinal hernia is more common than femoral in the female.

14. E Obturator hernia

Obturator hernia is six times more common in women. The pain of the hernia is referred along the geniculate branch of the obturator nerve to the knee. A swelling is not easily felt because the hernia is covered by the pectineus. A swelling is rarely obvious unless the limb is flexed, abducted and externally rotated; in this position, a hernia may be felt. On vaginal examination, a tender swelling may be felt in the region of the obturator foramen. A CT of the pelvis may be necessary, if the diagnosis is in doubt. Operation is the treatment of choice as strangulation in the form of a Richter's hernia is not uncommon.

Chapter 47

Upper gastrointestinal surgery

Questions

Theme: Gastric and duodenal conditions

Options for Questions 1–3:

A	Carcinoma of the stomach	E	Gastric outlet obstruction
B	Duodenal adenocarcinoma	F	Gastric ulcer
C	Duodenal diverticulum	G	Gastritis
D	Gastric lymphoma	H	Leiomyoma of the stomach

For each of the following situations, select the single most likely diagnosis. Each option may be used once, more than once or not at all.

1. A 60-year-old woman, a smoker, complains of bouts of epigastric pain for the past 8 months. The pain comes on 10–15 minutes after meals. Vomiting relieves her pain. Although her appetite is good, she is frightened to eat for fear of the pain. These bouts of pain are cyclical: there are periods when she is pain-free. From time to time she has taken over-the-counter medicines with some benefit. On examination, there is nothing to find except for some epigastric tenderness.

2. A 63-year-old man presents to his GP with intermittent non-bilious vomiting for the past couple of months. The vomitus is foul-smelling and contains undigested food taken a few days before. He has suffered from indigestion for many years for which he takes over-the-counter drugs. He has lost 12 kg in weight during this period. He looks dehydrated, unwell with a succussion splash and a visible gastric peristalsis.

3. A 55-year-old man complains of recent loss of appetite, epigastric pain, intermittent vomiting and weight loss for the last 6 weeks. The vomitus at times is dark red. He recently noticed that his left leg is swollen with a tender cord-like structure along his calf diagnosed as thrombophlebitis.

Theme: Oesophageal conditions

Options for Questions 4–9:

A	Achalasia	F	Oesophageal varices
B	Barrett's oesophagus	G	Pharyngeal diverticulum
C	Boerhaave's syndrome	H	Schatzki's ring
D	Carcinoma of the oesophagus	I	Scleroderma
E	Hiatus hernia		

For each of the following situations below, select the single most likely diagnosis. Each option may be used once, more than once or not at all.

4. A 50-year-old man complains of intermittent difficulty in swallowing (dysphagia) with food sticking in the lower retrosternal region for the past 8 weeks; the dysphagia is usually for solid foods. This was preceded by heart-burn for several months for which he underwent an oesophagogastroduodenoscopy (OGD) with biopsy and was put on proton pump inhibitors. He is due for another OGD after 6 weeks.

5. A 60-year-old woman complains of repeated bouts of coughing when lying in bed and a sensation of food material spilling over into her gullet. She suffers from recurrent chest infections for which she is treated with antibiotics. She has occasional dysphagia and is embarrassed by halitosis.

6. A 45-year-old man complains of dysphagia of almost 2 years' duration. This is more marked with liquids. Sometimes there is regurgitation of undigested food and foul-smelling frothy sputum. He suffers from intermittent cough, chest infections and retrosternal discomfort. He has lost 10 kg in weight in 6 months.

7. A 65-year-old man, a heavy smoker and drinker, complains of progressive dysphagia of 8 weeks' duration. He has difficulty swallowing solids, which tends to stick in the middle of his retrosternal region. He has lost so much weight that his belt has gone up two notches within the last 8 weeks and his clothes feel very loose.

8. A 55-year-old man, a chronic alcoholic, has been admitted as an emergency with sudden onset of blood-stained vomiting in the form of bright red blood and clots. He has previously had episodes of vomiting when he vomited up small amounts of dark blood and did not seek immediate help. On examination, he has a pulse rate of 110 bpm and his blood pressure is 100/60 mmHg. On abdominal examination, he has distended veins radiating from his umbilicus.

9. A 42-year-old man presents as an emergency with sudden onset of very severe retrosternal chest pain that came on after a severe bout of vomiting. The vomitus contained the alcohol and food that he had ingested a short while ago; it also contained streaks of bright red blood. On examination, he has a pulse of 130 bpm and blood pressure of 90/60 mmHg. There is crepitus in both supraclavicular areas.

Theme: Gastric and duodenal conditions

Options for Questions 10–12:

A Carcinoma of the stomach
B Duodenal adenocarcinoma
C Duodenal diverticulum
D Gastric lymphoma

E Gastric outlet obstruction
F Gastric ulcer
G Gastritis
H Leiomyoma of the stomach

For each of the following situations, select the single most likely diagnosis. Each option may be used once, more than once or not at all.

10. A 35-year-old woman complains of upper abdominal discomfort of 6 weeks' duration. She is otherwise well and has not been off work as a medical secretary. Her GP had a barium meal carried out and referred her for a surgical opinion.

11. A 65-year-old woman presented with undue shortness of breath of recent origin and intermittent vomiting of 3 months' duration. On examination, her GP found that she has iron deficiency anaemia with a haemoglobin of level of 80 g/L. She is jaundiced and complains of recent itching. The serum biochemistry shows a picture of obstructive jaundice.

12. A 70-year-old man presents to his GP, since he suddenly vomited blood clots and a couple of days later noticed that he had black tarry stools. The GP felt a vague lump in the epigastrium. The patient was not keen on hospital admission. Therefore, he had haematological tests carried out which showed haemoglobin of 100 g/L, and a barium meal showed a space-occupying lesion. He was then persuaded to be admitted to the surgical ward.

Answers

1. F Gastric ulcer

This patient has features of peptic ulceration in the stomach because the pain comes on shortly after food. Periodicity is a typical feature of the pain. She needs an oesophagogastroduodenoscopy (OGD) and multiple biopsies. A gastric ulcer should be regarded as malignant unless otherwise proven conclusively by an experienced endoscopist and histopathologist. In case of a benign gastric ulcer *Helicobacter pylori* infection should be sought for by doing the rapid urease test, or biopsy. *H. pylori* infection should be successfully eradicated. Advising on lifestyle changes, in particular stopping smoking, is essential. After the course of medical treatment an OGD should be done to confirm that the ulcer has healed. If the ulcer has not healed, a gastrectomy should be done (**Figure 47.1**). Very rarely a benign gastric ulcer can turn malignant.

H. pylori is responsible for type B gastritis. The types of gastritis are shown in **Figure 47.2**.

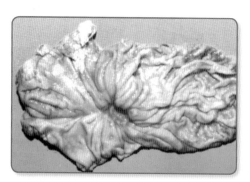

Figure 47.1 Stomach showing punched out ulcer with overhanging edge – a benign gastric ulcer.

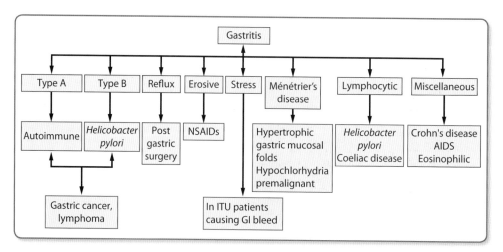

Figure 47.2 Types of gastritis.

2. E Gastric outlet obstruction

The features of indigestion for many years with vomiting, dehydration, weight loss, succussion splash and visible gastric peristalsis is typical of gastric outlet obstruction from a cicatrised, healed duodenal ulcer. The effects of dehydration are loss of skin turgor, dry tongue and sunken eyes. This patient will have serious metabolic effects of hypochloraemic, hypokalaemic, metabolic alkalosis. Long-standing alkalosis may cause reduction in the ionised serum calcium resulting in clinical tetany.

This patient will need resuscitation, confirmation of the diagnosis followed by definitive treatment. The patient should have vigorous intravenous rehydration using normal saline with added potassium; this is monitored by an indwelling urinary catheter and a central venous pressure line. The barium meal will show a huge stomach with a large amount of food residue. The stomach is washed out, an OGD is performed, followed by the definitive treatment of posterior, retrocolic, isoperistaltic gastrojejunostomy.

3. A Carcinoma of the stomach

Anorexia, asthenia and anaemia (the 3 As) are the hallmarks of cancer stomach. This man complains of abdominal pain, intermittent vomiting of blood and weight loss. He has Trousseau's sign, usually a sinister finding of visceral cancer.

The patient should have an OGD and biopsy followed by a staging CT scan. An endoluminal ultrasound at the same time as OGD will assess accurately the local extent. If investigations thus far indicate the possibility of a radical curative resection, then a laparoscopy and laparoscopic ultrasound as a staging procedure is appropriate.

When feasible, radical curative total gastrectomy is carried out. In distal growths, confined to the pylorus a subtotal gastrectomy can be carried out. Histologically two types are identified: intestinal type where the prognosis is better and diffuse anaplastic type, also called linitis plastica (**Figure 47.3**) which has a dismal outcome.

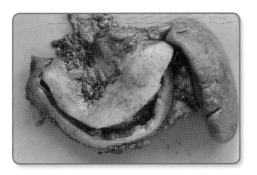

Figure 47.3 Linitis plastica. Courtesy of Dr James McPhie.

4. B Barrett's oesophagus

This patient has had heartburn for several months for which he underwent oesophagogastroduodenoscopy, biopsy and is now being treated medically. This is a typical history in gastro-oesophageal reflux disease (GORD). The patient's dysphagia could well be due to stricture within Barrett's oesophagus. The condition is a metaplastic response to chronic GORD. Here the squamocolumnar junction moves proximally where strictures can occur. Such patients should be under regular endoscopic surveillance to exclude dysplasia or in situ cancer. In the presence of intestinal metaplasia, the increased risk of adenocarcinoma is 25–30 times that of the general population. The relative risk of cancer increases with the increasing length of abnormal mucosa.

Management:

- balloon dilatation for strictures
- antireflux surgery for severe symptoms of GORD
- surveillance for dysplasia
- resection for severe dysplasia (some authorities consider severe dysplasia as in situ carcinoma) or carcinoma.

5. G Pharyngeal diverticulum (Zenker's diverticulum)

This patient has the classical symptoms of a pharyngeal diverticulum – recurrent chest infections from aspiration of food contents into the tracheobronchial tree, which occurs more when the patient is recumbent. Dysphagia is a late symptom. Very rarely when the diverticulum is large, it may be felt on the left side of the neck and the contents emptied with a gurgling sound.

The diverticulum occurs through a weakness between the oblique thyropharyngeus part and the circular cricopharyngeus part of the inferior constrictor muscle. The gap, triangular in shape, is called the Killian's dehiscence. It is thought to occur due to incoordination between the constrictor muscles of the pharynx and the cricopharyngeal sphincter.

Results from a barium swallow shows arrest of barium in a smooth pouch which may contain food residue shown as filling defects within the pouch (**Figure 47.4**). Endoscopic stapling diverticulotomy with cricopharyngeal myotomy is the treatment of choice.

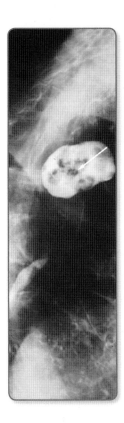

Figure 47.4 Barium swallow showing arrest of barium in a smooth pouch with food residue (arrow). This is typical of a pharyngeal diverticulum.

6. A Achalasia

Long-standing dysphagia, particularly for liquids, is the hallmark of achalasia. It may be associated with odynophagia (painful swallowing). Repeated chest infections from regurgitation of food, especially at night, is common. The condition is the result of the absence of ganglion cells in the myenteric plexus of Auerbach, which is situated between the muscle layers and forms part of the enteric nervous system. This causes failure of relaxation of the gastro-oesophageal junction resulting in massive dilatation of the proximal oesophagus with large amount of food residue.

Barium swallow shows a classical 'bird's beak' appearance distal to a massively dilated oesophagus containing food residue (**Figure 47.5**) with absence of the gastric air bubble. OGD should be carried out to exclude carcinoma, a complication that may occur in 3%. Depending upon the severity, balloon dilatation can be attempted initially. The definitive treatment is Heller's cardiomyotomy, carried out laparoscopically or thoracoscopically.

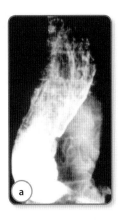
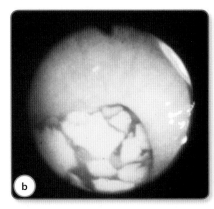

Figure 47.5 (a) Barium swallow shows a classical 'bird's beak' appearance distal to a massively dilated oesophagus containing food residue. (b) Oesophagogastro-dudenoscopy view showing food residue in oesophagus.

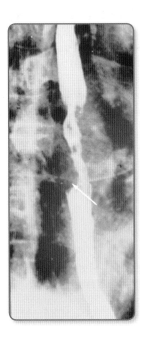

Figure 47.6 Barium meal showing shouldering (arrow) typical of carcinoma.

7. D Carcinoma of the oesophagus

This patient has typical features of oesophageal carcinoma. Clinical examination would not show much other than evidence of weight loss. There will be features of malnutrition and, if the condition is advanced, a secondary liver or a left supraclavicular lymph node may be felt.

A barium swallow will show an irregular stricture with shouldering (**Figure 47.6**). An urgent oesophagogastroduodenoscopy will show a polypoid growth; at the same time an endoluminal ultrasound (EUS) is done to assess the local extent of the growth and the state of mediastinal lymph node followed by biopsy. A CT of the chest and abdomen is carried out to stage the disease. If resection is regarded as a possibility then laparoscopy and laparoscopic ultrasound is carried out as a final staging procedure to exclude peritoneal secondaries.

If the carcinoma is resectable, then a two-stage Ivor-Lewis operation is done. Palliation consists of stenting and radiotherapy.

8. F Oesophageal varices

This patient has upper gastrointestinal haemorrhage from oesophageal varices. This is due to portal hypertension resulting from cirrhosis. Clinical examination of the patient may show caput medusa, spider naevi, mild jaundice, testicular atrophy, gynaecomastia and ascites. As a result of portal hypertension, several sites of porto-systemic anastomosis open up; caput medusa (**Figure 47.7**) and oesophageal varices being the obvious ones in this patient. Other sites are the gastro-oesophageal junction, the lower part of the rectum, the bare area of the liver, the retroperitoneum and the posterior surface of the pancreas. This patient must be immediately resuscitated. Once stable, OGD (**Figure 47.8**) is carried out to find the cause of the haematemesis. If the cause of bleeding is confirmed to be the varices they are treated by rubber band ligation and sent home on propranolol and isosorbide mononitrate.

In the emergency situation, if this initial intervention is not successful, because of technical reasons, oesophageal tamponade with a Segstaken-Blakemore tube (**Figure 47.9**) is attempted or a transjugular intra-hepatic porto-systemic stent shunt (TIPPS) (**Figure 47.10**) is inserted.

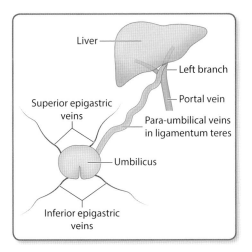

Figure 47.7 Formation of caput medusae as a result of portosystemic anastomosis on the anterior abdominal wall in portal hypertension.

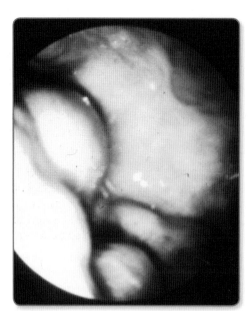

Figure 47.8 OGD showing large oesophageal varices.

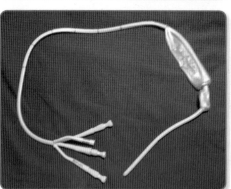

Figure 47.9 Sengstaken-Blakemore tube for oesophageal tamponade.

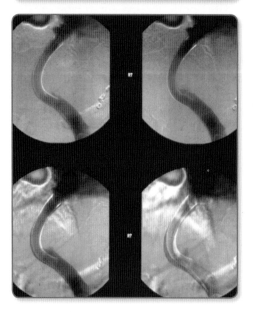

Figure 47.10 TIPPS stent for portal hypertension.

9. C Boerhaave's syndrome (Figure 47.11)

This patient has spontaneous rupture of the oesophagus. He has a typical history of forced vomiting followed by features of shock with bilateral surgical emphysema of the neck. The combination of vomiting, excruciating chest pain and subcutaneous emphysema called Mackler's triad should alert one to the diagnosis. If undiagnosed the patient rapidly develops septic shock from chemical and bacterial mediastinitis which can rapidly lead to multiorgan failure and death. The differential diagnosis is myocardial infarction, pericarditis, pneumothorax, pulmonary embolism.

The patient needs to be immediately resuscitated, followed by confirmation of diagnosis by CT scan with oral contrast. If the patient is seen within the first 24 hours, transthoracic repair with feeding jejunostomy and functional gastrostomy is carried out. In late diagnosis, the aim should be to prevent further soilage, with a view to initial salvage surgery followed by definitive surgery later. A suggested treatment regimen is given in **Figure 47.12**.

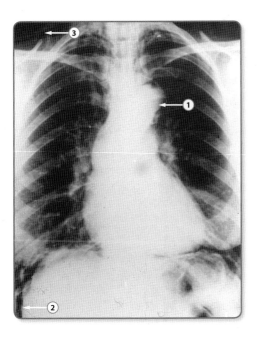

Figure 47.11 Chest X-ray in Boerhaave's syndrome. ① Pneumomediastinum ② surgical emphysema ③ surgical emphysema in neck.

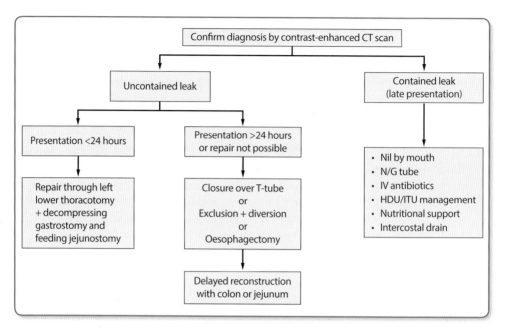

Figure 47.12 Suggested treatment regimen for Boerhaave's syndrome.

10. C Duodenal diverticulum

The barium meal shows the C of the duodenum with an outpouching of the contrast inside a smooth-lined pouch on the mesenteric border (**Figure 47.13**). This is typical of a congenital duodenal diverticulum. A congenital diverticulum is one where all the coats of the bowel – mucosa, muscularis and serosa – go to form the diverticulum. It is found at the entrance of the ampulla of Vater which is the junction of the foregut and hindgut and the site of maximum weakness.

These do not produce any symptoms. A duodenal diverticulum is regarded as 'a diagnostic scapegoat of the upper abdomen'. If a patient with upper abdominal symptoms has been found have a duodenal diverticulum on OGD, the clinician should look for other causes as the diverticulum is an innocent bystander. However, the condition has a clinical significance. It may be difficult to do an endoscopic retrograde cholangiopancreatography and hazardous to attempt papillotomy.

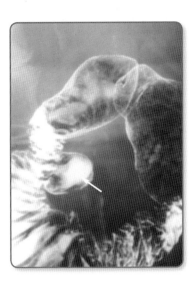

Figure 47.13 Barium meal showing duodenal diverticulum (arrow).

11. B Duodenal adenocarcinoma

This woman's presenting symptom of shortness of breath is due to anaemic hypoxia. She has intermittent vomiting and has been found to have clinical itching and biochemical features of obstructive jaundice. These features point to an obstruction in the duodenum causing block of the ampulla of Vater – a periampullary carcinoma. This is the commonest site of adenocarcinoma of the small bowel.

The management is confirmation of the diagnosis by oesophagogastroduodenoscopy and biopsy; a barium meal will show an 'apple-core' deformity with a hugely dilated stomach; staging is carried out by CT scan, chest X-ray, laparoscopy and laparoscopic ultrasound. If the growth is localised without any distant spread, curative resection (possible in 70%) is performed by Whipple's pancreaticoduodenectomy; the 5-year survival rate is about 20%. Palliation is carried out by stenting of the common bile duct to alleviate jaundice and an anterior gastrojejunostomy for gastric outlet obstruction.

12. H Leiomyoma of the stomach

Acute upper gastrointestinal tract haemorrhage is the classical presentation of a leiomyoma of stomach. The possibility of the presence of an epigastric mass may denote a gastric cancer; this is unlikely in the absence of weight loss. Oesophagogastroduodenoscopy (OGD) is the investigation of choice, but as the patient refused hospital admission initially, a barium meal was carried out. This shows a smooth filling defect in the body of the stomach, typical of a submucosal tumour (**Figure 47.14**). In the centre of the filling defect there is a patch of barium

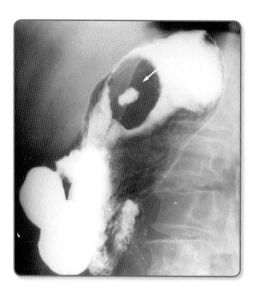

Figure 47.14 Barium meal showing smooth filling defect in the body of the stomach with mucosal ulceration, typical of a leiomyoma (arrow).

due to ulceration of the tumour which causes the acute bleeding – the typical presenting feature. These tumours are referred to as gastrointestinal stromal tumours.

The patient needs an urgent OGD which would show a tumour in the posterior wall of the stomach; this is followed by a CT. The treatment is local excision.

Chapter 48

Hepatobiliary and pancreatic surgery

Questions

Theme: Acute hepatobiliary presentations

Options for Questions 1–4:

A	Acute cholangitis	E	Liver fluke
B	Acute cholecystitis	F	Mirizzi's syndrome
C	Acute pancreatitis	G	Viral hepatitis
D	Gallstone ileus		

For each of the following situations, select the single most likely diagnosis. Each option may be used once, more than once or not at all.

1. A 59-year-old man presents with acute severe central abdominal pain radiating to the back. This had been preceded by several weeks of intermittent right upper quadrant pain. He has no significant past medical history, but is mildly obese.

2. A 72-year-old woman presents with symptoms of obstructive jaundice. She is known to have a solitary large gallstone, but it has been managed conservatively due to significant comorbidity.

3. A 45-year-old obese woman presents with severe constant right upper quadrant pain. Over the past 3 years she has been experiencing similar intermittent episodes which previously have always resolved spontaneously.

4. An 80-year-old woman presents with a 2-day history of increasing vomiting and abdominal distension. She has not passed any stool or flatus for 24 hours. This patient was diagnosed with a large solitary gallstone some years previously, but surgery was not performed due to severe comorbidity.

5. A 56-year-old woman who is on the waiting list for laparoscopic cholecystectomy presents with a 1-week history of worsening right upper quadrant pain, vomiting, fevers and rigors.

Theme: Classification of jaundice

Options for Questions 6–8:

A Blood transfusion jaundice	**E** Physiological jaundice
B Hepatic (hepatocellular)	**F** Posthepatic (cholestatic)
C Infective jaundice	**G** Prehepatic
D Mixed hepatic and posthepatic	

For each of the following situations, select the single most likely diagnosis. Each option may be used once, more than once or not at all.

6. A 74-year-old woman fell 2 weeks previously which resulted in a large haematoma on her left thigh. The haematoma has gradually reduced in size, however she has noticed that her skin has a yellow tinge. Blood tests show an isolated raised bilirubin with normal coagulation screen.

7. A 60-year-old woman has been admitted as an emergency with a 4-day history of severe right upper quadrant pain, vomiting, jaundice and intense pruritus. She is found to have a high temperature with rigors and hyperdynamic circulation.

8. An 18-year-old woman presents with jaundice and pallor. She reports that she has always looked pale and on previous blood tests she has been anaemic. Her anaemia was previously thought due to menorrhagia, although her periods have never been particularly heavy. On examination, her abdomen is soft and non-tender with a palpable spleen.

Theme: Hepatobiliary investigations

Options for Questions 9–11:

A Abdominal ultrasound scan	**E** Magnetic resonance
B Computerised tomographic scan	cholangiopancreatography
C Endoscopic ultrasound scan	**F** Operative cholangiogram
D Endoscopic retrograde	**G** Percutaneous transhepatic
cholangiopancreatography	cholangiogram

For each of the following situations, select the single most likely diagnosis. Each option may be used once, more than once or not at all.

9. A 46-year-old moderately obese woman presents with severe right upper quadrant pain which has gradually increased in severity. This episode was preceded by 6 months of intermittent right upper quadrant pain and nausea. On examination, she is pyrexial and Murphy's sign is positive. Liver function tests are normal.

10. A 68-year-old man presents with right upper quadrant pain and mildly deranged obstructive liver function tests. Abdominal ultrasound scan demonstrated gallstones in the gallbladder, but the common bile duct could not be seen.

11. A 53-year-old woman presents for elective cholecystectomy following a long history of intermittent right upper quadrant pain. Ultrasound scan had demonstrated gallstones within the gallbladder but no other significant abnormalities. Preadmission blood tests had shown mildly raised bilirubin, alkaline phosphatase and gamma-glutamyl transpeptidase. She is currently well and pain free.

Theme: Hepatobiliary tumours

Options for Questions 12–13:

A	Adenoma		D	Hepatocellular carcinoma
B	Angiosarcoma		E	Liver metastasis
C	Cholangiocarcinoma			

For each of the following situations, select the single most likely diagnosis. Each option may be used once, more than once or not at all.

12. A 43-year-old man with cirrhosis due to alcoholic liver disease presents with constant right upper quadrant pain which has increased over several months. On examination, the liver edge is palpable and found to be firm and irregular.

13. A 70-year-old man, who is a long-term smoker, presents with vague right upper quadrant pain. He has lost considerable weight over the past 6 months and for the past year has been experiencing worsening haemoptysis. On examination, an irregular liver edge is palpable.

Theme: Benign conditions

Options for Questions 14–15:

A Liver trauma
B Polycystic liver disease
C Primary biliary cirrhosis
D Primary sclerosing cholangitis
E Right heart failure

For each of the following situations, select the single most likely diagnosis. Each option may be used once, more than once or not at all.

14. A 42-year-old woman presents with fatigue, itch and constant mild right upper quadrant pain. These symptoms have been present for several months but have recently increased in severity.

15. A 56-year-old man is referred by his GP with an irregular palpable liver edge approximately 5 cm below the costal margin. He had presented for a routine check-up and had not complained of any abdominal discomfort. He is systemically well with no weight loss.

Answers

1. C Acute pancreatitis

Acute pancreatitis usually presents with upper/central abdominal pain radiating to the back. On examination, there may be Cullen's sign and Grey Turner's sign (**Figure 48.1**). It is more common in men. Aetiology varies across the world but gallstones and alcohol account for the majority of presentations. The key blood test is serum amylase which would typically be elevated greater than three times normal in an episode of pancreatitis. Amylase levels rise within 2–12 hours of onset of abdominal pain and peak after 1–3 days. It should be noted that in patients presenting late, the amylase level may be falling. Serum lipase level may remain elevated for longer and can be a useful addition to the investigation profile. Levels of these enzymes do not provide prognostic information. The clinical course in acute pancreatitis may be protracted with risks of subsequent complications related to the systemic inflammatory response. Mild acute pancreatitis usually results in pancreatic oedema followed by complete resolution. At the more severe end of the scale pancreatic necrosis may occur with varying degrees of local tissue destruction. Scoring systems are used in an attempt to predict those patients who are likely to deteriorate. These include the Glasgow scoring system and Ranson's criteria. Pancreatic necrosis may become infected or an abscess may develop, risking generalised sepsis, multiorgan failure and death. A fluid collection may develop in the lesser omental sac known as a pseudocyst. This may resolve with time, or persist and become infected.

The main differential here is acute cholecystitis, however the pain is central suggesting pancreatitis as a more likely diagnosis. Gallstone ileus would likely present with signs of obstruction.

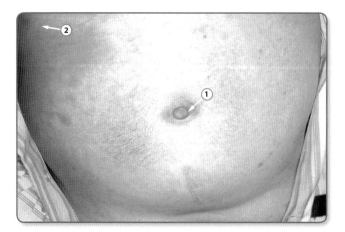

Figure 48.1 Patient with acute severe pancreatitis showing bruising around the umbilicus (Cullen's sign, ① and bruising of the flanks (Grey Turner's sign, ②.

2. F Mirizzi's syndrome

A single large gallstone will be unlikely to pass through the cystic duct into the common bile duct. However, the stone within the gallbladder may cause pressure on the common hepatic duct leading to biliary obstruction and jaundice (**Figure 48.2**). In the chronic setting a fistula may develop between the gallbladder and common hepatic duct. A fistula can also develop between the gallbladder and small bowel. If a large stone passes into the small bowel then gallstone ileus may occur as the stone can lead to small bowel obstruction.

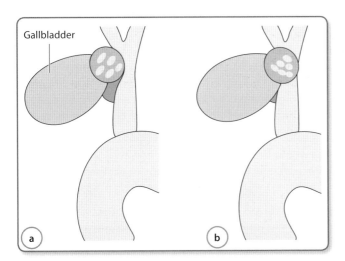

Gallbladder

a   b

Figure 48.2 The two types of Mirizzi's syndrome. (a) Type I Mirizzi's syndrome with a large gallstone pressing on the common hepatic duct. (b) Type II, progression of Mirizzi's syndrome with the gallstone fistulating into the common hepatic duct.

3. B Acute cholecystitis

This is inflammation of the gallbladder causing acute pain in the right upper quadrant and sometimes round to the epigastrium. The pain may have variable presentations, including sharp, dull, constant or cramp-like pain, which radiates to the back or to the right scapula. In the overwhelming majority, this is associated with gallstones; however acute cholecystitis can occur without gallstones, and is termed acalculous cholecystitis. This may occur as a manifestation of severe illness rather than a primary condition. On examination, Murphy's sign may be positive. This sign is elicited by the examiner placing their hand below the right costal margin and asking the patient to breathe in. If the gallbladder is acutely inflamed, inspiration will lead to inferior displacement of the gallbladder which comes into contact with anterior abdominal wall, causing exacerbation of pain and the patient to 'catch their breath'. For a positive test the examiner should also test below the left costal margin for absence of pain. Ultrasound scan is generally the favoured imaging modality for diagnosis, enabling assessment of gallbladder wall thickness, presence of gallstones and calibre of the common bile duct. The gallbladder becomes distended with mucus and can present with similar symptoms to acute cholecystitis. Carcinoma of the gallbladder is rarely found. Given the possibility of carcinoma, it is important to avoid perforation during cholecystectomy. If the gallbladder is perforated there is a risk of disseminating the malignancy.

It is important to understand the difference between cholecystitis and cholangitis. The latter describes ascending infection within the biliary tree. Patients can deteriorate rapidly, requiring prompt diagnosis and intervention.

4. D Gallstone ileus

Gallstone ileus is an infrequent complication of gallstones. It develops in a chronic setting where a fistula develops between the gallbladder and duodenum. The gallstone then passes into the duodenum. If the stone is large it may obstruct the ileum. The stone passes down to the ileocaecal valve where it finally obstructs the small bowel. Although most gallstones are radio-opaque, occasionally this unusual cause for obstruction may be seen on an abdominal radiograph. The original fistula may enable gas to enter the biliary tree causing pneumobilia. This is seen as gas in the right upper quadrant (**Figure 48.3**). Larger gallstones are predominantly cholesterol based (around 80%); pigment stones are smaller consisting primarily of bilirubin and calcium salts. Stones can also be of mixed composition.

The main differential here would be acute pancreatitis; however, the history of a solitary large gallstone makes this less likely. Abdominal distention may be a feature of acute pancreatitis but patients are unlikely to be completely obstructed.

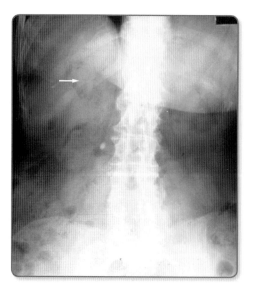

Figure 48.3 Pneumobilia. Gas is seen in the right upper quadrant (arrow), within the biliary tree. This has been caused by a fistula developing between the gallbladder and duodenum. A radio-opaque gallstone is also seen in the duodenum.

5. A Acute cholangitis

Acute cholangitis or ascending cholangitis occurs when bacteria from the duodenum ascends upwards in the biliary tree causing an infection. It occurs when the bile duct is occluded by gallstone(s) or secondary to an infected biliary stent. Acute cholangitis can be life-threatening. Acute cholangitis presents with right upper quadrant pain, jaundice and fever. This is also known as Charcot's triad. Definitive management after resuscitation with fluids and antibiotics is ERCP + sphincterotomy to extract the gallstone followed by cholecystectomy.

6. G Prehepatic

In the presence of a large haematoma which is resolving the most likely cause is the increased breakdown of haem. This produces unconjugated bilirubin. This is conjugated by hepatocytes and excreted with bile into the duodenum. In addition to serum bilirubin a range of tests can be used to determine the underlying cause of jaundice. Liver function tests classically include alkaline phosphatase, gamma-glutamyl transpeptidase and aminotransferase. While these are essentially markers of damage to hepatocytes and biliary epithelium, they are often useful in delineating the cause. This patient has an isolated raised bilirubin. This is most likely a prehepatic aetiology but disorders of bilirubin metabolism should be considered. In hepatocellular jaundice aminotransferase is likely to be greatly elevated, with alkaline phosphatise and gamma-glutamyl transpeptidase less markedly so. In cholestatic jaundice alkaline phosphatase and gamma-glutamyl transpeptidase are usually increased with aminotransferase less elevated. A coagulation screen (prothrombin time) can provide an indicator of synthetic liver function and will be prolonged in cases of considerable impairment. Especially in elderly patients it is important to consider medications that may cause jaundice.

7. D Mixed hepatic and posthepatic

This patient has the typical features of cholangitis. This is most likely caused by a gallstone within the common bile duct, known as choledocholithiasis. Patients developing cholangitis may deteriorate rapidly due to overwhelming sepsis. The classical symptoms of fever, jaundice and right upper quadrant tenderness are known as Charcot's triad. While choledocholithiasis is the commonest cause patients with biliary obstruction due to another cause may also develop these symptoms. The sepsis that has ensued following bile duct obstruction may result in a mixed liver function test picture (i.e. raised aminotransferase, gamma-glutamyl transpeptidase, and alkaline phosphatase) although the underlying cause is posthepatic.

8. G Prehepatic

A palpable spleen in the presence of jaundice suggests a haemolytic process; this is supported by the presence of pallor. The history suggests that anaemia has been a long-standing issue. The underlying aetiology may be autoimmune haemolytic anaemia or hereditary spherocytosis. The direct antiglobulin test can distinguish between the two; the former being positive and the latter negative. Autoimmune haemolytic anaemia is caused mainly by IgG or IgM antibodies directed against red blood cells. Hereditary spherocytosis is a condition which results in spherical rather than biconcave red blood cells. These spherical cells are more prone to haemolysis and given these patients are prone to gallstones. Splenectomy prevents anaemia and should be performed when symptomatic or when significant evidence of the disease is present.

9. A Abdominal ultrasound scan

This overweight, middle aged woman appears to be conforming to the classical picture of a patient with symptomatic gallstones. Biliary colic is caused by the gallbladder contracting against a gallstone in the neck of the gallbladder. This is usually intermittent with the patient generally pain free between episodes. The gallbladder may become inflamed with increasing constant pain in the right upper quadrant. Ultrasound scan would be the most appropriate first investigation and should provide an indication of the thickness of the gallbladder wall (suggesting inflammation), the presence of stones and the dimensions of the common bile duct.

10. E Magnetic resonance cholangiopancreatography

Sometimes the common bile duct may not be visualised by ultrasound, which is most often due to overlying bowel gas obscuring the view. As the patient has mildly deranged liver function tests a gallstone obstructing the bile duct should be contemplated. Magnetic resonance imaging in the form of magnetic resonance cholangiopancreatography can provide excellent views of the biliary tree and visualise filling defects which may represent a stone. The majority of gallstones are radiolucent and so would not be see on CT. Endoscopic retrograde cholangiopancreatography could be used to image the biliary system, but this is an invasive procedure exposing the patient to risks that would not necessarily be justified at this stage. In some centres the patient may go straight to laparoscopic cholecystectomy with intraoperative cholangiogram to assess for choledocholithiasis.

11. F Operative cholangiogram

This mildly deranged liver function tests in this case could indicate biliary obstruction. If the patient was symptomatic or if the derangement was marked, it would be appropriate to delay surgery and arrange further investigation. Given the patient is currently well and pain free, it may be a small stone has been passed through the common bile duct and no further intervention is required. However, it would be appropriate to perform intraoperative cholangiogram to investigate the possibility of a stone in the common bile duct. This procedure requires cannulation of the biliary tree, usually via the cystic duct. It can be performed during laparoscopic or open procedures. If a stone is demonstrated, there are two main choices: (1) laparoscopic exploration of the common bile duct if the team is experienced in this technique or (2) complete the cholecystectomy laparoscopically and then electively perform endoscopic retrograde cholangiopancreatography and endoscopic papillotomy.

12. D Hepatocellular carcinoma

This may arise spontaneously but more frequently occur on a background on liver cirrhosis. The tumour may either form a large single mass or occur as multiple foci throughout the liver. Patients may present with hepatomegaly, ascites and distant metastases. Deterioration may be rapid and patients usually present late. Some patients may be suitable for surgical resection but due to risks of decompensation patients with cirrhosis are not usually resected. In this instance, the patient may be considered for liver transplantation. Chemoembolisation of large tumours may improve the preoperative condition of selected patients.

The main differential here is liver metastasis. However, with the background of cirrhosis hepatocellular carcinoma is most likely.

13. E Liver metastasis

This patient appears to have a malignant process underlying his current condition. The most likely cause for his right upper quadrant pain is hepatic metastases secondary to lung cancer. Increasing tumour bulk causes stretch on the liver capsule, leading to pain. Metastatic hepatic malignancy is 20 times more common than primary liver malignancy. Common primary sites include the gastrointestinal tract, breast, lung, genitourinary system, melanoma, and sarcoma. However essentially all solid malignancies with metastatic potential may involve the liver.

14. C Primary biliary cirrhosis

This is an autoimmune disease of the liver characterised by progressive destruction of bile canaliculi eventually leading to fibrosis and cirrhosis. The disease classically affects middle aged women between the age of 30 and 65 years. Patients may present with fatigue, jaundice, itch and right upper quadrant pain. Late presentation may reveal the complications of cirrhosis and portal hypertensions such as ascites, varices and hepatic encephalopathy. Liver function tests show a cholestatic picture with abnormal immunological investigations. Immunology includes antimitochondrial antibodies (in 95% of patients), smooth muscle antibodies in 50%, IgM elevated in at least 80% of patients, and antineutrophil cytoplasmic antibody negative. Ursodeoxycholic acid may help reduce cholestasis and liver damage, cholestyramine can reduce itch. As the disease progresses liver transplantation may be the only option although the disease can recur in around 15% of patients. Primary biliary cirrhosis should be contrasted with primary sclerosing cholangitis which affects extrahepatic bile ducts, can lead to stricture formation and is associated with inflammatory bowel disease.

15. B Polycystic liver disease

Most patients with this condition are asymptomatic. It is often associated with polycystic kidney disease. Liver function is usually normal, but the hepatomegaly, potential bleeding into cysts, or obstruction of the venous or biliary drainage of the liver lead to complications. Most patients are managed conservatively unless symptoms are significant in which case laparoscopic deroofing of large cysts can be performed. Unusually, liver transplantation may be necessary where multiple cysts cannot be treated by resection.

Chapter 49

Surgery of the small and large bowel

Questions

Theme: Colon and rectum

Options for Questions 1–3:

A	Angiodysplasia	D	Pneumatosis intestinalis
B	Carcinoma of caecum	E	Rectal prolapse
C	Carcinoma of rectum	F	Ulcerative colitis

For each of the following situations, select the single most likely diagnosis. Each option may be used once, more than once or not at all.

1. A 60-year-old man complains of alteration in his bowel habit having to wake up in the morning earlier than usual with an intense desire to open his bowels. He rushes to the toilet only to find that he passes considerable amount of wind, some watery stools and blood. He has lost some weight. His GP found that there are several masses in the left iliac fossa; rectal examination was normal.

2. A 60-year-old woman complains of undue shortness of breath when walking upstairs and carrying out her daily household work for the last couple of months. Her GP found that she had a mass in the right iliac fossa, haemoglobin was 75 g/L and faecal occult blood tests were positive. An oesophagogastroduodenoscopy carried out in an open access endoscopy clinic was normal.

3. A 40-year-old woman complains of diarrhoea for 3 months. This takes the form of several loose motions a day (anything up to six), with slime and bright red blood. She feels lethargic with vague left-sided abdominal pain. She is anaemic without any abdominal signs; rectal examination shows blood and slime on the examining finger. Her C-reactive protein is 125 mg/L.

Theme: Small intestine and appendix

Options for Questions 4–7:

A Acute appendicitis	**E** Ileocaecal tuberculosis
B Acute small bowel obstruction	**F** Jejunal diverticulosis
C Carcinoid tumour	**G** Meckel's diverticulum
D Crohn's disease	**H** Small bowel lymphoma

For each of the following situations, select the single most likely diagnosis. Each option may be used once, more than once or not at all.

4. A 70-year-old woman complains of colicky generalised abdominal pain, abdominal distension and vomiting of 2 day's duration. The vomitus was bilious to start with but immediately prior to admission it became faeculent in nature. She has a blood pressure of 100 mmHg systolic with a pulse rate of 120 beats per minute and a distended abdomen with high-pitched bowel sounds. She also has pain radiating down the inside of her left thigh down to the knee which is exacerbated by coughing. A plain X-ray (**Figure 49.1**) and CT scan (**Figure 49.2**) of her abdomen is shown.

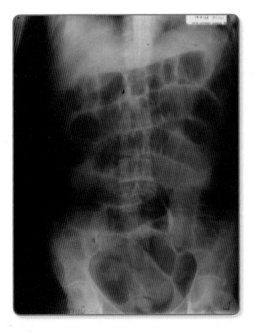

Figure 49.1 Plain X-ray of abdomen showing acute distal small bowel obstruction.

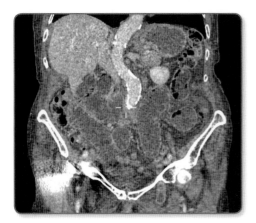

Figure 49.2 CT scan of abdomen showing left obturator hernia.

5. A 45-year-old woman complains of alternating constipation and diarrhoea for 6 months. The diarrhoea takes the form of 4–6 loose motions a day often associated with colicky abdominal pain and aching in the right iliac fossa. She has episodes of feeling unwell. Recently, she noticed a couple of painful, bluish-red nodules on her shin. Her GP felt a vague mass in the right iliac fossa, and diagnosed the lumps on her shin as erythema nodosum.

6. A 28-year-old woman complains of pain in the right iliac fossa of 18 hours' duration. The pain, initially started around the umbilicus, has now settled in the right lower abdomen; it is exacerbated by coughing. It is associated with nausea, vomiting, anorexia and several bouts of watery diarrhoea. On examination, she is afebrile with tenderness, rigidity and rebound tenderness in her entire lower abdomen.

7. A 50-year-old woman complains of increasing diarrhoea of several weeks duration. She is a sufferer of coeliac disease and has been on a gluten-free diet for almost 5 years. The present episode of diarrhoea is different from her usual bouts that she experiences from her coeliac disease. Recently, she has started developing colicky abdominal pain with episodes of fever and has noticed she has been losing weight.

Theme: Colon, rectum and anal canal

Options for Questions 8–14:

A	Acute diverticulitis	F	Colovesical fistula
B	Acute large bowel obstruction	G	Familial adenomatous polyposis
C	Anal carcinoma	H	Fistula-in-ano
E	Carcinoma of descending colon	I	Ischaemic colitis

For each of the following situations, select the single most likely diagnosis. Each option may be used once, more than once or not at all.

8. A 70-year-old slightly obese woman complains of pain in her left lower abdomen spreading to the rest of the abdomen for the past 10 days. She has had loose stools for 3 days. She has rigors and is pyrexial and has tenderness rigidity and rebound tenderness over the entire lower abdomen. Rectal examination reveals a tender mass felt in the pelvis through the rectal wall.

9. A 60-year-old man complains of frequency of micturition, suprapubic discomfort and passing very foul-smelling urine. He has been treated for repeated attacks of urinary tract infection by several courses of antibiotics. Recently, he has noticed passing air bubbles in urine. He has been constipated for many years. Clinical examination revealed no abnormality.

10. A 68-year-old man complains of generalised colicky abdominal pain of 48 hours' duration; in between the attacks of colic he is left with a dull ache. He has been constipated over the past few months, his last bowel action being 3 days ago. His abdomen is distended, mainly in the peripheral part, and tympanitic; the rectum is hollow.

11. A 25-year-old man, recently moved to the area, presented to his new GP with loose stools with blood and mucus of 8 weeks' duration. In the past, he was seen for regular camera examination of his large bowel once a year ever since he was a teenager. He is very concerned as his father died of cancer of the large bowel when he was 45 years old.

12. A 68-year-old man complains of dull aching left-sided abdominal pain for almost 6 months. This is often associated with the passage of blood-stained diarrhoea. Almost 2 years ago he had a myocardial infarct as a result of which he suffers from angina for which he is on medication. On examination, he is not shocked and has tenderness on the left side of the abdomen along the descending colon.

13. A 55-year-old man who has a renal transplant complains of 'piles'. He has noticed a lump around his anus which is constantly present, painful and bleeds on and off. This has been going on for the past 4–5 months. On examination, he has a fleshy ulcerated mass with raised and everted edges.

14. A 48-year-old man, a known patient of Crohn's disease, developed perianal pain with seropurulent discharge 6 weeks ago. When the discharge is significant, the pain is much less. It started when he felt an acute pain, which was relieved when there was a significant discharge.

Answers

1. C Carcinoma of rectum

This 60-year-old man has altered bowel habit in the form of early morning spurious diarrhoea, tenesmus and feeling of incomplete evacuation of his bowels. This is typical of a low rectal carcinoma. The masses felt in the left iliac fossa are inspissated faecal matter proximal to an annular growth causing impending obstruction. He needs a sigmoidoscopy and biopsy followed by a barium enema which may show a 'napkin-ring'-appearance (**Figure 49.3**), an annular carcinoma in the rectosigmoid. A synchronous carcinoma, which occurs in up to 10%, should always be excluded by a colonoscopy.

The carcinoma should be accurately staged by a contrast-enhanced CT scan, MRI of the pelvis and endoluminal ultrasound. After confirmation of the diagnosis and staging, definitive treatment is instituted after discussion with a multidisciplinary team, followed by anterior resection. Very low growths may require abdominoperineal excision of the rectum.

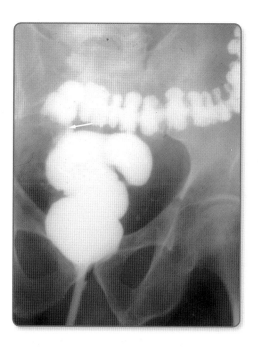

Figure 49.3 Barium enema of the upper rectum showing a 'napkin-ring' deformity (arrow) typical of annular carcinoma.

2. B Carcinoma of the caecum

This woman suffers from anaemic hypoxia and is unable to carry out her daily routine activities without becoming breathless. She is bleeding from her lower gastrointestinal tract as her faecal occult blood test is positive. With no alteration in her bowel habit and a mass in the right iliac fossa, a carcinoma of the caecum should be suspected. A barium enema (**Figure 49.4**) shows an irregular filling defect in the caecum, typical of a polypoid carcinoma. Caecal carcinoma can also present as an emergency with acute distal small bowel obstruction due to obstruction to the ileocaecal junction by the growth; another emergency presentation is when the condition masquerades as 'acute appendicitis' because of obstruction to the lumen of the appendix by the cancer.

After confirmation of diagnosis and a staging CT scan, a right hemicolectomy is carried out with ileotransverse anastomosis. If the postoperative staging shows a Dukes' C cancer, then adjuvant chemotherapy is given.

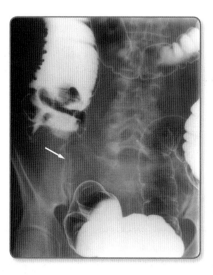

Figure 49.4 Barium enema showing an irregular filling defect (arrow) in the caecum, typical of a polypoid carcinoma.

3. F Ulcerative colitis

This young woman presents with clinical features of ulcerative colitis – several loose motions a day with blood and slime, lethargy, left-sided abdominal pain, raised inflammatory markers and anaemia. She requires a colonoscopy and biopsy to confirm the diagnosis. The colonoscopic findings are red, inflamed mucosa that bleeds easily on touch, purulent discharge, small ulcers and regenerative nodules called pseudopolyps. Biopsy shows increased inflammatory cells, numerous crypt abscesses and depletion of goblet cells. Barium enema shows complete loss of haustration, granular mucosa and narrow contracted 'lead-pipe' colon (**Figure 49.5**). The complications are shown in **Table 49.1**. Patients who have a stricture should be colonoscoped and biopsied for an underlying carcinoma. The mainstay of treatment is medical with surgical indications shown in **Table 49.2**. Proctocolectomy and ileostomy is one of the operations carried out.

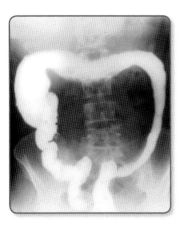

Figure 49.5 Barium enema showing complete loss of haustration, granular mucosa, and narrow contracted colon, likened to a 'lead-pipe'.

Table 49.1 Local and systemic complications of ulcerative colitis	
Local complications	**Systemic (remote or distant) complications**

• Acute dilatation or toxic megacolon (10%)
• Perforation (2%)
• Massive haemorrhage (3%)
• Benign stricture (10%)
• Inflammatory polyposis
• Carcinoma (5%)
• Anorectal complications (15%):
  – Fissure
  – Anorectal abscess and fistula
  – Rectovaginal fistula
	• Arthritis
	• Ankylosing spondylitis
	• Skin lesions :
	  – Erythema nodosum
	  – Pyoderma gangrenosum
	• Eye lesions
	• Liver and biliary tract disease:
	  – Sclerosing cholangitis
	• Stomatitis
	• Oesophagitis

Table 49.2 Indications for emergency/urgent and elective operations for ulcerative colitis	
Indications for emergency/urgent operations	Failure of medical treatment during an acute exacerbation Perforation Acute toxic megacolon Severe haemorrhage
Indications for elective operations	Intractability and chronic invalidism Risk (or actual development) of malignant change Retardation of growth and development Local anorectal complication Remote or systemic complications

4. B Acute small bowel obstruction

This patient has the hallmarks of distal small intestinal obstruction. Faeculent vomiting or aspirate is a sinister symptom. It denotes distal ileal obstruction where the bowel is incarcerated or about to strangulate. This patient has tell-tale signs of dehydration – sunken eyes, dry tongue and loss of skin turgor. The plain abdominal

X-ray (**Figure 49.1**) confirms the mechanical obstruction as shown by the valvulae conniventes of distended jejunum and characterless ileum. The CT scan (**Figure 49.2**) confirms the cause as an incarcerated obturator hernia. Clinically this diagnosis should be suspected with features of distal small intestinal obstruction in a female who complains of pain radiating down the inner side of the thigh to the knee. This is because the hernia presses along the geniculate branch of the obturator nerve and is referred to as Howship–Romberg sign. This patient should be resuscitated and should have an immediate operation.

5. D Crohn's disease

This woman, with altered bowel habit, abdominal pain, generally feeling unwell, suggestion of a mass in the right iliac fossa and erythema nodosum, has inflammatory bowel disease, Crohn's disease being the most likely. The perianal region should be thoroughly examined (**Figure 49.6**) for other manifestations such as fistulae.

Figure 49.7 shows gross narrowing of the terminal ileum as it enters the caecum – the classical 'string sign of Kantor'. It also shows strictures, mucosal fissuring with radiating spicules, skip lesions, entero-cutaneous fistula and cobblestone mucosa.

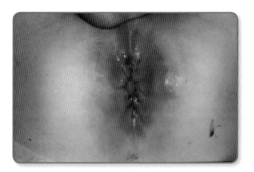

Figure 49.6 Perianal Crohn's disease.

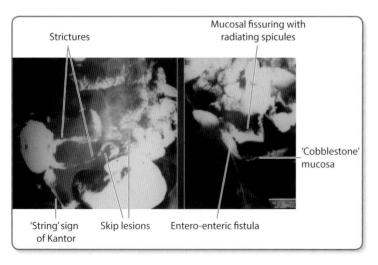

Strictures

Mucosal fissuring with radiating spicules

'Cobblestone' mucosa

'String' sign of Kantor

Skip lesions

Entero-enteric fistula

Figure 49.7 Barium enema showing radiological appearances in Crohn's disease.

The macroscopic pathology (**Figures 49.8**) shows aphthoid and serpiginous ulcers, strictured lumen, gross thickening from transmural inflammation and cobblestone mucosa from oedema between ulcers. The next investigation should be a colonoscopy to look for lesions in the large bowel which affects 30% of cases. Classical non-caseating giant cell granuloma is seen in 60% (**Figure 49.9**). Complications are shown in **Table 49.3**.

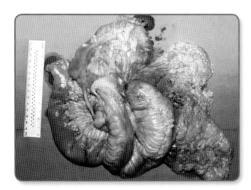

Figure 49.8 Right hemicolectomy specimen showing characteristic macroscopic features in Crohn's disease – thickened, oedematous ileum, mesenteric fat over-riding bowel wall, enteroenteric fistula.

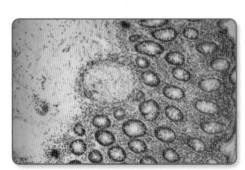

Figure 49.9 Histopathology in Crohn's disease: transmural inflammation with non-caseating granuloma.

Table 49.3 Local and distant complications of Crohn's disease	
Local complications	**Distant (metastatic) complications**

• External fistulae:
  – Enterocutaneous
  – Colocutaneous
  – Enterovaginal
  – Colovaginal
  – Perianal
• Internal fistulae:
  – Enteroenteric
  – Enterocolic
  – Enterovesical
  – Colovesical
• Abscesses
• Stricture
• Carcinoma
• Haemorrhage
• Perforation
• Toxic megacolon
	Infected
	Skin:
	• Pyoderma gangrenosum
	• Erythema nodosum
	Eyes:
	• Keratitis
	• Episcleritis
	Joints:
	• Septic arthritis
	• Septicaemia
	• Psoas abscess
	Non-infected
	• Polyarthropathy
	• Venous thrombosis
	• Physical retardation
	• Hepatobiliary disease
	• Ureteric strictures

6. A Acute appendicitis

This patient has some of the typical features of acute appendicitis – the visceral-somatic sequence of periumbilical colic settling in the right iliac fossa combined with nausea, vomiting and anorexia. The diarrhoea would suggest a pelvic position of the appendix. The classical signs in acute appendicitis are not present in all patients. They are: the 'pointing sign', when the patient points to the umbilicus as the site of origin of the pain and the right iliac fossa as the site where the pain has settled. The other signs described are: Rovsing's sign, the 'psoas sign' and the 'obturator sign'.

The diagnosis of acute appendicitis is clinical. Women pose a greater challenge to the diagnosis. Whilst there are scoring methods and imaging techniques available to come to an accurate diagnosis, in practice, a diagnostic laparoscopy gives a definitive diagnosis. Emergency appendicectomy, either laparoscopic or open, is the treatment of choice.

7. H Small bowel lymphoma

This patient, known to have coeliac disease, has developed colicky abdominal pain with increasing diarrhoea, a symptom distinctly different from her usual diarrhoea of coeliac disease. Patients with coeliac disease have an increased chance of developing small bowel lymphoma. Her colicky abdominal pain is suggestive of intermittent small bowel obstruction. The diagnosis can be confirmed by small bowel enema and CT scan. The treatment is small bowel resection and end-to-end anastomosis. Accurate staging of the disease is carried out followed by appropriate postoperative chemotherapy.

Often the diagnosis is made at laparotomy, carried out as an emergency for intestinal obstruction or perforation. Lymphoma supervening on coeliac disease is of the T-cell type. Another type, which is a part of non-Hodgkin's B-cell lymphoma, is an annular ulcerative lesion which may present as obstruction, haemorrhage and perforation. These tumours are referred to as mucosa-associated lymphoid tissue tumours (MALTomas).

8. A Acute diverticulitis

This 70-year-old woman has the clinical features of acute diverticulitis – pain in the left lower abdomen, passage of loose stools, fever, nausea and abdominal distension with tenderness, rigidity and rebound tenderness in the left iliac fossa. Moreover, on rectal examination a tender mass is felt in the pouch of Douglas through the rectal wall – the inflamed mass of sigmoid diverticulitis. Routine haematological tests should show polymorphonuclear leucocytosis and increase in inflammatory markers. After blood cultures are taken, she is treated with intravenous metronidazole and cefuroxime, intravenous fluids and analgesics. The diagnosis is confirmed by ultrasound or CT.

Once the patient has recovered, thorough imaging is carried out by barium enema and colonoscopy. A significant stricture may show on barium enema (**Figure 49.10**) . The complications are shown in **Table 49.4**. If the acute diverticulitis does not settle, it may result in a pericolic abscess.

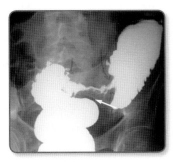

Figure 49.10 Barium enema showing stricture of sigmoid colon from diverticular disease (arrow).

Table 49.4 Presentation of diverticular disease		
Types of diverticular disease	**Notes**	**Complications**
Diverticulosis	Asymptomatic Symptomatic	Fistulae: • Colovesical • Coloenteric • Colocutaneous • Colovaginal • Colocolic
Painful diverticular disease	Due to excessive segmentation	Obstruction (mimics carcinoma) Abscess Perforation (purulent or faecal peritonitis)
Acute diverticulitis	Also referred to as left-sided appendicitis	Haemorrhage (almost always stops with conservative management)

9. F Colovesical fistula

This patient has repeated attacks of urinary tract infection and pneumaturia, a classical method of presentation of colovesical fistula. Some patients may complain of faecaluria. Colovesical fistula most commonly occurs from diverticular disease, other causes being Crohn's colitis and colorectal carcinoma.

This patient requires a barium enema to confirm the diagnosis of diverticular disease and gas in the urinary bladder (**Figure 49.11**) or rarely barium in the urinary bladder. A flexible sigmoidoscopy or colonoscopy and biopsy must be carried out to exclude an unsuspected carcinoma in the midst of the diverticular segment. Full colonoscopy may not be possible in view of the strictured sigmoid colon, a common occurrence.

Surgical treatment consists of resection of the fistulous tract and the affected segment of colon, closure of the hole in the bladder and end-to-end colocolic anastomosis.

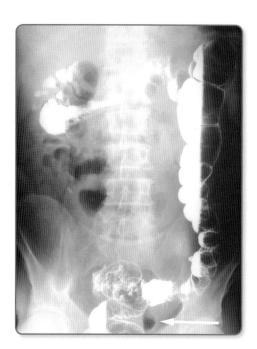

Figure 49.11 Barium enema showing air in the urinary bladder (arrow).

10. B Acute large bowel obstruction

This patient has the features of acute closed-loop large bowel obstruction – colicky abdominal pain with persisting dull ache in between colics, increasing constipation, peripheral abdominal distension and a hollow rectum. As he has not vomited, his problem is one of closed-loop obstruction where there is a competent ileocaecal valve with no distension of the small bowel. With a history of increasing constipation, the cause should be presumed to be a left colonic carcinoma until proven otherwise.

This patient needs to be resuscitated. Once stabilised, the site and cause of obstruction is established. Plain abdominal X-rays (**Figure 49.12**) followed by CT colonography or lower gastrointestinal endoscopy are carried out.

Once optimised and the cause and site of obstruction established, definitive treatment is instituted. Of several choices, stenting the growth with subsequent resection is one of them. A Hartmann's operation or a subtotal colectomy with ileorectal anastomosis are others.

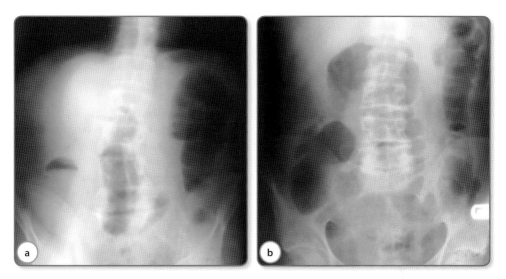

Figure 49.12 Plain abdominal X-rays showing acute closed-loop large bowel obstruction. (a) X-ray taken in an upright position, which reveals multiple fluid levels. (b) X-ray taken in a supine position, which shows that the caecum, transverse colon and descending colon are massively distended.

11. G Familial adenomatous polyposis

This young man with loose stools combined with blood and mucus and colicky abdominal pain with a family history of large bowel cancer should arouse the suspicion of familial adenomatous polyposis. The fact that his father died at a young age of cancer and he was under annual colonoscopic surveillance in his previous place of residence since he was a teenager, makes the diagnosis very probable. He needs urgent imaging with full colonoscopy and a barium enema with genetic studies carried out. An oesophagogastroduodenoscopy is also carried out to exclude polyps in the duodenum and a barium meal and follow through to detect any small bowel polyps.

If the diagnosis is established the patient should be offered surgical treatment in the form of:

- Colectomy and ileorectal anastomosis
- Restorative proctocolectomy with ileoanal anastomosis.

The condition is inherited as an autosomal dominant inherited disease from mutation of the adenomatous polyposis colic gene.

12. I Ischaemic colitis

This patient suffers from ischaemic colitis. In chronic cases, the underlying pathology is usually a thrombotic episode that allows collateral circulation to form resulting in fibrosis and stricture. Plain abdominal X-ray or contrast imaging may show 'thumbprinting' with narrowing of the affected bowel. Confirmation is by colonoscopy which would show heaped-up, oedematous, bluish purple mucosa with ulceration and contact bleeding. Rarely, the condition progresses to gangrene or to a late stricture when a limited resection needs to be carried out. Three types of ischaemic colitis are recognised: gangrenous type, transient ischaemic type, type with stricture formation. Conservative supportive treatment results in recovery in the vast majority.

13. C Anal carcinoma

This patient says that he can feel a painful lump that is constantly present and bleeds should arouse the suspicion that he does not suffer from piles. Moreover, as a renal transplant patient he has a 100 times increased risk of developing anal carcinoma. Other predisposing causes are human papilloma virus infection, anal intraepithelial neoplasia, HIV infection and anal sexual practices. The physical findings of an ulcerated mass with raised everted edges are clinically diagnostic of squamous cell carcinoma. The disease should be confirmed, staged and treated.

Confirmation is carried out by biopsy under general anaesthetic. At the same time an examination under anaesthetic, which is a useful method of clinical staging, is carried out. A CT scan and MRI should complete the staging. Chemoradiotherapy is the mainstay of treatment.

14. H Fistula-in-ano

This patient, who is a sufferer from Crohn's disease, has perianal symptoms suggestive of fistula-in-ano which has occurred as a complication of a burst perianal abscess 6 weeks ago.

He now needs the fistula thoroughly evaluated. Clinical assessment of the function of the anal sphincter by resting tone and voluntary squeeze is made; this is complemented by more accurate assessment by anal manometry and endoanal ultrasound. Finally, an MRI and examination under anaesthesia using a probe is essential to look for secondary extensions. Surgical treatments will depend on whether the internal opening is above the anal sphincter (high anal fistula) or below the anal sphincter (low anal fistula).

A high anal fistula will require a staged procedure of fistulotomy and use of a Seton. while a low anal fistula may be treated by fistulectomy. The patient also requires immunotherapy.

Chapter 50

Endocrine and breast

Questions

Theme: The thyroid gland

Options for Questions 1–3:

A Anaplastic carcinoma
B Colloid goitre
C Differentiated thyroid cancer
D Diffuse toxic goitre (Grave's disease)
E Multinodular goitre
F Thyroid incidentaloma
G Toxic multinodular goitre

For each of the following situations, select the single most likely diagnosis. Each option may be used once, more than once or not at all.

1. A 27-year-old woman presents with weight loss and palpitations of 2 months' duration. She has a good appetite and a preference for cold weather. Recently her periods have been irregular. She has also noticed a swelling occupying most of the front of her neck. On examination she looks restless and excitable with a regular pulse rate of 98 bpm. She has a diffuse goitre which feels warm and vascular with a bruit.

2. A 32-year-old woman presents with a solitary thyroid nodule of 2 months' duration. On clinical examination a 2 cm nodule is found in the left lobe. She is euthyroid. Ultrasound demonstrates a mixed solid and cystic lesion. US-guided fine-needle aspiration cytology from the solid part of the lesion reads 'malignancy cannot be excluded'.

3. A 60-year-old woman with a large multinodular goitre of 20 years' duration complains of hoarseness of voice, dysphagia and dyspnoea lasting 6 weeks. She also has stridor and a sensation of heaviness and choking in her throat.

Theme: Hypercalcaemia/hyperparathyroidism

Options for Questions 4–6:

A Familial hypocalciuric hypercalcaemia	**E** Parathyroid hyperplasia
B Hyperthyroidism	**F** Secondary hyperparathyroidism
C Hypercalcaemia of malignancy	**G** Sarcoidosis
D Parathyroid adenoma	**H** Tertiary hyperparathyroidism

For each of the following situations, select the single most likely diagnosis. Each option may be used once, more than once or not at all.

4. A 72-year-old woman presents with marked thirst, aches and pains all over her body and a feeling of nausea. Routine blood biochemistry shows a serum calcium of 2.9 mmol/L. She underwent a mastectomy 6 years ago for carcinoma.

5. A 30-year-old man complains of lethargy, abdominal pain and generally feeling unwell for the past couple of months. He has had two typical attacks of ureteric colic, once on each side. On routine biochemistry his serum calcium is found to be 3.1 mmol/L.

6. A 50-year-old woman who suffered from chronic renal failure for many years underwent a renal transplant 1 year ago. She felt very well after her transplant for a few months. Thereafter, she started feeling lethargic and generally unwell although her renal function remained stable. Her serum calcium is 2.9 mmol/L, and she has a raised serum phosphate.

Theme: The adrenals/neuroendocrine tumours

Options for Questions 7–9:

A	Addison's disease	D	Gastrinoma
B	Conn's syndrome	E	Multiple endocrine neoplasia
C	Cushing's syndrome	F	Pheochromocytoma

For each of the following situations, select the single most likely diagnosis. Each option may be used once, more than once or not at all.

7. A 38-year-old man has been admitted as an emergency with acute haematemesis. After resuscitation, an oesophagogastroduodenoscopy (OGD) showed a gastric ulcer at the gastro-oesophageal junction with hypertrophied gastric rugae. He has also had intermittent diarrhoea for several months. He underwent closure of a perforated duodenal ulcer 8 months ago. For some years he has had indigestion and heartburn for which he has been on proton pump inhibitors (PPI).

8. A 38-year-old man presents with paroxysmal headaches, palpitations and sweating. He has attacks of dyspnoea and bitterly complains of feeling generally unwell and weak. His GP has noted that he has intermittent episodes of labile hypertension.

9. A 40-year-old woman presents with recurrent attacks of ureteric colic that have been treated conservatively. Since the age of 30 years, she has been diagnosed with duodenal ulcers, which are also treated conservatively and she has been on continuous medical treatment. Recently, she has been embarrassed by the onset of milk secretion from her breasts. She is found to have hypercalcaemia.

Theme: The breast

Options for Questions 10–12:

A   Abscess
B   Aberration of normal
    development and involution
    (ANDI)
C   Carcinoma

D   Fat necrosis
E   Fibroadenoma
F   Mondor's disease
G   Phyllodes tumour

For each of the following situations, select the single most likely diagnosis. Each option may be used once, more than once or not at all.

10. A 21-year-old woman who is 5 weeks' post-partum complains of a painful lump in her right breast which came on 2 days ago after breast feeding her new-born baby. She has throbbing pain over a red tender lump deep to her areola. On examination, she has a firm, red, tender lump extending to the lower outer quadrant of her right breast.

11. A 38-year-old woman complains of generalised pain in her right breast, often associated with her periods. She sometimes feels a lump, the size of which tends to vary. On examination, she has a tender lump in the upper outer quadrant of her right breast.

12. A 55-year-old woman complains of a lump in her left breast that appeared about 4 months ago and has been rapidly growing. It is painful. On examination, she has a mobile, slightly tender, 12 cm irregular lump, the surface of which is bosselated with the overlying skin stretched and about to ulcerate.

Answers

1. D Diffuse toxic goitre (Grave's disease)

This woman has diffuse toxic goitre. This condition presents with symptoms which are protean in nature due to a raised level of thyroid hormones; simultaneously there is a diffuse enlargement of the thyroid gland (**Tables 50.1** and **50.2**). This occurs mostly in women between the ages of 20 and 40 and is the result of excessive circulating thyroxine. Almost 75% have eye signs but only a minority develop exophthalmos. Myopathy and eye signs such as ophthalmoplegia may be seen.

The diagnosis is confirmed by performing thyroid function tests which show a reduced TSH and increased T_3 and T_4; an ultrasound will show a diffuse enlargement of the thyroid gland. Treatment is with antithyroid drugs: carbimazole and propylthyouracil often supplemented by β-blockers to combat cardiovascular effects. Surgery, total or near total thyroidectomy, is considered for pressure symptoms, cosmesis and failure of drug compliance.

Table 50.1 Clinical features of primary thyrotoxicosis					
General	**Cardiovascular system**	**CNS and eyes**	**GI tract**	**Skin**	**Hormones**
Weight loss Fatigue Sweating Heat intolerance Smooth goitre Thrill and bruit over goitre Myopathy	Palpitations Tachychardia Atrial fibrillation Vasodilation	Tremor Anxiety Emotional lability Psychosis Agitation Exophalmos Lid lag Chemosis Proptosis	Diarrhoea Increased appetite Vomiting	Hot, moist palms Pre-tibial myxoedema Thyroid acropachy Onycholysis	Oligomenorrhoea Amenorrhoea Reduced libido
CNS, central nervous system; GI, gastrointestinal.					

Table 50.2 Clinical diagnoses of thyrotoxicosis		
Primary thyrotoxicosis	**Toxic multinodular goitre**	**Toxic nodule**
Goitre and hyperthyroidism appear together Female:male ratio = 10:1 Age group 20-40 years Due to TSH antibodies IgG Predominantly CNS and eye features Thyroid uniformly enlarged, vascular with thrill and bruit	Hyperthyroidism supervenes on a long-standing goitre Goitre is nodular Age group > 40 years Predominantly affects CVS Due to autonomous overproduction of thyroxine	Solitary over-active nodule Female:male ratio = 9:1 60% present with the nodule 40% present because of toxicity Diagnosed by isotope scan
CNS, central nervous system; CVS, cardiovascular system; TSH, thyroid-stimulating hormone.		

2. C Differentiated thyroid cancer

This young woman, presenting with an euthyroid solitary nodule, has a differentiated thyroid cancer (papillary or follicular or one of their variants; see **Table 50.3**) unless otherwise proven. Ultrasound of the nodule shows a solid and cystic lesion whilst the result of the fine-needle aspiration cytology was equivocal. In this situation, this patient requires a hemithyroidectomy to obtain proper histology. Before this is done, the patient should have a chest X-ray and MRI of the neck to detect lymphadenopathy.

The facility to do a frozen section, if available, is useful. This is because if the frozen section show a follicular carcinoma, then the surgeon should proceed to total thyroidectomy. If it shows a papillary carcinoma, the appropriate surgery can be carried out (total or hemi-thyroidectomy with node dissection) depending upon the scoring of the cancer. Follicular carcinoma can only be diagnosed in the presence of vascular and capsular invasion, hence the need for histology.

Table 50.3 Classification of thyroid neoplasms		
Benign	**Malignant**	
Follicular adenoma	Primary	Secondary (3–4%)
Colloid nodule		
Cyst	Papipallary carcinoma (60%)	Breast
	Follicular carcinoma (20%)	GI tract
	Anaplastic carcinoma (10%)	Kidney
	Medullary carcinoma (5%)	Local infiltration
	Lymphoma (5%)	

3. A Anaplastic carcinoma

This woman has the typical features of an anaplastic (undifferentiated) carcinoma – a long-standing goitre with recent onset of tracheal compression and recurrent laryngeal nerve infiltration. This type of thyroid cancer constitutes 10% of thyroid cancers and occurs most often in areas of endemic goitre. It spreads by local infiltration, lymphatics and blood stream. The diagnosis is confirmed by fine-needle aspiration cytology or core biopsy; the tumour shows spindle-shaped and giant cells with polypoid nuclei and numerous mitoses. After staging the disease with a CT scan and chest X-ray, external beam radiotherapy is the treatment of choice. Respiratory embarrassment may require tracheal decompression by isthmusectomy. The prognosis is extremely poor, with the majority of patients succumbing to the disease within 6 months of the diagnosis being made.

4. C Hypercalcaemia of malignancy

This woman, who underwent a mastectomy for carcinoma 6 years ago, now has generalised features of hypercalcaemia. This is a paraneoplastic complication arising from skeletal metastases. It affects 10% of all cancer patients. In a minority hypercalcaemia may occur without any bony metastases. The cause of malignant hypercalcaemia is the secretion of a parathormone-like peptide by the tumour. It also occurs from osteoclastic activity; other causes may be the production of prostaglandins, vitamin D metabolites, tumour growth factor-α (TGF-α) and tumour growth factor-β (TGF-β). The treatment is to palliate the patient by rehydration and the use of bisphosphonates.

5. D Parathyroid adenoma

This man has the features of hypercalcaemia. The classical description of 'stones, moans, abdominal groans and psychic moans' are an exception rather than a rule. Most often this condition is discovered by hypercalcaemia on routine biochemical screening for some unrelated complaint. Patients may develop symptoms from a peptic ulcer or suffer from recurrent attacks of pancreatitis, acute or chronic. Clinically usually there are no signs.

These patients need to be thoroughly investigated. Corrected serum calcium level is calculated; if elevated, serum parathormone level is assayed. A raised serum calcium in the presence of elevated parathyroid hormone confirms primary hyperparathyroidism. The cause in 90% of such patients is a parathyroid adenoma. Next the adenoma should be localised by performing US and technetium-labelled sestamibi scan. The latter is particularly important to exclude an adenoma in an ectopic gland such as in the mediastinum. Once localised, the adenoma is excised.

6. H Tertiary hyperparathyroidism

This patient who has had a renal transplant after suffering from chronic renal failure for many years has tertiary hyperparathyroidism. This condition arises after many years of chronic renal failure resulting in hypocalcaemia and increased serum phosphate. This causes increased secretion of PTH resulting in functional hyperplasia of the parathyroids. Normally the condition is reversed after renal transplantation.

However, occasionally hyperfunction continues in an autonomous manner even after renal transplantation. This results in continued parathyroid hyperplasia. In such instances one or more of the glands may become autonomous producing an adenoma. This requires full assessment followed by parathyroidectomy for the adenoma or hyperplasia, depending on the case.

7. D Gastrinoma

This patient has a history of recurrent peptic ulcer complications (perforation, bleeding) along with indigestion, for which he has been on PPIs. The patient shows a clear ulcer diathesis in the stomach and duodenum. Such patients are also prone to developing peptic ulcer in atypical sites. The cause is a non-β cell tumour of the pancreas called a gastrinoma, first described in 1955 by Zollinger and Ellison. These tumours account for a fifth of pancreatic endocrine tumours (PETs) and the vast majority are situated within the gastrinoma triangle formed above by the junction of the cystic duct and the common bile duct, on the lower right by the junction of the second and third parts of the duodenum and the lower left by the junction of the body and neck of the pancreas (**Figure 50.1**). The characteristic feature is recurrent peptic ulceration particularly at atypical sites. More than 60% are malignant by the time the diagnosis is made. Clinical manifestations (emergency or elective) of peptic ulcer disease and gastro-oesophageal reflux disease (GORD) is the presentation in more than three-quarters of these patients. Diarrhoea is a common symptom due to excessive gastric acid secretion.

Diagnosis is made when a gastric pH is below 2.5 and a serum gastrin concentration above 1000 pg/mL (normal <100 pg/mL). Preoperative localisation of pancreatic gastrinomas are made by EUS whereas dudodenal gastrinomas, because of their small size, are difficult to localise preoperatively. Treatment is surgical removal for tumours that are benign or have not metastasised.

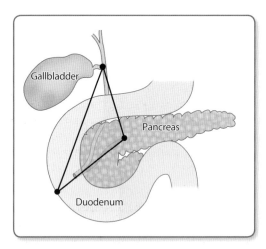

Figure 50.1 The gastrinoma triangle.

8. F Pheochromocytoma

This patient has the features of a pheochromocytoma – labile hypertension with palpitation, sweating and headache resulting from episodic catecholamine release from the tumour. This may be precipitated by physical activity. Undetected for a long time, there may be harmful effects of catecholamine on the heart collectively referred to catecholamine cardiomyopathy. 10% of these tumours are bilateral, 10% occur in children, 10% are extra-adrenal, 10% are malignant and 10% are inherited.

Initially the biochemical diagnosis is made by two separate 24-hour urinary levels of metanephrines, catecholamines and vanillylmandelic acid. This is followed by localisation of the tumour. For this, MRI is the investigation of choice particularly to localise a tumour in an extra-adrenal site. It is also a safer investigation than a CT scan because use of contrast during CT may provoke a hypertensive crisis. The overall management has to be a team effort between the cardiologist, anaesthetist, surgeon and radiologist.

9. E Multiple endocrine neoplasia

This woman has hypercalcaemia, peptic ulcer and galactorrhoea. This should alert one to the diagnosis of multiple endocrine neoplasia syndrome 1 consisting of primary hyperparathyroidism (pHPT), gastrinoma (pancreatic endocrine tumour) and a prolactinoma (pituitary tumour). Hypercalcaemic symptoms are usually the initial presentation. This is due to parathyroid hyperplasia for which she needs to be investigated. A gastrinoma producing Zollinger–Ellison syndrome is the cause of her recurrent and refractory peptic ulcer.

Serum gastrin estimation and the secretin test followed by localisation of the tumour within the gastrinoma triangle are done. CT scan, MRI, and endoscopic and intraoperative ultrasound are the localisation techniques. The pituitary tumour is a prolactin-secreting microadenoma (prolactinoma). As it is a small tumour, it does not produce pressure symptoms but causes endocrine dysfunction; in some patients there may be no endocrine disturbance. Diagnosis is confirmed by elevated blood prolactin levels and localisation done by MRI.

10. A Abscess

This patient has lactational breast abscess. It usually spreads from the infant who harbours staphylococci in the nasopharynx. The causative organism is *Staphylococcus aureus*. Infection usually starts from a sore and a cracked nipple with lactiferous ducts becoming blocked by epithelial debris causing stasis. The organism causes clotting of milk with the organisms multiplying within the clot. The affected segment of the breast shows the classical signs of acute inflammation with the pain being severe and throbbing. A cellulitis forms first which is then replaced by an abscess.

Antibiotic treatment during the cellulitic stage may prevent progression to an abscess. If an abscess has formed, aspiration (repeated if necessary under ultrasound guidance) is performed; this may enable the patient to continue breast feeding. If the condition does not settle in spite of repeated aspiration under antibiotic cover, incision and drainage should be carried out.

11. B Aberration of normal development and involution (ANDI)

This woman suffers from aberration of normal development and involution (ANDI), a term coined by Cardiff Breast Clinic to encompass several terms used in the past to denote various aspects of benign breast disease such as fibroadenosis, chronic mastitis, benign mammary dysplasia, cystic mastopathy and fibrocystic disease. This condition affects one-third of women between the ages of 20 and 50 years. It occurs as a result of the effect of cyclical patterns of female hormones on breast tissue. This is influenced by menstrual cycle, pregnancy, the contraceptive pill and hormone replacement therapy. The clinical changes are a reflection of these hormonal changes on the tissues of the breast – lobules, ducts, stroma and epithelium lined by apocrine cells. Cysts form wherein the fluid is thin and dark giving a blue hue – hence the term 'blue-dome' cyst. The management should follow the usual triple assessment.

12. G Phyllodes tumour

This woman has a phyllodes tumour also called serocystic disease of Brodie (described by Sir Benjamin Brodie in 1840) and cystosarcoma phyllodes (although it is not cystic and very rarely sarcomatous). The name of the tumour is derived from the Greek word 'phyllo' meaning 'leaf' and macroscopically the tumour has a leaf-like appearance. The clinical features in this woman may easily be mistaken for an advanced carcinoma. It is a benign tumour which may have a very low malignant risk, the latter showing hypercellular stroma. Some tumours are termed borderline malignant.

Imaging by mammography will show a well circumscribed or lobulated lesion; US shows hyperechoic areas within a hypoechoic mass. Treatment in the majority is enucleation or wide local excision depending upon the size. Mastectomy may be necessary when the tumour is massive or in case of malignancy.

Chapter 51

Vascular surgery

Questions

Theme: Arterial disorders of the lower limbs

Options for questions 1–3:

A	Aortoiliac occlusive disease	E	Femoropopliteal occlusive disease
B	Critical limb ischaemia	F	Popliteal aneurysm
C	Femoral artery aneurysm	G	Thromboangiitis obliterans
D	Femoropopliteal embolism		

For each of the following cases select the single most likely diagnosis. Each option may be used once, more than once or none at all.

1. A 62-year-old man, a heavy smoker, presents with aching pain in his left buttock and thigh of 6 months' duration. This comes on after walking 200 metres although the distance is less when he tries to walk faster or uphill. On examination, he has a much weaker femoral pulse on the left side. A systolic bruit can be heard in the left ilia fossa. He is unable to do his work as a self-employed builder.

2. A 45-year-old woman presents with a pulsating mass in her right groin of 3 months' duration. She had arterial blood samples taken from the right groin over several weeks whilst in the ITU. The lump appeared a few weeks after discharge from the ITU. She has marked wasting of her thigh muscles.

3. A 76-year-old man, a smoker for over 60 years, complains of severe, constant pain in his right lower limb for the past 3 weeks. The pain is worse at night and he tries to get relief by sleeping in a chair. On examination, the skin is shiny, the veins are guttered, the skin is hairless, without any pulses below the femoral; one of his toes has become black.

Theme: Arterial disorders of the abdomen

Options for questions 4–6:

A   Abdominal aortic aneurysm
B   Abdominal compartment syndrome
C   Ischaemic colitis
D   Mesenteric ischaemia
E   Renal artery stenosis

For each of the following cases select the single most likely diagnosis. Each option may be used once, more than once or none at all.

4.   A 31-year-old woman complains of headaches, giddiness, dyspnoea and an episode of epistaxis over the last month. Her blood pressure is 150/100 mmHg. Anti-hypertensive treatment by her GP has made very little effect. A systolic bruit is present in the left lumbar area.

5.   A 72-year-old woman presents as an emergency complaining of sudden onset of very severe abdominal pain with vomiting and bloody diarrhoea. The pain is generalised with abdominal tenderness and rigidity. She has atrial fibrillation following a myocardial infarction 4 weeks ago.

6.   A 66-year-old man complains of throbbing backache for 6 weeks. This is associated with abdominal pain and the patient complains of a 'feeling of thumping heart beat in his stomach'. Examination reveals a pulsatile mass in the epigastrium.

Theme: Arterial disorders of the head and neck

Options for questions 7–9:

A   Berry aneurysm
B   Carotid artery stenosis
C   Carotid body tumour
D   Cirsoid aneurysm
E   Subclavian steal syndrome
F   Thoracic outlet syndrome

For each of the following cases select the single most likely diagnosis. Each option may be used once, more than once or none at all.

7.   A 45-year-old woman complains of pain in the distal part of her left hand which feels cold and tips of the fingers look blue and ischaemic. Her symptoms disable her as she is left-handed. She has a weak radial pulse which becomes weaker on hyperabduction and hyperextension of the arm. There is a systolic bruit in the left supraclavicular area.

8.   A 66-year-old man who suffers from angina complains of sudden episodes of blindness in his right eye which lasts for a few seconds. It feels as though a curtain falls momentarily in front of his eye and makes him feel giddy and at the same time there is weakness of his left upper limb and temporary loss of speech. Examination reveals a systolic bruit in the right anterior triangle of the neck.

9.   A 53-year-old man, a home decorator by profession, complains of attacks of giddiness and fainting while doing his work particularly painting ceilings and walls when he stretches his right upper limb. The feeling subsides once he stops stretching his arm.

Theme: Venous disorders

Options for questions 10–12:

A Chronic venous insufficiency	**C** Klippel–Trénaunay syndrome
B Deep vein thrombosis	**D** Varicose veins

For each of the following cases select the single most likely diagnosis. Each option may be used once, more than once or none at all.

10. A 27-year-old woman, a mother of three, complains of heaviness in her left leg which she has had for almost 3 years. For the last 2 years on the inner side of the leg she noticed the appearance of a large vein that has been getting larger and causing her distress from the cosmetic point of view. She seeks advice both for relief of her symptom and cosmesis.

11. A 76-year-old man presents with an ulcer on the medial side of his left ankle which has been present for almost 11 months. It started a few years ago with a swollen lower limb which in due course became hard and then produced an ulcer which has not healed so far. He has chronic pain in his limb.

12. A 53-year-old woman underwent an emergency Hartmann's operation for perforated diverticular disease. Two days after her operation she complains of pain in her right calf. On examination, she is pyrexial, has a swollen, tender right calf with shiny skin.

Answers

1. A Aortoiliac occlusive disease

This patient who has thigh and buttock claudication has the typical features of aortoiliac occlusive disease due to atherosclerosis. He has a limited claudication distance which is affecting his livelihood. Therefore, intervention needs to be carried out while at the same time he should be strongly advised to give up smoking. As intervention is planned, an angiogram is carried out.

Intervention should be considered when the three Ls are affected – limb threatened, livelihood threatened, life-style affected. When intervention (surgical or radiological) is to be performed, an angiogram is mandatory to show the site, length and number of obstructions and run off. Once, during the angiogram the length of obstruction is seen, the vascular team can decide whether to do an interventional procedure such as percutaneous transluminal subintimal angioplasty with stenting or an open operation such as a bypass procedure.

2. C Femoral artery aneurysm

This patient has an aneurysm of the femoral artery (**Figure 51.1**) brought on by repeated trauma caused by needle punctures. The aneurysm is partly thrombosed. This is a false aneurysm. This has resulted in wasting of the thigh muscles. The patient needs an angiogram followed by repair. This patient underwent exploration of the femoral artery and revascularisation using her own reversed long saphenous vein.

The most common cause of femoral artery aneurysm is atherosclerosis, usually being a part of a generalised arterial dilatation, the other causes being trauma, infection due to injection of drugs and false aneurysms that occur at the site of a graft anastomosis. The majority are symptomless but may be a source of distal emboli. The popliteal artery is the second most common site of aneurysms, causing 70% of all peripheral aneurysms.

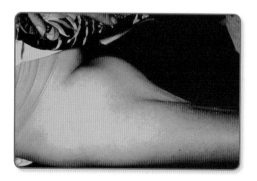

Figure 51.1 Femoral artery aneurysm.

3. B Critical limb ischaemia

This patient has critical limb ischaemia which is very important to recognise because if the limb is not revascularised immediately the patient will lose the limb. It is mandatory to exclude diabetes. Although the condition of critical ischaemia should be clinically obvious (**Figure 51.2**), the general consensus on critical limb ischaemia enunciates certain criteria to define the condition:

- Persistently recurring rest pain requiring regular analgesia for >2 weeks
- Ulceration or gangrene of the foot or toes plus ankle systolic pressure <50 mmHg
- Toe systolic blood pressure <30 mmHg
- Absence of arterial pulsations in big toe
- Marked structural or functional changes of the skin capillaries in the affected area

This patient should undergo an angiogram and attempt at limb salvage should be made at the earliest. In view of co-morbid conditions, extra-anatomic bypass grafts (axillo-femoral or femoro-femoral) may be necessary.

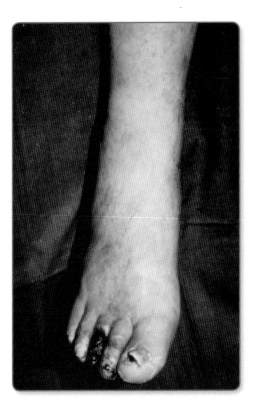

Figure 51.2 Critical limb ischaemia.

4. E Renal artery stenosis

This young patient has uncontrolled hypertension with a systolic bruit in the region of her kidney. She has renal artery stenosis causing renovascular hypertension. It can also result in renal failure in the long term. Renovascular hypertension can be due to one of two causes:

- Atheromatous renovascular disease: occurs in those over 50 years; renal ostium is involved in 85%. It is the cause in almost two-thirds of cases
- Fibromuscular hyperplasia accounts for about a third. It occurs in young women and the ostium is not involved

The diagnosis of renovascular hypertension must be suspected if there is a relatively short history of symptoms and there is presence of an abdominal bruit. An angiogram should be carried out to find out the cause. The treatment is percutaneous transluminal angioplasty with stenting. Aortorenal vein bypass is the open surgical treatment. The various causes of surgically remediable hypertension are shown in **Table 51.1**.

Table 51.1 Surgically remediable causes of hypertension			
Renal	**Vascular**	**Endocrine**	**Miscellaneous**
Renal artery stenosis Atherosclerosis Fibromuscular hyperplasia	Coarctation of aorta	Phaechromocytoma Cushing's syndrome Conn's syndrome	Paraneoplastic syndroms Hypernephroma

5. D Mesenteric ischaemia

This patient has acute mesenteric ischaemia, the most likely cause being superior mesenteric artery (SMA) embolism. In view of the sudden onset, with the patient having had a recent myocardial infarction and has atrial fibrillation (AF), embolism rather than thrombosis is the most likely cause. In the clinical presentation of ischaemic disease, the symptoms are out of proportion to the signs, the patient's pain being excruciating while the signs of rigidity and peritonism are less marked and delayed. Vomiting and bloody diarrhoea follow. Occlusion at the origin of the SMA is usually from thrombosis whilst emboli arrest at the origin of the middle colic artery. Ischaemia of the inferior mesenteric artery produce minimal symptoms because of the copious collateral circulation.

Confirmation is by mesenteric angiography followed by embolectomy, thrombolysis or bowel resection which may be extensive and may require parenteral nutrition in the long term.

6. A Abdominal aortic aneurysm

This patient has typical features of abdominal aortic aneurysm [AAA; **Figure 51.3**)] the throbbing backache being caused by the AAA eroding into the front of the lumbar vertebra. 95% of AAA are infrarenal and atherosclerotic in origin. They present either as an emergency from a leak or rupture or electively from a variety of symptoms or asymptomatically picked up at aneurysm screening. The presentation of AAA is shown in **Figure 51.4.**

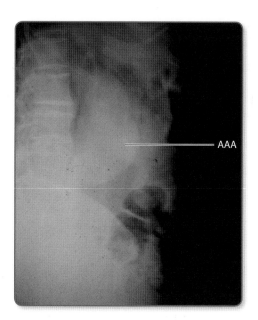

Figure 51.3 Plain abdominal X-ray lateral view showing abdominal aortic aneurysm.

AAA

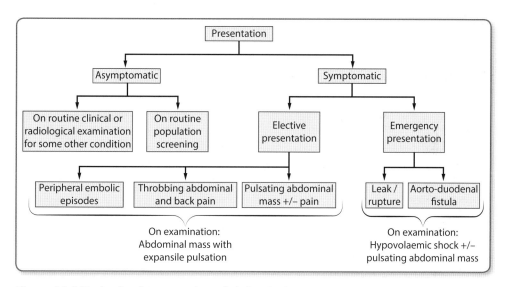

Figure 51.4 Methods of presentation of abdominal aortic aneurysm.

The elective patient should be investigated. The initial investigation is an ultrasound to assess the size. Asymptomatic patients whose AAA is <5.5 cm in diameter, are observed by US periodically. Symptomatic patients or those whose aneurysm is >5.5 cm should be investigated with a view to intervention, their general condition permitting, either by open surgery or endovascular repair (EVAR). An algorithm for investigating an AAA that presents electively is given in **Table 51.2**.

Table 51.2 Investigations for AAA	
Routine	**Specific (when endovascular repair is considered)**
Haematology Biochemistry Chest X-ray ECG Pulmonary function tests Echocardiography	Ultrasound (US) scan CT scan Contrast enhanced spiral CT MR angiography

In asymptomatic patients, if the US scan shows the aneurysm to be <5.5 cm, the patient is observed. In symptomatic patients or those with size ≥5.5 cm surgical intervention is advised, in which case the above investigations are carried out.

7. F Thoracic outlet syndrome

This patient has features of thoracic outlet/inlet syndrome. The condition typically has vascular, neurological and local clinical features which are listed in **Figure 51.5**. Whilst one of them predominate as the presenting feature, various anatomical abnormalities may be the cause of the compression:

- a complete cervical rib
- a partial rib to which is attached a fibrous band
- an incomplete rib ending in an irregular bony lump
- a sharp edge of the scalenus anterior muscle
- a complete fibrous band extending from the C7 transverse process to the first rib

The vascular features may be due to obstruction of the subclavian vessels, arterial obstruction causing ischaemia, venous obstruction causing swelling of the limb, or axillary vein thrombosis. Neurological features may be due to compression of the lower cord of brachial plexus (C8 and T1) mainly affecting the ulnar nerve. Disabling clinical features will require surgery.

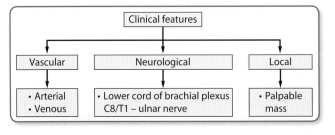

Figure 51.5 Clinical features of thoracic outlet/inlet syndrome.

8. B Carotid artery stenosis

This patient has typical features of carotid artery stenosis as evidenced by his presentation of transient ischaemic attacks (TIAs), amaurosis fugax and reversible intermittent neurological deficit (RIND). The presence of a systolic bruit on the carotid artery clinically confirms the diagnosis. The degree of stenosis should be assessed by a duplex scan followed by a digital subtraction carotid angiography **(Figure 51.6)** with a view to surgical intervention.

Symptomatic patients and those who are asymptomatic with a stenosis of more than 70% should be considered for operation of carotid endarterectomy or carotid angioplasty and stenting. The latter procedure is reserved for those considered unsuitable for open operation such as: a high carotid bifurcation, symptomatic restenosis following endarterectomy, or those who have had previous radiotherapy to the neck. Those with coronary artery disease may be considered for both procedures at the same time. A carotid body tumour **(Figure 51.7)** can also give rise to similar symptoms.

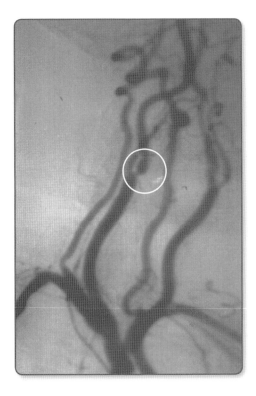

Figure 51.6 Right internal carotid artery stenosis with post-stenotic dilatation (circled).

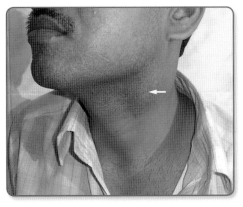

Figure 51.7 Carotid body tumour.

9. E Subclavian steal syndrome

This patient suffers from subclavian steal syndrome. This condition results when there is obstruction (stenosis or occlusion) of the subclavian artery proximal to the origin of the vertebral artery. As a result, when the arm is being used excessively, resulting in increased workload, there is greater demand of blood; this is met by retrograde flow of blood from the ipsilateral vertebral artery causing vertebrobasilar insufficiency. The subclavian artery thus stealing blood from the vertebrobasilar system to supply the distal territory of the obstructed subclavian artery (**Figure 51.8**). This reversal of flow causes ischaemia to the brain supplied by the basilar artery resulting in dizziness, vertigo, syncope, ataxia, visual changes, dysarthria, weakness and sensory disturbances.

An arterial duplex scan and CT angiogram helps to confirm the diagnosis. PTA with stenting should be the first option of treatment.

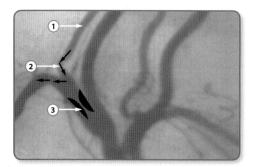

Figure 51.8 Subclavian steal syndrome. ① Vertebral artery. ② Blood being stolen by the subclavian artery from the vertebral artery. ③ Occlusion of the subclavian artery proximal to the vertebral artery.

10. D Varicose veins

This young mother of three has primary varicose veins of the long saphenous system. The acronym CEAP is used to classify (**Table 51.3**) and assess progression and indication for intervention in venous disorders (Clinical, aEtiology, Anatomy, Pathophysiology). The long saphenous vein (LSV) is the longest superficial vein arising anterior to the anterior edge of the medial malleolus and terminating into the anterior surface of the femoral vein after perforating the cribriform fascia in the femoral triangle.

This patient should be clinically examined to determine the anatomical distribution of the varicose veins and the presence of saphenofemoral incompetence. Varicose veins in the medial thigh and calf suggest long saphenous incompetence whereas anterolateral thigh and calf varicosities indicate isolated incompetence of the proximal anterolateral long saphenous tributary. Prior to any intervention, a Duplex scan should be carried out. The 'C' component of CEAP is widely used as a guide for intervention.

Component	Description
	Table 51.3 Description of CEAP classification
C0	No evidence of venous disease
C1	Telangiectasia or reticular veins
C2	Simple varicose veins
C3	Ankle oedema of venous origin
C4a	Skin pigmentation or eczema
C4b	Lipodermatosclerosis
C5	Healed venous ulcer
C6	Open venous ulcer

CEAP, Clinical, aEtiology, Anatomy, Pathophysiology.

11. A Chronic venous insufficiency

This elderly man suffers from chronic venous insufficiency and its aftermath. Chronic venous insufficiency (CVI) results from a deep vein thrombosis following which the venous system does not recanalise resulting in chronic venous hypertension. The combined effect is often called post-thrombotic or post-phlebitic syndrome which clinically results in chronic leg pain limiting activity, oedema and leg ulcers. The patient complains of aching pain, heaviness, swelling, cramp and itching or tingling. Examination of the limb shows perimalleolar oedema, telangiectasia, brown pigmentation and venous eczema. Thickening of the subcutaneous tissues occurs

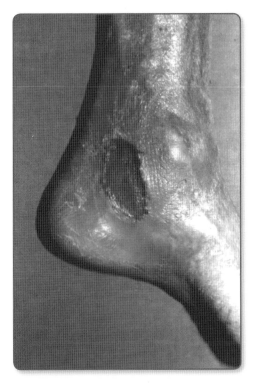

Figure 51.9 Venous ulcer from chronic venous insufficiency.

due to the formation of a pericapillary fibrin cuff from the leakage of fibrin and red blood cells. Red blood cell leakage results in haemosiderin deposition which is the cause of the pigmentation. The pericapillary fibrin cuff causes tissue anoxia, lipodermatosclerosis and ulceration (**Figure 51.9**). In a long-standing venous ulcer one should be aware of a Marjolin's ulcer.

12. B Deep vein thrombosis

This patient has developed deep vein thrombosis (DVT). The diagnosis must be confirmed by Duplex Doppler ultrasound to assess flow and presence of thromboses. D-Dimer, which detects the breakdown products of a thrombus, is a useful negative predictor of thrombosis and can be used as a screening tool.

Once diagnosed treatment is commenced immediately with intravenous heparin, followed by warfarin 48 hours later, each hospital having its own protocol. The warfarin is monitored by taking an international normalised ratio (INR) maintained at about 2.5 to 3.

Patients at risk of developing a pulmonary embolus should have an inferior vena cava filter inserted ideally through the right internal jugular vein. The predisposing risk factors are shown in **Table 51.4**. A protocol for DVT prevention is shown in **Table 51.5.**

Table 51.4 Risk categorisation of deep vein thrombosis		
Low	**Moderate**	**High**
DVT < 10%	DVT 10–40%	DVT 40–80%
Proximal DVT < 1%	Proximal DVT 1–10%	Proximal DVT 10–30%
Fatal PE 0.01%	Fatal PE 0.1–1%	Fatal PE 1–10%
Minor surgery (<30 min)	Major surgery	Major surgery for cancer
Major surgery, age < 40 years	Age > 40 years	Major surgery, trauma or illness +
Minor trauma or medical illness	Caesarean section	risk factors
	Major medical illness	Joint replacement
	Major trauma / burns	Major amputations
	Minor surgery + past	
	History of PE, DVT, thrombophilia, paraplegia	
	Joint replacement	
DVT, deep vein thrombosis; PE, pulmonary embolism		

Table 51.5 Prevention of deep vein thrombosis		
Pre-operative	**Intra-operative**	**Post-operative**
Pre-operative	Use heel pads	Early mobilisation
Reduce risk factors (stop OCP, lose weight)	Pneumatic calf compression + TED stockings	Physiotherapy
TED stockings	Optimal hydration	TED stockings
Low-molecular weight heparin		Low-molecular-weight heparin
Consider IVC filter to prevent PE in high risk		Optimal hydration
IVC, inferior vena cava; OCP, oral contraceptive pill; PE, pulmonary embolism; TED, thromboembolism deterrent.		

Chapter 52

Genitourinary surgery

Questions

Theme: Urological investigation

Options for Questions 1–3:

A Bone scan	**D** Plain intravenous urography
B Kidney, ureters and bladder X-ray	**E** Renal tract ultrasound scan
C Non-contrast CT kidney, ureters and bladder	**F** Triple phase contrast enhanced CT abdomen and pelvis

For each of the following situations, select the single most appropriate investigation. Each option may be used once, more than once or not at all.

1. A 29-year-old man presents with sudden onset of left loin pain which radiates to his left testis. He has tenderness in the left loin but an otherwise unremarkable examination. Urinalysis reveals microscopic haematuria only. Full blood count and renal function are normal. Renal colic is suspected.

2. A 35-year-old man presents to the emergency department having been stabbed with a kitchen knife in the left loin. He is haemodynamically stable but has passed frank haematuria. His abdomen is soft and non-tender. He has no significant past medical history.

3. A 25-year-old woman is referred to the urology department with recurrent urinary tract infections. A flexible cystoscopy is undertaken to ensure the patient does not have a bladder stone or fistula and to assess for urethral stenosis. The cystoscopy is normal. She requires further investigation to exclude a renal cause of her infections.

Theme: Urolithiasis

Options for Questions 4–6:

A	Conservative management	**D**	Percutaneous nephrolithotomy
B	Extracorporeal shockwave lithotripsy	**E**	Rigid ureteroscopy and stone fragmentation
C	Nephrectomy	**F**	Ureteric stent insertion

For each of the following situations, select the single most appropriate treatment. Each option may be used once, more than once or not at all.

4. A 32-year-old woman has right loin to groin pain with fevers. She has associated nausea and vomiting. Inflammatory markers are raised and she has a polymorphonuclear leucocytosis. Renal function is normal. She has no significant past medical history. Imaging confirms a 7 mm distal right ureteric calculus with proximal hydronephrosis. She is commenced on analgesia, intravenous hydration and antibiotics but she continues to spike fevers.

5. A 49-year-old man, a football coach, has recurrent episodes of left loin pain which is controlled with diclofenac. A CT confirms the diagnosis of urolithiasis with a 7 mm right upper pole calculus with a density of 600 Hounsfield units. It is visible on plain abdominal X-ray.

6. A 47-year-old man with recurrent urinary tract infections is found to have a left staghorn calculus on CT kidneys, ureters and bladder. A dimercapto-succinic acid renogram confirms the split function to be 45% on the left and 55% on the right.

Theme: Scrotal swellings

Options for Questions 7–8:

A	Direct inguinal hernia	**D**	Indirect inguinal hernia
B	Epididymal cyst	**E**	Testicular tumour
C	Hydrocele	**F**	Varicocele

For each of the following situations, select the single most likely diagnosis. Each option may be used once, more than once or not at all.

7. A 27-year-old man presents with a 6-month history of scrotal swelling. There is no associated pain. He has no systemic upset. He does suffer from chronic constipation. The swelling is reducible and has a cough impulse. It is distinct from the testis.

8. A 64-year-old man with a recent diagnosis with a left renal tumour attends for his preoperative assessment and mentions to the junior doctor that he has a recent left scrotal swelling. It is a soft swelling, more obvious on standing but is not painful and feels separate to the testis. It does not trans-illuminate.

Theme: Bladder cancer

Options for Questions 9–10:

A Course (six doses) of intravesical *Bacillus* Calmette–Guérin vaccine
B Cystectomy
C Percutaneous needle biopsy
D Radical pelvic radiotherapy
E Transurethral resection of bladder tumour
F Conservative management

For each of the following situations, select the single most appropriate treatment. Each option may be used once, more than once or not at all.

9. A 57-year-old woman is referred by her GP after 2 days of frank painless haematuria. She is otherwise well with significant co-morbidities. At haematuria clinic she has an ultrasound which is normal and a flexible cystoscopy which reveals a papillary tumour on the right lateral bladder wall.

10. A 69-year-old man with a history of ulcerative colitis and G3pT1a bladder cancer has his initial course of intravesical *Bacillus* Calmette–Guérin therapy. At follow-up cystoscopy there is a recurrent tumour which is resected. There is a mobile mass palpable on examination under anaesthetic. Pathology of the re-resection reveals disease progression to at least G3pT2a disease. Staging CT chest, abdomen and pelvis reveals no evidence of metastatic disease.

Theme: Prostate cancer

Options for Questions 11–12:

A Active surveillance
B Androgen deprivation
C Cryotherapy
D High intensity focussed ultrasound
E Radical prostatectomy
F Radical radiotherapy

For each of the following situations, select the single most appropriate treatment. Each option may be used once, more than once or not at all.

11. A 65-year-old man with Gleason 3 + 3 = 6 prostate cancer and a presenting prostate-specific antigen of 8 µg/L. He has had previous radiotherapy for testicular cancer but is otherwise very fit. He is keen on a radical treatment for this prostate cancer.

12. A 90-year-old man presents with urinary retention, a stony hard prostate which is fixed, and a prostate-specific antigen of 567 µg/L. He has a bone scan which confirms sclerotic bone metastases.

Theme: Bladder outlet obstruction

Options for Questions 13–14:

A	Finasteride (5-α-reductase inhibitor)	C	Open prostatectomy
B	Observation	D	Tamsulosin (α-blocker)
		E	Transurethral resection of prostate

For each of the following situations, select the single most appropriate treatment. Each option may be used once, more than once or not at all.

13. An 81-year-old man presents to the emergency department with poor urinary flow, passing very little in the urine over the last few days, and nocturnal incontinence. He is very fit with minimal past medical history. He has a palpable bladder, a large (90 g) but smooth prostate. The bladder scanner reveals > 999 mL residual volume. He is catheterised and has a residual volume of 1.5 L. His urea and electrolytes show a creatinine of 627 μmol/L (the baseline value 2 weeks previously was 94 μmol/L).

14. A 70-year-old man has severe lower urinary tract symptoms. He has been on tamsulosin and finasteride for 18 months with no improvement. On rectal examination, the prostate is very large and transrectal ultrasound confirms the volume to be 130 cm³. Flexible cystoscopy is normal with the exception of a large occlusive prostate. His urinary flow rate is impaired. He wishes further treatment.

Answers

1. C Non-contrast CT kidney, ureters and bladder

Non-contrast CT kidney, ureters and bladder (CTKUB) is the gold standard investigation for diagnosis of urinary tract calculi with a sensitivity >97%, while plain intravenous urography and kidney, ureters and bladder X-ray have sensitivities of 85 and 50% respectively. CTKUB has the advantage that intravenous contrast is not required thus avoiding associated complications and CT may diagnose other causes of flank pain.

2. F Triple phase contrast-enhanced CT abdomen and pelvis

Triple phase CT is the imaging of choice for suspected renal injury. This allows accurate assessment of the degree of parenchymal, collecting system and vascular disruption. Indications for imaging include any penetrating renal injury or blunt injury with at least one of the following conditions:

(i)   frank haematuria

(ii)   microscopic haematuria and any haemodynamic instability

(iii)   pre-existing anatomical abnormality

(iv)   paediatric patients, or

(v)   a significant mechanism of injury.

Most cases of renal injury are managed conservatively. Interventional radiology and selective embolisation for ongoing bleeding can be used and occasionally surgical intervention is required.

3. E Renal tract ultrasound scan

An ultrasound is the investigation of choice to ensure there are no upper urinary calculi or associated hydronephrosis. An ultrasound is ideal in this young female patient as is it non-invasive and there is no exposure to X-rays.

4. F Ureteric stent insertion

An infected, obstructed kidney is a urological emergency and prompt decompression is important for resolution of sepsis. This can be done by either nephrostomy or ureteric stent insertion. Following resolution of sepsis the patient can have definite stone management. Stones <1 cm may pass spontaneously but with these complications, it is likely to be impacted and require active intervention. Extracorporeal shockwave lithotripsy, and ureteroscopy and stone fragmentation are possibilities in the proximal ureter; ureteroscopy and stone fragmentation is more appropriate in the distal ureter.

5. B Extracorporeal shockwave lithotripsy

This patient has a symptomatic stone, which therefore requires treatment. Renal stones can be treated with extracorporeal shockwave lithotripsy (ESWL), flexible ureteroscopy and stone fragmentation or percutaneous nephrolithotomy (PCNL). ESWL would be the treatment of choice for most renal stones <1 cm, with a stone-free rate of approximately 85%. It is less effective for larger stones (>1 cm), harder stones (>1000 HU), stones in the lower pole of the kidney and distal ureter and in those with obesity. In such cases flexible ureteroscopy and stone fragmentation may be an alternative. Note rigid ureteroscopy is not possible in the kidney as ureteroscopic deflection is required for stone localisation. PCNL is generally reserved for patients who have stones resistant to ESWL or ureteroscopy, large stones >2 cm or staghorn calculi.

6. D Percutaneous nephrolithotomy

A staghorn calculus should be treated if the patient if fit enough. Left untreated mortality renal related mortality as a result of the stone is 30%. Standard treatment would be percutaneous nephrolithotomy. This is the most effective form of treatment for complete stone clearance, which will preserve renal function as well as preventing infection. In cases when the kidney is non-functioning, there is no need to preserve the kidney for function and the patient is best served by nephrectomy.

7. D Indirect inguinal hernia

A hydrocele often does not allow palpation of the testis if large and transilluminates without a cough impulse, unlike the hernia presented here. This is an indirect hernia as it follows the inguinal canal into the scrotum. Surgical repair is indicated to prevent complications. Chronic constipation is a risk factor and this should be managed appropriately to prevent recurrence.

8. F Varicocele

A varicocele is a dilatation of the veins (pampiniform plexus) around the testis. It is more common on the left as these veins combine to form the testicular vein which drains perpendicularly into the left renal vein. On the right the testicular vein drains into the vena cava. Varicoceles are typically idiopathic. They can be described as 'a bag of worms' on examination and often reduce in size or disappear on lying flat. They are largely asymptomatic. In this case, the varicocele is a likely complication of the known renal cancer which may involve the left renal vein and obstruct testicular venous drainage.

9. E Transurethral resection of bladder tumour

Initial treatment of bladder cancer is transurethral resection which allows local staging. In those patients which superficial disease is suspected a single dose of mitomycin C is given postoperatively to prevent disease recurrence. At diagnosis

50% patients have superficial disease (pTa); 20% have superficially invasive (pT1) and 30% have muscle invasive disease (pT2–4). In those patients with pTa or pT1 disease trans-urethral resection of bladder tumour may be definitive treatment although risk of disease recurrence and progression can be stratified pathologically and further intravesical immunotherapy (*Bacillus* Calmette–Guérin) or chemotherapy (mitomycin C) given.

10. B Cystectomy

This man has muscle invasive disease with no evidence of metastasis. Local endoscopic treatment or intravesical chemotherapy and immunotherapy will not be sufficient for disease control. Options include radical radiotherapy or cystectomy. Although there are no randomised controlled trials and the evidence is debated by some, cystectomy may have a survival benefit over radiotherapy for those fit enough to undergo such major surgery. In this case inflammatory bowel disease would also make radiotherapy less attractive.

11. E Radical prostatectomy

This man is most likely to have localised prostate cancer (low prostate-specific antigen and moderately differentiated prostate cancer). As such, his treatment options are active surveillance, brachytherapy, radical radiotherapy and radical prostatectomy. In view of previous pelvic radiotherapy he would not be suitable for further radiotherapeutic treatment. As such the only suitable treatment available to choose from here is radical surgery. Radical prostatectomy can be performed by open, laparoscopic or robotic means. The more minimally invasive treatments offer reduced blood transfusion requirements and more rapid hospital discharge.

12. B Androgen deprivation

This patient has metastatic prostate cancer; tissue is not required for confirmation. Men with this condition should be offered androgen deprivation therapy in the form of luteinising hormone releasing hormone agonist injections (usually every 3 months), with initial androgen receptor blocker treatment for 3 weeks to prevent testosterone flare. This therapy will prevent pathological fracture rates and reduce the prostate-specific antigen (PSA) in the vast majority of patients. Eventually the prostate cancer will escape control (PSA will rise) and an androgen receptor blocker will be required in addition to a luteinising hormone releasing hormone agonist. Once the PSA rises again, so-called castration-resistant prostate cancer (CRPC) has developed. At this stage in younger, higher performance patients chemotherapy can provide approximately 3 months survival advantage. Median survival in CRPC is 12–18 months.

13. E Transurethral resection of prostate

This patient has chronic urinary retention due to his increasing difficulty passing urine, with nocturnal incontinence (pathognomic of this condition) and the residual volume of >800 mL. This man has high pressure chronic retention in view of his new onset renal failure. As such he should not be treated with conservative or medical treatment, otherwise this problem will reoccur. He should have a transurethral resection of prostate, long term catheter or possibly intermittent self catheterisation, if he is motivated to do so.

14. C Open prostatectomy

This man has severe lower urinary tract symptoms secondary to bladder outflow obstruction. Medical therapy has been unsuccessful. Surgical treatment is indicated. As the prostate is large (>100 g) open prostatectomy is the procedure of choice.

Chapter 53

Transplantation

Questions

Theme: Types of transplant graft

Options for Questions 1–4:

A	Autograft	D	Piggy-back graft
B	Allograft	E	Split graft
C	Isograft	F	Xenograft

For each of the following situations below, select the single most likely graft type. Each option may be used once, more than once or not at all.

1. A 65-year-old man has end-stage liver disease due to alcohol induced cirrhosis. Following appropriate work up a liver transplant is performed using the right lobe of his son's liver. Postoperatively both patients progressed well.

2. A 50-year-old woman of rare blood type requires a major surgical procedure. Two weeks prior to the procedure the patient donates blood which is stored in the event that it is required in the perioperative period.

3. A 28-year-old fire-fighter was caught in a fire and suffered third degree burns to his forearm. The plastic surgeons scheduled him for surgery to treat the burns.

4. A 16-year-old boy was involved in a road traffic accident and sustained severe injuries to his liver. He was managed conservatively with embolisation. One week later he became septic and required liver transplant. His identical twin brother consented to partial liver transplant.

Theme: Principles of transplantation

Options for Questions 5–7:

A	Brainstem death	D	Living–unrelated
B	Cross-species	E	Non-heart beating
C	Living–related		

For each of the following situations, select the single most likely option. Each option may be used once, more than once or not at all.

5. A 49-year-old man with chronic renal failure of unknown aetiology has been on long term dialysis and awaits kidney transplantation. At clinic review the patient is keen to discuss options for transplantation and is concerned about receiving a transplant from an accepted donor source which is associated with the least favourable outcome.

6. A 58-year-old man with alcohol-related cirrhosis of the liver presents with acute-on-chronic liver failure. Given the severity of his condition he requires urgent liver transplantation. After waiting for several days, organ transplantation is performed from a donor source which is most commonly used for this type of transplantation.

7. A 32-year-old fit and well woman wants to donate one of her kidneys to her spouse who is currently on the transplant waiting list. She attends the pre-transplant counselling clinic today for counselling. She is concerned about her fertility as she plans to have children in the future.

Theme: Basic principles of transplant immunology

Options for Questions 8–11:

A	Acute rejection	D	Delayed-graft function
B	Acute-on-chronic rejection	E	Hyperacute rejection
C	Chronic rejection		

For each of the following situations, select the single most likely rejection type. Each option may be used once, more than once or not at all.

8. A 55-year-old man received a renal transplant 2 months previously for renal failure of unknown aetiology. After initially functioning well his renal function has now deteriorated considerably.

9. A 64-year-old man received a renal transplantation for diabetic nephropathy 3 years previously. Over the past 18 months his creatinine clearance has been slowly deteriorating. He has noticed his urine output has reduced recently.

10. A 67-year-old woman with decompensated chronic liver failure undergoes liver transplantation. Soon after the vasculature is anastomosed the organ becomes congested and dusky. The transplant surgeon is concerned about the viability of the organ.

11. A 34-year-old woman who underwent uneventful kidney transplant 1 week ago has been feeling unwell with rising creatinine. Nursing staff have been reporting persisting low urine output which has been tailing off over the last few hours. She now requires dialysis.

Theme: Renal replacement therapy

Options for Questions 12–16:

A   Arterio-venous fistula   D   Haemofiltration
B   Fluid resuscitation   E   Peritoneal dialysis
C   Haemodialysis

For each of the following situations, select the single most likely therapy. Each option may be used once, more than once or not at all.

12. A 78-year-old woman patient has developed renal failure secondary to long standing hypertension. She has been placed on the transplant waiting list but requires renal replacement therapy until a donor kidney becomes available.

13. A 39-year-old professional man has developed renal failure. He is diabetic but this has been well-controlled, despite the deterioration in renal function. He requires renal replacement therapy but hopes to maintain his career during the wait for a donor organ.

14. A 60-year-old diabetic woman is recovering on the intensive care unit following major abdominal surgery. Several days following the procedure has developed significant fluid overload in the context of oliguria and hyperkalaemia.

15. An 89-year-old woman is reviewed on the orthopaedic ward 4 days following hemiarthroplasty for fracture neck of femur. She is found to be severely dehydrated. Blood tests are sent urgently which show markedly elevated urea and creatinine with a potassium level of 6.0 mmol/L.

16. A 79-year-old woman on continuous ambulatory peritoneal dialysis (CAPD) was admitted for abdominal pain and sepsis and treated for peritonitis secondary to peritoneal dialysis. Her renal function is raised and she now requires a temporary form of dialysis.

Answers

1. B Allograft

This refers to graft tissue from a donor of the same species. Liver transplantation is performed for a range of acute, chronic and malignant conditions (**Table 53.1**). While the majority of organs originate from deceased donors, living donor liver transplantation is becoming more frequent. Here the right (or sometimes left) lobe of the donor's liver is removed (55–70% of total liver volume) with the remaining liver regenerating over several weeks to months.

Table 53.1 Indications for liver transplantation	
Reason for liver transplant	**Cause**
Acute hepatic failure	Viral hepatitis Paracetamol overdose Other drug/toxin induced acute liver failure
Chronic hepatic failure	Hepatitis B or C cirrhosis Primary biliary cirrhosis Primary sclerosing cholangitis Biliary atresia Alcoholic cirrhosis Autoimmune chronic active hepatitis Budd–Chiari syndrome Hemochromatosis
Malignancy	Non-resectable hepatoblastoma which is chemosensitive Hepatocellular carcinoma according to the Milan criteria Epithelioid haemangioendothelioma (Note: metastatic liver disease is NOT an indication for transplantation)
Inborn errors of metabolism	Crigler–Najjar type 1 Primary oxalosis Urea cycle defects Familial amyloid polyneuropathy

2. A Autograft

Patients with rare blood groups may be able to donate blood preoperatively to enable transfusion if required intraoperatively. This may reduce complications associated with blood transfusion in these patient groups but its use is dependent on the centre.

During major abdominal surgery, such as aortic aneurysm repair, where high blood loss can occur a system to reinfuse blood lost into the abdominal cavity can be employed.

Other examples of an autograft include bone graft to aid repair of complex fractures and tissue transfer for plastic surgery procedures.

3. E Split graft

Split-skin graft involves taking the epidermis and part of the dermis from either the donor or the host. The graft is obtained from a mesher. Advantages of the split graft is that is covers large areas of up to nine times its size and its rate of autorejection is low. Common donor sites include thigh, buttock, back, upper arm, forearm and abdominal wall.

4. C Isograft

An isograft refers to transplantation of tissues between two genetically identical individuals. Hence, rejection is almost impossible.

5. E Non-heart beating

In the context of a predictable cardiac arrest in a controlled setting such as intensive care unit non-heart beating donors may be considered for renal transplantation. However, organs from this donor source who do not meet the criteria for brainstem death confer the worst prognosis. Minimising the length of time between cardiac arrest and organ retrieval is crucial to optimise long-term graft viability. Alive related and alive unrelated donors offer the best graft outcomes given suitable tissue and blood typing match.

6. A Brainstem death

Patients who fulfil the criteria for brainstem death (**Table 53.2**) and are ventilated in the intensive care unit may be considered for organ donation. At present this is commonest source of donated livers. It is preferable to non-heart beating donors

Table 53.2 Criteria for brainstem death

Preconditions

1. No doubt that the patient's conditions due to irreversible brain damage of known aetiology
2. No evidence that this state is due to depressant drugs
3. Primary hypothermia must be excluded
4. Potential reversible circulatory, metabolic and endocrine disturbances must be excluded
5. Reversible causes of apnoea, such as muscle relaxants and cervical cord injury must be excluded

Definitive criteria

1. Fixed pupils
2. No corneal reflexes
3. Absent oculovestibular reflex
4. No response to supraorbital pressure
5. No cough reflex to bronchial stimulation or gagging response to pharyngeal stimulation
6. No respiratory effort in response to disconnection of the ventilator to ensure elevation of the arterial partial pressure of carbon dioxide to at least 6.0 kPa (6.5 kPa in patients with chronic carbon dioxide retention)

as brainstem dead donors have a shorter warm ischaemic time, which corresponds to a more favourable outcome. With recent developments in techniques to treat organs in transit as well as improved immunosuppressive regimens outcomes are improving.

Living related donations have increased in recent years and they are often associated with the best outcomes.

7. D Living–unrelated

Living–unrelated kidney transplant is transplanting kidneys from a live, unrelated donor, in this case a spouse. This form of transplant avoids the need of the recipient to be on a waiting list and allows for a planned elective transplant. The donor can return back to their life once recovered from the surgery.

8. A Acute rejection

Acute rejection usually presents within 3 months but can occur up to 6 months following organ transplantation. It is detected by graft dysfunction. Acute rejection is a T-cell mediated process, with lymphocyte infiltration in the interstitium and later the vessel walls. Given the fact that human leukocyte antigens are polymorphic it is extremely unlikely that a perfect match will occur.

The diagnosis can be confirmed by biopsy, although is difficult to distinguish from acute tubular necrosis or drug nephrotoxicity. The incidence of acute rejection can be reduced by maintenance immunosuppressive regimens and if/when acute rejection does occur it may be reversible with episodic use of high dose steroids.

9. C Chronic rejection

This can occur anytime from months to years following transplantation and is defined as an alloimmune response leading to gradual deterioration in organ function. It involves both humoral and cell mediated responses.

At biopsy renal tubular atrophy, glomerular basement membrane thickening and vascular changes may be noticed. There is no treatment and chronic rejection is not reversible.

In addition to the phenomenon of immune mediated rejection other major factors which determine long-term graft function include donor age, preservation/reperfusion related graft injury, tissue quality and posttransplant stressors in the recipient such as infection, drug toxicity and comorbidity. A constellation of these factors can contribute to chronic allograft dysfunction, where the underlying alloimmune response seen in chronic rejection is less evident. Chronic allograft nephropathy is characterised by renal insufficiency, progressive vasculopathy and non-specific pathology occurring at least 3–6 months following renal transplantation.

10. E Hyperacute rejection

Hyperacute rejection can occur immediately or within minutes to hours of transplantation. It occurs where there are preformed antibodies in the serum of the recipient against donor antigens, eliciting a humoral immune response. Antibodies attach to class 1 antigens on the vascular endothelium leading to complement activation, intravascular coagulation and subsequent impaired tissue perfusion. Thrombotic occlusion then leads to graft necrosis and loss of the graft.

Antibodies involved in hyperacute rejection include ABO blood group antigens, histocompatibility antigens and vascular endothelial antigens. The treatment for hyperacute rejection is immediate removal of the organ. Patients who have had multiple pregnancies, multiple blood transfusions or previous transplants are more likely to have developed antibodies to transplant antigens.

11. D Delayed graft function

Delayed graft function is a type of acute kidney injury that occurs between 7–10 days post kidney transplantation. This form of ischaemic-reperfusion injury requires dialysis post-transplantation.

12. C Haemodialysis

A percutaneous large bore cannula is sited to enable access to a central vein. Blood is pumped into the dialysis machine where a semi-permeable membrane separates the blood from the dialysis fluid. The blood and dialysis fluid run in different directions, known as counter current circulation. Diffusion of substances occurs across the membrane. Haemodialysis requires the patient to attend the haemodialysis centre around three times per week. For patients with work or childcare commitments this can be a considerable burden, and peritoneal dialysis may be more appropriate.

13. E Peritoneal dialysis

Here dialysis fluid is infused into the peritoneal cavity via an access port in the abdominal wall. The osmotic pressure within the dialysis fluid leads to ultrafiltration due to osmotic pressure and diffusion to replace the renal excretory functions. Peritoneal dialysis can be performed independently by the patient at home, rather than having to attend a dialysis centre and may prove a more practical solution. In patients with poorly controlled diabetes peritoneal dialysis is contraindicated due to the risk of infection.

Peritoneal filtration is not a recognised practice.

14. C Haemofiltration

This is a short-term solution for the management of renal failure. Haemofiltration relies on a positive hydrostatic pressure enabling water and solutes to pass across a semipermeable membrane. Fluid is replaced in isotonic form to account for water and electrolytes removed. The rate of solute removal is related to the pressure gradient applied, which can be adjusted to account for the clinical situation. Haemofiltation is mainly used in the critical care environment where temporary support of renal function can be provided.

Haemodialysis and peritoneal dialysis are long-term options which would not be appropriate here as the patient's renal function will hopefully recover.

15. D Haemofiltration

See above.

16. A Arterio-venous fistula

AV fistula is an abnormal communication between an artery and a vein. AV fistula can occur congenitally or formed surgically under local anaesthetic. In patients with end-stage renal failure requiring haemodialysis, blood flows from the artery to the haemodialysis machine and then back into the vein. It can take up to 2–3 months for the fistula to mature before the fistula can be used. Surgical complications encountered with AV fistula include risk of failure of fistula to mature, aneurysms, stenosis and thrombosis.

Chapter 54

Head and neck

Questions

Theme: Oral cavity and tongue

Options for Questions 1–3:

A Assessment of HIV status	**G** Incisional tissue biopsy
B CT scanning	**H** Lateral neck X-ray
C Epstein–Barr virus serology	**I** MRI scanning
D Excision tissue biopsy	**J** Oral swab for microscopic analysis
E Fine needle aspiration biopsy	**K** Saliva sample for microscopic
F Human papilloma virus serology	analysis

For each of the following situations, select the single most appropriate investigation. Each option may be used once, more than once or not at all.

1. A 64-year-old man presents with a 6-week history of loose teeth and ulceration of the gum. He has an 80 pack-year history of cigarette smoking. Examination reveals a 2 cm ulcerated lesion over the left mandible and no palpable lymph nodes in the neck.

2. A 75-year-old woman presents with a 3-month history of oral discomfort. Her past history includes non-insulin dependent diabetes mellitus and chronic obstructive pulmonary disease, for which she uses a steroid inhaler. On removal of her dentures, examination reveals white plaques involving the hard palate and buccal mucosa. Gentle brushing dislodges the plaques to reveal reddened mucosa.

3. A 59-year-old man presents with a neck mass. He has a 50 pack-year history of smoking. Examination of the neck reveals a 2 cm firm mass in the anterior triangle without fixation to the skin. Examination of the mouth reveals poor dentition without any identifiable primary lesion.

Theme: Nose and sinuses

Options for Questions 4–7:

A	Acute sinusitis	F	Nasal fracture
B	Chronic sinusitis	G	Nasal polyposis
C	Congenital syphilis	H	Nasal septal deviation
D	Midline T cell lymphoma	I	Squamous cell carcinoma
E	Nasal foreign body	J	Wegner's granulomatosis

For each of the following situations, select the single most likely diagnosis. Each option may be used once, more than once or not at all.

4. A 45-year-old man presents with a 1-year history of anosmia (loss of sense of smell) and bilateral nasal obstruction. He has a history of asthma. Examination of the nose reveals bilateral obstruction with greyish masses visible on both sides of the nasal cavity.

5. A 23-year-old woman who works as a teacher presents with a 2-week history of right sided rhinorrhoea (nasal discharge) and facial pain, which followed a recent viral upper respiratory tract infection. On examination, she is pyrexial (38.5°C) with tenderness over the left cheek, periorbital and frontal regions, with green discharge visible in the right nostril.

6. A 45-year-old woman presents with symptoms of nasal obstruction and discharge. She has renal and pulmonary dysfunction. Examination reveals a nasal septal perforation and significantly abnormally thickened erythematous nasal mucosa.

7. A 4-year-old boy presents with a 1-month history of unilateral nasal discharge. He is well, but has profuse discharge from the left nostril which is foul-smelling.

Theme: Salivary glands

Options for Questions 8–10:

A	Auriculotemporal nerve	E	Parotid duct
B	Facial nerve	F	Parotid gland
C	Lingual nerve	G	Sublingual gland
D	Minor salivary gland of the hard palate	H	Submandibular duct
		I	Submandibular gland

For each of the following situations, select the single most primary structure involved. Each option may be used once, more than once or not at all.

8. A 55-year-old woman presents with recurrent pain and swelling inferior her right mandible. The symptoms are related to eating and have been present for 3 months. On examination she has no palpable abnormality in the neck, however a hard 5 mm mass is palpable in the right floor of mouth.

9. A 72-year-old man presents with a 3-year history of a slowly enlarging mass inferior to the left ear. The mass is painless, and there is no history of weight loss. On examination there is an 8 cm mass overlying the left angle of mandible. The overlying skin is normal and facial nerve function is not affected.

10. A 72-year-old man presents with a 3-month history of a rapidly enlarging mass over the right cheek. The mass is painful and is associated with weakness of the right face. Examination confirms a mass over the angle of the right mandible which is 5 cm, firm with indurated overlying skin and associated weakness of the muscles of facial expression on the right side of the face.

Theme: Ear disease

Options for Questions 11–12:

A	Acute mastoiditis	E	Otitis externa
B	Bullous myringitis	F	Squamous cell carcinoma of
C	Cholesteatoma		postnasal space
D	Chronic otitis media with effusion		

For each of the following situations, select the single most likely diagnosis. Each option may be used once, more than once or not at all.

11. A 6-year-old boy presents with a 1-week history of fever and right ear pain, which has not responded to antibiotics. On examination he is well, but has a temperature of 38.5°C. Examination of his left ear is normal, but the skin behind the right ear is erythematous and fluctuant. Examination of the ear canal shows a bulging, red ear drum.

12. A 76-year-old man, a smoker, presents with a 1-month history of left sided deafness. Examination of the ears shows normal ear canals, with a fluid level visible on the left ear drum.

Answers

1. G Incisional tissue biopsy

The most likely diagnosis here is squamous cell carcinoma. The disease is strongly associated with smoking, and tends to present in patients in their 60s and 70s. Confirmation of the diagnosis is best achieved with an incisional biopsy. Treatment will depend on the size of the primary lesion (determined by examination and imaging), the presence of nodal metastases and any evidence of distant metastases (usually pulmonary). Although excisional biopsy would allow a diagnosis to be made, it would be likely to require a major operation including sacrifice of part of the mandible. It would be inappropriate to undertake such major surgery without first confirming the diagnosis and staging the disease to allow treatment planning.

2. J Oral swab for microscopic analysis

Oral candidiasis often presents with pain. Examination reveals the characteristic white plaques which can be removed by brushing with a moist swab. Predisposing factors include diabetes, dentures, as well as corticosteroid and antibiotic use. Treatment would include oral solutions containing nystatin, or for resistant cases, systemic therapy such as fluconazole. In addition to these treatments this patient should be advised in regards to oral hygiene, and also encouraged to rinse her mouth following use of her steroid inhaler to remove residue from the oral mucosa. Although oesophageal candidiasis is related to HIV infection and considered an AIDS defining illness, oral candidiasis is common and not an indication for assessment of HIV status.

3. E Fine-needle aspiration biopsy

Patients with a significant history of smoking are at risk of head and neck cancer. Although a primary lesion in the mouth would be expected in such a patient, the absence of one does not exclude squamous cell carcinoma. The most appropriate investigation would be fine-needle aspiration of the neck node, which would ideally be done under ultrasound guidance to maximise the chance of a diagnostic sample. Although Epstein–Barr virus and human papilloma virus have both been shown to be related to cancers of the head and neck, serology would not be diagnostic and so are less useful than cytology in this case. Having made a diagnosis of small cell carcinoma, cross-sectional imaging would be appropriate, and in most cases CT scanning is employed. It is quick, cheap and more readily available than MRI, although in cases where dental amalgam results in significant artefact on CT scanning, MRI can be particularly useful.

4. G Nasal polyposis

This patient presents with the classical symptoms of nasal polyps. Inflammation of the sinonasal mucosa results in oedematous tissue which eventually bunches out to obstruct the airway, thereby interfering with smell. There is thought to be an allergic component, and nasal polyps are common in asthmatics. Symptoms tend to be bilateral, and indeed unilateral nasal polyps should be considered as malignant until proven otherwise. Examination of inflammatory nasal polyps reveals insensate greyish polypoid mucosa, although in extreme cases where mucosa approaches the nasal vestibule the superficial mucosa may become hypertrophic. Treatment of these patients starts with steroids, often topically applied in an attempt to shrink the polyps. Although surgery may be used for non-responders, it does not cure the condition, but rather debulks tissue which reduces symptoms and allows for more effective delivery of steroids to affected mucosa.

5. A Acute sinusitis

Acute sinusitis occurs when the sinus ostia (drainage pathways of the sinuses in to the nose) become blocked. This tends to result from infection. The sinus then becomes a closed system and mucus which builds up can become infected. Patients present with pain, fever and ipsilateral nasal discharge. Although the maxillary sinus is most commonly affected, the relationship of the sinus drainage pathways means that a pan-sinusitis often develops. Such patients were classically investigated with plain X-ray imaging, however such films add little to management and with the advent of low radiation dose CT scanning, cross-sectional imaging has replaced standard X-rays as the investigation of choice. Treatment includes decongestion of the nasal mucosa and antibiotic therapy, with surgical drainage reserved for the occasional patient that does not respond. Complications of acute sinusitis are rare but can be life-threatening and include the spread of infection to the cranial cavity and orbit.

6. J Wegener's granulomatosis

Wegener's granulomatosis is a vasculitis which can affect many systems, but commonly involved are renal and pulmonary with associated airway problems. The mucosa of the nose can be affected by granulomas which over time can result in perforation of the nasal septum, and collapse of the dorsum of the nose. Although this can also occur in congenital syphilis, she is in the wrong age group. Malignancy would also be possible, and although unlikely a biopsy could be performed to exclude small cell carcinoma or T-cell lymphoma. Wegener's is most commonly treated with systemic steroids and surgical input is rarely required for nasal symptoms. The upper airway can also be affected at the level of the subglottis, which can result in airway obstruction from inflamed mucosa. Although it is rare, this is an occasional indication for tracheostomy.

7. E Nasal foreign body

This presentation is typical for a nasal foreign body. Often a child inserts the object and does not inform the parents. Such objects can remain without symptoms and signs for long periods before resulting in infection with associated discharge. Organic materials and sponge result in a particularly offensive smell. Treatment requires removal, either with or without general anaesthetic depending on cooperation of the child. Specific foreign bodies including batteries and magnets applied to both sides of the nasal septum require urgent removal, whereas incidental foreign bodies such as this can be removed on the next available theatre list.

8. H Submandibular duct

This patient presents with symptoms which are typical of submandibular duct obstruction. The examination findings confirm the presence of a stone within the duct which is causing obstruction. A plain X-ray of the floor of the mouth confirms the diagnosis (**Figure 54.1**). Although the submandibular gland swells within its capsule, causing pain, the pathology is located within the duct. The submandibular gland produces a constant flow of saliva however during mastication, saliva production increases, hence the association of symptoms with eating.

Salivary stones most commonly affect the submandibular rather than the parotid duct. This may relate to the fact that drainage against gravity tends to result in salivary stasis. Floor-of-mouth X-ray will demonstrate submandibular stones in 80% of cases. Transoral resection under local or general anaesthetic with marsupialisation of the duct to prevent subsequent stenosis should allow removal of this stone. The duct runs in close proximity to the lingual nerve; in fact, the two loop around one another and care must be taken not to damage the nerve both in transoral and transcervical approaches to the submandibular duct.

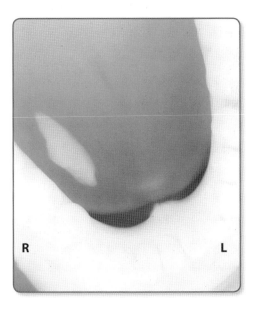

Figure 54.1 Floor-of-mouth X-ray demonstrating a radio-opaque stone in the right submandibular duct.

9. F Parotid gland

Although many students expect parotid lesions to present in the cheek, the most common site to find a small parotid lesion is inferior to the ear lobe in the tail of the parotid. This elderly man presents with symptoms which suggest a benign neoplasm of salivary tissue. The most common diagnosis here would be pleomorphic adenoma, although Warthin's tumour (also called papillary cystadenoma lymphomatosum) would be in the differential diagnosis also. Both of these tumours more commonly affect the parotid than the submandibular salivary gland. Malignancy of the parotid is less likely, particularly in the absence of features such as pain, facial nerve dysfunction and overlying skin changes.

Investigation of salivary masses starts with fine-needle aspiration biopsy, and many clinicians would also order cross-sectional imaging (ideally MRI). Although fine-needle aspiration biopsy is not 100% accurate, a biopsy suggesting malignancy would alter preoperative work up, consent, and the extent of surgical resection.

10. F Parotid gland

This man presents in a similar fashion to the preceding case but with some specific differences. The mass is growing rapidly, is painful and associated with both skin change and facial nerve dysfunction. These are all hallmarks of malignancy. Although the facial nerve is involved, this is much more likely to be parotid pathology than a primary of the facial nerve. The most commonly involved structure would be the parotid gland itself, which can be affected by conditions including mucoepidermoid carcinoma, adenocarcinoma, adenoid cystic carcinoma and carcinoma ex-pleomorphic adenoma (**Figure 54.2**). Although primary parotid pathology should be suspected, this could also represent a metastatic intraparotid lymph node, which highlights the need for a full head and neck examination

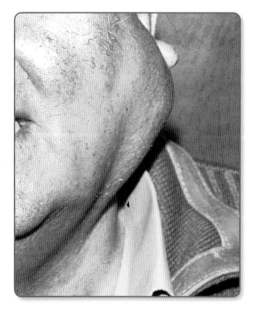

Figure 54.2 Classical parotid swelling.

with particular reference to the skin of the scalp, the lymphatic drainage of which includes these nodes. The next stage in management here would involve fine-needle aspiration cytology followed by imaging of the lesion (probably with MRI) and the neck to identify any involved cervical lymph nodes.

11. A Acute mastoiditis

This child has acute mastoiditis with a subperiosteal abscess. Acute otitis media is very common, with up to 80% of children experiencing at least one episode. In the event that an episode of acute otitis media does not resolve without complication, the tympanic membrane may rupture, allowing the pus under pressure to escape. The mastoid air cells drain in to the middle ear, and infection of the middle ear space results in mucosal oedema which can obstruct this outflow. The closed system which results from this obstruction may harbour infection that will ultimately discharge, either into the soft tissues over the bone as in this case, or superiorly in to the cranial cavity, putting the child at risk of meningitis or intracranial abscess.

Investigation of this child should involve contrast enhanced CT to visualise the mastoid air cell system and to identify any intracranial abscess. Management is guided by imaging, but assuming there is no collection in the brain, incision and drainage of the collection should be performed.

12. F Squamous cell carcinoma of postnasal space

Unilateral deafness in an elderly patient who smokes is a red flag for cancer. The ear drains in to the postnasal space via the Eustachian tube. If occluded, the serous fluid produced by the middle ear mucosa is trapped and will lead to a conductive hearing loss. This patient requires nasendoscopy to exclude a lesion in the postnasal space. Assuming there is an abnormality, urgent biopsy should be arranged with imaging to stage local, regional and distant disease.

Chapter 55

Surgical conditions of the skin

Questions

Theme: Benign skin lesions

Options for Questions 1–5:

A Acrochordon	E Pilomatricoma
B Dermoid cyst	F Pyogenic granuloma
C Erythema nodosum	G Seborrhoeic keratosis
D Keratoacanthoma	H Sebaceous (epidermal) cyst

For each of the following cases, select the single most appropriate diagnosis. Each option may be used once, more than once or not at all.

1. A 30-year-old woman who recently started on the contraceptive pill presents to the GP with painful lesions on both her lower legs.

2. A 50-year-old avid gardener presents to the GP with a solitary, friable nodular lesion over the dorsum of his left middle finger. He reckons that he injured his finger whilst gardening 5 days ago.

3. A distressed mother brings her 7-year-old daughter to the GP since she has been teased at school due to a lesion on her forehead. She is otherwise fit and healthy. On examination, there is a 2 cm, hard, mobile, solitary nodule on the forehead with a very faint green, bluish discolouration of the overlying intact skin.

4. A 40-year-old woman presents to the 2-week referral to the plastic surgery outpatient clinic with a short history of a rapidly growing lesion on her right temple, which she said has stopped increasing in size. On examination, there is a dome shaped 2 cm nodule with a central keratin plug.

5. A 5-year-old girl is brought to the GP with a cystic lesion on the lateral aspect of her right outer eyebrow. On examination, the lesion does not transilluminate. There is no punctum and it is attached to underlying tissue.

Theme: Premalignant and malignant skin lesions

Options for Questions 6–9:

A	Actinic keratosis	E	Marjolin's ulcer
B	Bowen's disease	F	Pyogenic granuloma
C	Cutaneous horn	G	Seborrhoeic naevus
D	Giant congenital melanocytic naevus		

For each of the following cases, select the single most appropriate diagnosis. Each option may be used once, more than once or not at all.

6. A 46-year-old woman who sustained a full thickness burn to her left leg 20 years ago presents to the burns out-patient clinic with a rapidly growing friable lesion on her previous burn scar that is foul smelling.

7. A 66-year-old retired builder presents with a crusty lesion over the nape of his neck. It does not give him any trouble but he has noticed that it comes and goes spontaneously. On closer examination, there is a rough erythematous lesion with overlying fine keratosis. There are similar lesions across his forehead and cheeks (**Figure 55.1**).

8. A 35-year-old woman presents to the outpatient clinic with a well-defined, erythematous patch on the dorsum of her right hand that measures 2 cm in diameter. She states that it ulcerates occasionally. She is currently undergoing chemotherapy for non-Hodgkin's lymphoma (**Figure 55.2**).

9. A 70-year-old man presents to the outpatient clinic with a lesion over his right upper eyelid. He wants it to be removed. He is upset that his grandchild is afraid of his appearance and has commented that he has 'antlers'.

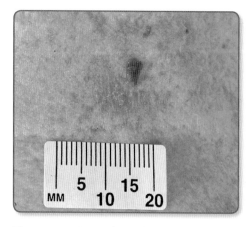

Figure 55.1 A rough erythematous lesion.

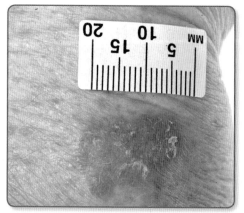

Figure 55.2 Erythematous patch on the hand of a patient with non-Hodgkin's lymphoma.

Theme: Premalignant and malignant lesions

Options for Questions 10–14:

A   Actinic keratosis
B   Basal cell carcinoma
C   Bowen's disease
D   Giant congenital melanocytic naevus

E   Lentigo maligna
F   Mycosis fungoides
G   Sebaceous naevus
H   Squamous cell carcinoma

For each of the following cases, select the single most appropriate diagnosis. Each option may be used once, more than once or not at all.

10. A 47-year-old woman presents to the plastic surgery outpatient clinic with the lesion shown in **Figure 55.3** on her left cheek.

11. A 50-year-old renal transplant patient presents with a lesion on the left lower leg that occasionally bleeds spontaneously (**Figure 55.4**).

12. A 65-year-old woman with a lesion shown in **Figure 55.5** on the left side of her nose that she has had for a few years.

13. A 14-year-old boy is brought by his mother to the outpatient clinic since they are concerned about a large pigmented hairy mole on his back that he has had since birth. They are worried that this hairy mole might be malignant.

14. A 15-year-old boy has had a yellow, velvety plaque on his scalp since birth. He has come to the clinic because he has noticed it increasing in size since reaching puberty.

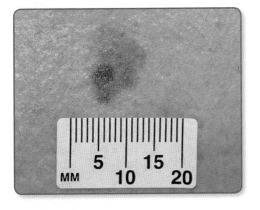

Figure 55.3 Lesion on left cheek.

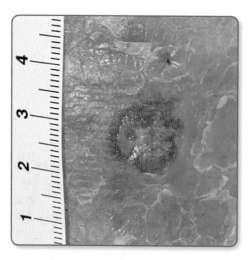

Figure 55.4 A lesion on the left lower leg that occasionally bleeds spontaneously.

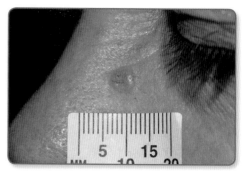

Figure 55.5 A long-term nasal lesion.

Theme: Types of melanoma

Options for Questions 15–17:

A   Acral lentiginous melanoma
B   Amelanotic melanoma
C   Desmoplastic melanoma
E   Lentigo maligna

F   Mucosal melanoma
G   Nodular melanoma
H   Superficial spreading melanoma

For each of the following cases, select the single most appropriate diagnosis. Each option may be used once, more than once or not at all.

15. A 57-year-old Asian man presents to his GP with a discoloured nail on his right thumb. He initially thought it was caused by trauma but now is slightly concerned as it seems to be darkening. On examination, epitrochlear and axillary lymphadenopathy are palpable.

16. A 35-year-old Caucasian man presents to the outpatient clinic with a mole on the right buttock that he noticed while having a shower. It measures 7mm in diameter and has an irregular border. Dermoscopy examination of the mole demonstrates a colour variegation.

17. A 40-year-old labourer presents to the GP with weight loss and a 2–3-week history of a bleeding, nodular lesion over the right forehead.

Theme: Management of skin and soft tissue cancers

Options for Questions 18–24:

A   Core biopsy
B   Electrochemotherapy
C   Excisional biopsy
D   Fine needle aspiration
E   Isolated limb perfusion
F   Mohs micrographic surgery
G   MRI scan

H   MRI scan with contrast
I   Punch biopsy
J   Radiotherapy
K   Sentinel lymph node biopsy
L   Staging CT scan
M   Ultrasonography

For each of the following cases, select the single most appropriate investigation or management plan. Each option may be used once, more than once or not at all.

18. A 65-year-old fit and healthy man presents with a rapidly growing, painless mass on the left anterior thigh that is fixed to the underlying fascia. Ultrasound suggests a possibility of soft tissue sarcoma. What would be the next most appropriate investigation?

19. A 2 mm excision biopsy of proven recurrent basal cell carcinoma on the left lower eyelid revealed incomplete excision of the deep margin.

20. A 37-year-old woman with a pigmented naevus on her back which she noticed has grown larger and changed colour. On clinical examination, melanoma is suspected.

21. A 60-year-old man had a superficial malignant melanoma completely excised from his back. Histology results reveal a 6 mm Breslow thickness. Clinical examination did not reveal any regional or systemic lymphaedenopathy. In addition to a wide local excision what other procedure could be performed in the same sitting?

22. A 45-year-old man with a previously excised melanoma on the anterior chest who is now currently under 5-year surveillance attends his 3-monthly follow-up clinic. On clinical examination, there was hepatomegaly. Which initial investigation would be most appropriate?

23. A 55-year-old man with previously excised 8 mm Breslow thickness nodular melanoma from the left lower leg presents with multiple cutaneous metastases on the left lower leg. He has previously had adjuvant radiotherapy. Past medical history of note includes peripheral vascular disease. Which treatment modalities can be considered?

24. A 34-year-old estate agent presents with soft, asymptomatic, mobile 3 cm lesion on the left flank which she has had for years. The mass is non-pulsatile and does not transilluminate. She is not keen on surgery if the lesion is benign. What would be the most ideal investigation?

Theme: Depth of burn injury

Options for Questions 25–27:

A	Deep dermal burn	F	Mid dermal burn
B	Epidermal burn	G	Second degree burn
C	First degree burns	H	Superficial dermal burn
D	Fourth degree burn	I	Third degree burn
E	Full thickness burn		

For each of the following cases, select the single most appropriate description of the burn injury. Each option may be used once, more than once or not at all.

25. A 27-year-old man presents to the emergency department after his trousers caught fire during Bonfire Night. Describe the burn as shown in **Figure 55.6**.

26. A 4-year-old boy accidentally pulled a cup of freshly made tea onto his left forearm. His mother reports that blisters formed immediately and the nurse in the emergency department has deroofed them. On examination, the scald looks shiny and wet and there is capillary refill. Describe the burn as shown in **Figure 55.7**.

27. A 67-year-old man suffered a mechanical fall and briefly lost consciousness. On regaining consciousness, he found that he had spilled a freshly made hot water bottle across his abdomen. Describe the burn as shown in **Figure 55.8**.

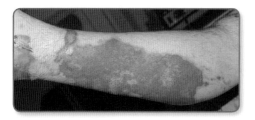

Figure 55.6 Left calf burn, as a result of a Bonfire Night accident.

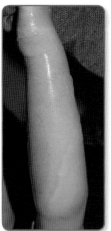

Figure 55.7 Forearm burn on a 4-year-old boy.

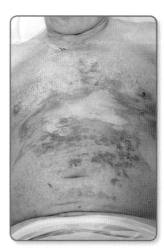

Figure 55.8 Abdominal burn following spillage from a hot water bottle.

Theme: Fluid resuscitation in acute burns

Options for Questions 28–31:

A	4.1 L	F	6–8 L
B	3.6 L	G	10–14 L
C	4.2 L	H	2.5–3 L/hour
D	2–4 L	I	1.8–2.4 L/hour
E	5–7 L		

For each of the following cases, select the single most appropriate estimate of resuscitation fluid requirements. Each option may be used once, more than once or not at all.

28. A 48-year-old woman is brought to the emergency department after she suffered an epileptic fit and fell against the radiator. Her burn injuries were estimated to be 30% TBSA. She weighs 70 kg. What is the total volume of intravenous fluid that should be given over 24 hours?

29. An 80-year-old man sustains 75% TBSA flame burn and weighs 45 kg. How much fluid should be administered intravenously within the first 8 hours?

30. A 30-year-old woman with 80% TBSA flame burn and weighs 60 kg. Injury occurred 4 hours ago. What is the ideal rate for intravenous fluid resuscitation within the next 4 hours?

31. A 12-year-old child with 16% TBSA scald and weighs 32 kg. How much maintenance fluid should be administered intravenously over 24 hours?

Theme: Management of burns injuries

Options for Questions 32–37:

A	Arterial blood gas	E	Escharotomy
B	Bronchial lavage	F	Fasciotomy
C	10% calcium gluconate	G	Fluorescein dye
D	Electrocardiogram	H	pH testing

For each of the following cases, select the single most appropriate investigations. Each option may be used once, more than once or not at all.

32. A 45-year-old man is brought to emergency department after he accidentally sustained an electrical burn while at work. He has full thickness burn to the tip of his left index finger and you note another wound over his right wrist. Clinical observations are as follows: respiratory rate 16/min, oxygen saturation 100% room air, pulse rate 130/min, blood pressure 120/60 mmHg. What important investigation would you like to arrange on patient's arrival to the department?

33. A 34-year-old builder attends the emergency department and reports of pain in both his knees. On examination, there are deep dermal burns over the anterior aspect of his knees. He informs you that he was working with cement for six hours before noticing the pain. What important investigations should be arranged?

34. A 19-year-old man is brought to the emergency department after he tried to light the living room fire with some petrol. He appears flushed and confused with slurred speech. In addition, his hair is singed and there is soot in his nostrils. Oxygen saturation is 98% on room air. The anaesthetist on call is on his way to review the patient. What important investigation would be useful in this scenario?

35. A 34-year-old man is brought in to the regional burns centre intubated on arrival. He suffered severe facial and trunk burns following self-immolation with petrol. The anaesthetist is having trouble achieving adequate ventilation for the patient. What procedure should be considered in this scenario?

36. A 14-year-old boy sustained a flash burn to his face after throwing an aerosol can into a bonfire. He now reports of blurry vision to his left eye.

37. A 45-year-old factory worker sustained TBSA 1% burn on the right forearm from hydrofluoric acid.

Answers

1. C Erythema nodosum

Erythema nodosum is the most common inflammatory disorder of the subcutaneous fat (panniculitis) and can be acute or chronic. The lesions are tender and primarily occur over the anterior lower legs. Early eruptions are red, slightly raised and shiny. They later flatten and turn into a deeper purplish colour, resembling a bruise. Erythema nodosum is associated with Crohn's disease (less commonly, ulcerative colitis), Behçet's syndrome, sarcoidosis, tuberculosis and certain drugs (i.e. oral contraceptives, hormonal replacement therapy, sulfonamides). Treatment is mainly conservative and targeted towards the underlying trigger.

2. F Pyogenic granuloma

Pyogenic granulomas are nodular, compressible, highly friable lesions that often occur at sites of trauma and areas that are often exposed, i.e. hands, forearms or face. The lesion is most common in children but can occur at any age. The colour can vary from red to bluish-black. Treatment includes curettage followed by destruction of base with silver nitrate or surgical excision.

3. E Pilomatricoma

Pilomatricoma (or benign calcifying epithelioma of Malherbe) is a hamartoma arising from hair matrix cells. It is asymptomatic, firm, often solitary (multiple may suggest association with certain inherited conditions) and the overlying skin usually shows epidermal atrophy. It has a bimodal age distribution, being most commonly found in patients in the first and sixth decades. They can occur in any part of the body but are most commonly found on the face or upper limbs. Lesions may demonstrate the 'tent' sign on stretching, which is usually multi-faceted. One should always consider pilomatricoma as an important differential in children presenting with firm nodular lesions since they rarely get epidermal cysts.

4. D Keratoacanthoma

Keratoacanthoma often occurs on sun-exposed areas and has a classic history of rapid growth for 4–6 weeks and reaching a plateau in size for another 4–6 weeks before spontaneously involuting over a period of few months. Clinically, they present as dome-shaped nodular lesions with a very well-defined border and often have a keratin plug in the centre. Histologically, it can be challenging to distinguish it from a well-differentiated squamous cell carcinoma. Watchful observation with serial measurements and photography can be considered only in cases that demonstrate a clear natural history. However, most clinicians would err on the side of caution and perform an excision biopsy, and most certainly so for lesions that fail to reduce to half its size within 4–6 weeks.

5. B Dermoid cyst

Dermoid cysts can occur due to entrapment of the epidermis during embryonic development and hence, arises at sites of embryonic closure zones. In the face, these sites include the region just above the lateral canthus of the eyebrows (angular dermoid), the glabella region and midline extending from the occipital scalp to the nasal root. Dermoid cysts can be found along the spine and might be associated with occult spina bifida. They are non-pulsatile, firm, cystic lesions that are lined with keratinizing stratified squamous epithelium (and may contain skin appendages like hair). Dermoid cysts are found in the subcutaneous tissue and, on occasion, present with a punctum. Differential diagnoses include lipoma and epidermal cyst. These cysts may have a deep intracranial extension and preoperative imaging using CT or MRI is required.

6. E Marjolin's ulcer

Marjolin's ulcer refers to malignant change within chronic inflammatory skin lesions or pre-existing scar tissue although its exact pathophysiology remains uncertain. However, there is a long latency period of 11–75 years with SCC being the most common phenotype. These lesions are most commonly found in the lower limbs and old burn scars are still the most common cause. Classical features include the formation of a nodule, induration and ulceration within the site of an old scar. Other features include rapid growth, a foul odour and everted margins. Multiple punch biopsies should be considered for any chronic, non-healing ulcer.

7. A Actinic keratosis

Actinic keratosis (or solar keratosis) is the most common epithelial dysplasia and arises from chronic sun exposure. They are often relatively small (most less than <6 mm in diameter), erythematous and covered with an adherent scale which gives it a roughened surface (sometimes they are more easily felt than seen). Commonly found on the sun-exposed areas (i.e. head, neck, dorsal hands), 20% of these regress spontaneously and rarely develop into SCCs (<1 in 1,000 annually). Treatment options include topical chemotherapy treatment using 5-fluorouracil or imiquimod cream, cryotherapy or laser resurfacing.

8. B Bowen's disease

Bowen's disease or squamous cell carcinoma in situ, often presents as a sharply defined erythematous patch with a scaly appearance. They are often mistaken to be psoriatic plaques or seborrheic keratosis. Only a small number of Bowen's disease (3–5%) become invasive. However, SCCs that originate from Bowen's disease have a greater propensity for metastasis. SCC in situ of the glans penis is termed erythroplasia of Queyrat. Treatment of choice is surgical excision. Medical options include topical chemotherapy agents, cryotherapy, curettage or cauterisation.

9. C Cutaneous horn

Cutaneous horns are yellowish, hard, protuberant 'horns' of hyperkeratosis occurring on the hands, face, ears and penis. Approximately 20–30% of these may overlie a malignant lesion such as SCC or BCC. Risk of cutaneous horns overlying a premalignant or malignant lesion is higher in elderly individuals with a fair complexion. Histologically, there is a compact proliferation of keratin and macroscopically it may have several antler-like divisions. Due to its association with malignancy, it is treated as a pre-malignant lesion and surgical excision is recommended.

10. E Lentigo maligna

Lentigo maligna, or Hutchinson's freckle, most often begins as a tan coloured macule that gradually darkens, often unevenly over a long period of time. These lesions often occur on sun damaged skin. After a period of radial growth for 5–20 years, it can progress to the vertical growth phase of invasive melanoma. At this stage, it is termed lentigo maligna melanoma. A palpable nodule arising within the lesion is the most suggestive feature of possible malignant change.

11. H Squamous cell carcinoma

Cutaneous squamous cell carcinoma is the second most common skin cancer (15–20% of skin cancers). Risk factors include age, Fitzpatrick skin types I–II, prolonged sun exposure (UVA and UVB are both implicated), chronic inflammation or irritation (Marjolin's ulcer and burns, respectively), exposure to arsenic and hydrocarbons and long term immunosuppression. Well-differentiated lesions typically are firm, erythematous papules with overlying keratinization whereas poorly differentiated lesions tend to be soft, granulomatous and may be associated with ulceration and necrosis. Patients on long-term immunosuppression are at higher risk of de novo SCCs which has a 14% metastatic rate.

12. B Basal cell carcinoma

This is the most common skin cancer worldwide (80%). Risk factors include skin type, sun exposure, exposure to arsenic or hydrocarbons, smoking, human papilloma virus (HPV), previous radiation and long-term immunosuppression. There are 27 different phenotypes of BCCs, with nodular BCC being the most common. Typical features of a nodular BCC include a dome-shaped papule with a pearly surface, rolled edges and overlying telangiectasia. The centre may present with ulceration.

13. D Giant congenital melanocytic naevus

Giant congenital melanocytic naevus (giant hairy naevus) are pigmented, hairy naevus that is present at birth and grows proportional with the body. These naevi are considered 'giant' if they measure >20 cm in diameter or has a TBSA of >5%. These giant naevi commonly occur on the trunk and 2–15% of these undergo malignant change. They account for a significant proportion of melanoma in children (40%) with axially based lesions posing the greatest risk for malignant change. Axial lesions also increase the risk of neurocutaneous melanosis (the presence of melanocytes within the central nervous system), which can undergo malignant change into leptomeningeal melanoma. Unlikely other types of malignant melanoma which arise from the dermoepidermal junction, malignant change in giant congenital melanocytic naevus occurs in the dermis or even deeper. Individuals with such lesions are considered at greatly increased risk of melanoma (8–10 times more that the general population) and require a lifetime of follow-up. Surgical options include serial excision and considering the use of tissue expanders or skin grafting to reconstruct large wound defects.

14. G Sebaceous naevus

Sebaceous naevus (naevus sebaceous of Jadassohn) are well-circumscribed plaques that are present since birth and are most commonly found on the scalp (50%). They can become much more pronounced and cerebriform-like during puberty due to hyperplasia of the sebaceous components and often get misdiagnosed as acanthosis nigricans or sebaceous keratosis. Larger sebaceous naevus (>10 cm) in association with ocular colobomas, epilepsy, and occasionally mental retardation raises the possibility of Schimmelpenning syndrome (sebaceous naevus syndrome). They have malignant potential and neoplasms that arise from these lesions are commonly trichoblastomas and syringocystadenoma papiliforms. There have been reports of malignant change into basal cell carcinomas but this phenomenon invariably occurs in adulthood. Hence, children with sebaceous naevi can be provided with the option for watchful waiting and excision in the future, if symptomatic. Serial excision is the surgical method of choice, as these lesions are often considerable in size and alopecic.

15. A Acral lentiginous melanoma

Often misdiagnosed as onychomycolysis, subungal haematoma, paronychia or even Kaposi's sarcoma, acral lengtinous melanoma often present with regional metastasis due to the delay in diagnosis. It is the most common type of melanoma in dark-skin and Asian populations and involve the hands (commonly thumb or hallus) or feet (people of African origins). These lesions tend to have indistinct margins with other clinical signs include melanonychia striata (a black discolouration of the proximal nail fold at the end of a pigmented streak), periungual hyperpigmentation, and Hutchinson's sign (pigmentation of the nail fold).

16. H Superficial spreading melanoma

Superficial spreading melanoma affects adults of all ages with no preference for sun-damaged skin. Lesions may arise de novo (40%) or in association with a pre-existing naevus. Risk factors for melanoma include: premalignant lesions, previous melanoma, ethnicity, Fitzpatrick type I skin, atypical naevus syndrome, a family history of more than three family members with malignant melanoma or pancreatic cancer in the (>10 times risk of melanoma of general population), and a history of prolonged sun exposure (occupational, excessive sun bed use).

17. G Nodular melanoma

Most aggressive phenotype of melanoma and often arises de novo without a clinically apparent radial growth phase. Nodular melanoma is more commonly found in men, and has a predilection for the head, neck and trunk.

18. G MRI scan with contrast

Soft tissue sarcomas are rare and often present at a late stage due to diagnostic difficulties. Ultrasonography is relatively inexpensive and non-invasive imaging modality that is useful as a first line investigation for a soft tissue mass. It is excellent in differentiating between cystic and solid lesions. Detailed characterization of a soft tissue mass by ultrasound is poor and MRI is the preferred imaging modality for this purpose. MRI is superior to CT scan in terms of tumour detection, image quality, and in delineating anatomical boundaries of lesions. The use of an intravenous contrast agent (gadolinium) provides more information regarding tumour morphology. Soft tissue sarcomas characteristically have a peripherally enhancing zone with a non-enhancing necrotic centre. A CT scan is a useful alternative for patients who are contraindicated for MRI imaging. If MRI proves inconclusive, a core biopsy can be used to obtain histological diagnosis. Previous NICE guidelines recommended that any palpable lesion that:

1. is rapidly growing
2. measures more than 5 cm in diameter)
3. is deep to fascia, fixed or immobile
4. painful or painless and
5. recurs after previous excision should be referred under the 2-week wait for suspected soft tissue sarcoma

The most recent 2015 NICE guidelines reported that none of the above five red flags have a predictive value of >3% and therefore only recommend 2-week wait referrals of ultrasound imaging with inconclusive results. Nonetheless, the five red flags are useful when evaluating soft tissue masses.

19. E Mohs micrographic surgery

Mohs micrographic surgery is a tissue sparing surgical excision method that utilises fresh frozen sections to achieve surgical margin clearance. The entire surgical margin is evaluated through horizontal sections (rather than vertical sections in standard histopathology). Mohs micrographic surgery is useful for recurrent or incompletely excised non-melanoma skin cancers, tumours with a poorly defined margin are more aggressive phenotypes (i.e. morpheaform BCC) and those tumours situated at aesthetically or functionally important regions such as the face, genital, perianal and hand. The other non-operative for this case scenario includes radiotherapy.

20. C Excisional biopsy

Narrow margin excision biopsy (2 mm lateral margin of healthy skin) is the preferred surgical method for excising suspected melanomas. The lesion should be photographed prior to excision and the longitudinal axis of the excision should be placed in a way that would be amenable to primary closure if a further wide local excision is warranted. Other excision methods for diagnosing melanoma such as shave biopsy and partial excision are not recommended due to sampling errors. It also interferes with pathological staging (Breslow thickness) of the lesion. Incisional biopsy or punch biopsy could be utilised for lentigo maligna or acral melanoma but only at the recommendation of a skin cancer multidisciplinary team. Patients with confirmed melanomas undergo a further wide local excision to ensure complete removal of the primary tumour and any existing microsatellites. The recommended lateral margins for wide local excision is dependent on the Breslow thickness of the melanoma itself. Breslow thickness is a staging system that measures melanoma depth starting from the granular epidermis to the deepest malignant cell, to the nearest 0.1 mm. It differs from Clark's staging system and carries prognostic value.

21. I Sentinel lymph node biopsy

Sentinel lymph node refers to the first lymph node that receives lymphatic drainage from the tumour itself. Patients with AJCC stage IB or above (in this case, patient is stage IIB, which is Breslow thickness 1.01–2 mm with ulceration or 2.01–4 mm with no ulceration) and no clinically palpable lymph nodes should be offered sentinel lymph node biopsy (SNLB). It is important to be aware that SNLB is not a curative treatment but rather a staging procedure. Five-year survival of patients with Breslow thickness 1.2–3.5 mm and a negative SNLB is 90% compared to those with the same Breslow thickness but who have a positive SNLB (75%). Twenty percent of patients who proceed to a complete regional lymph node dissection after a positive SLNB have pathological evidence of metastases. Risks of SNLB include failure of locating the sentinel node (5%) and a false negative result. In patients with palpable lymph nodes, an ultrasound-guided fine needle aspiration cytology should be considered.

22. K Staging CT scan

In this case scenario, the patient might have developed distant metastasis. Staging CT scan of the head, chest, abdomen and pelvis is useful to assess extent of metastasis and also assess suitability for surgery. Patients with metastases are classed to have stage IV melanoma and a measurement of serum lactate dehydrogenase (LDH) is recommended. PET CT scan is useful if further imaging is required or if there is an unknown primary tumour. It also provides clinicians with the ability to assess the presence of metastasis in the lower limbs (staging CT scans only image up to the perineal region).

23. B Electrochemotherapy

Electrochemotherapy is an emerging method for palliative treatment and locoregional control of metastatic melanoma especially in patients with cutaneous metastasis. The procedure is performed under local anaesthesia and delivers brief, intense electric pulses through an electrode that is placed within the tumour (intratumour) after intravenous administration of the chemotherapy drug (bleomycin). The electric pulses disrupt the tumour cell membranes, increasing its permeability and hence susceptibility to chemotherapy drugs. Isolated limb perfusion (ILP) and isolated limb infusion (ILI) can be considered for patients presenting with recurrent limb metastases or in patients who are not suitable for surgical excision, but possess good peripheral circulation. This procedure involves delivering chemotherapy drugs (actinomycin D and melphalan) directly to the affected limb intravenously under tourniquet isolation. All three methods are available in supraregional centres that treat melanoma. Whenever possible, surgical excision of solitary subcutaneous metastasis remains the treatment of choice.

24. M Ultrasonography

This patient is likely to have a lipoma. As explained in question 18, ultrasonography is a relatively inexpensive imaging method.

25. A Deep dermal burn

First, second and third degree burns are descriptions of burns that are not used in the UK. In this case scenario, the patient has deep dermal burns. The burn injury appears blotchy red, capillary refill is absent (fixed staining) and they usually don't form blisters (blisters are formed in superficial dermal burns). The fixed staining is due to extravasation of haemoglobin from damaged red blood cells indicating injury to the dermal vascular plexus. As nerve endings arise at the dermal level, these burns are insensate. The clinical distinction between mid-dermal and deep dermal burns is that mid-dermal burns have sluggish capillary refill, they appear a darker pink than superficial dermal burns and is not a dark blotchy red like deep dermal burns. These burns may be numb to light touch, but the surrounding area which may have a superficial burn will still be painful.

26. H Superficial dermal burn

Superficial dermal burns involve the epidermal and the papillary dermis (which is the superficial layer of the dermis). At this level, burns form blisters and as the nerve endings are exposed these burns are often extremely painful. Superficial dermal burns are moist (giving it a shiny appearance), pale pink in colour and there is capillary refill. Superficial dermal burns, usually treated conservatively, are capable of healing within 14 days with minimal scarring.

27. E Full thickness burn

Full thickness burns involve complete destruction of both epidermis and dermis. They appear white, leathery, insensate and may form an eschar. Full thickness burns will not heal and require surgical excision.

28. F 6–8 L

An ATLS approach should be adopted for the initial management of patients with burns. The total volume of resuscitation fluid required is calculated using the Parkland's formula which is 3–4 mL x TBSA (%) x weight (kg). Half of the calculated total volume is given over the first 8 hours after the time of initial injury, and the remaining half given over 16 hours. The fluid of choice is a crystalloid solution (Hartmann's). Burns >TBSA 15% in adults and >10% in children <12 years of age require fluid resuscitation. End organ function such as urine and cardiac output are often closely monitored and adjustments made to the rate of fluid administration as required.

Parkland's formula: 3–4 mL x TBSA (%) x weight (kg) = 3–4 mL x 30 x 70 = fluid resuscitation required is between 6,300 mL to 8,400 mL.

29. E 5–7 L

Parkland's formula: 3–4 mL x TBSA (%) x weight (kg) = 3–4 mL x 75 x 45 = fluid resuscitation required is between 10,125–13,500 mL. Half of the calculated volume is given over the first 8 hours starting from the time of injury: 10,125–13,500 mL/2 = 5,062.5 mL to 6,750 mL.

30. I 1.8–2.4 L/hour

Parkland's formula: 3–4 mL x TBSA (%) x weight (kg) = 3–4 mL x 80 x 60 = fluid resuscitation required is between 14,400–19,200 mL. Half of the calculated volume is given over the first 8 hours starting from the time of injury: 14,400 to 19,200 mL/2 = 7,200 mL to 9,600 mL. The volume of 7,200 mL to 9,600 mL will need to be given over 4 hours which is 7,200 mL to 9,600 mL /4 = 1,800 mL to 2,400 mL/hour aiming for a urine output of 0.5 mL–1 mL/kg/hour (for children this would be 1–2 mL/kg/hour).

31. A 4.1 L

Apart from fluid resuscitation, children with major burn injuries would also require maintenance fluids. This is calculated as 100 mL/kg/hour for the first 10 kg, 50 mL/kg/hour for the next 10 kg and 20 mL/kg/hour for each kg body weight over 20 kg. In a child who weighs 32 kg, this would be 100 mL + 50 mL + 22 mL = 172 mL/hour. The total volume of maintenance fluid that would be required in 24 hours will be 172 mL x 24 kg = 4,128 mL. 0.45% sodium chloride + 5% dextrose solution is the fluid of choice for maintenance fluids.

32. D Electrocardiogram

Electrical burn injuries are either low voltage (<1000 volts), high voltage (>1000 volts) or rarely, lightning strike. Tissue damage is mainly due to heat generation and this is dependent on the resistance of the tissue, duration of contact and the surface area at the point of contact. Bone has the most resistance with nerves and blood being the least resistant. Muscle injury post burn injury can result in rhabdomyolysis and subsequent acute kidney injury. All patients with an electrical burn injury should have an electrocardiogram performed immediately on admission. Any patient who had a cardiac arrest or the possibility of the electric current passing through the thorax should be monitored closely with telemetry as they are at high risk of dysrhythmias even if they present with an initial normal ECG trace.

33. H pH testing

Chemical burns could be from either acid or alkali and it is important to ascertain during history taking which type of chemical was involved and the duration of contact as they cause damage to tissues in different ways. Acidic chemicals cause coagulative necrosis. There is immediate tissue destruction with protein hydrolysis resulting in a tough, leathery eschar. The resultant eschar limits further spread of the chemical. Unlike acidic agents, alkalis have a more insidious pattern of injury causing saponification of fat cells in a process called liquefaction necrosis. Free alkali molecules have the ability to penetrate deeper into the wound, causing further damage. The initial management of chemical burns involve copious irrigation with water ('dilution is the solution to pollution') and regular pH testing (normal pH of skin is 4.5–6.2). It is important to note that chemical burns involving elemental sodium, potassium and lithium should not be treated with water irrigation as it will cause ignition.

34. A Arterial blood gas

In this case scenario, the patient is at high risk of inhalation injury. The singed facial hair suggests facial burns, and decreased GCS suggests carbon monoxide (CO) intoxication. Careful examination of each burns patient with the intent to rule out inhalation injury is imperative and an aesthetic review is warranted. Clinical signs and symptoms suggestive of inhalation injury include: carbonaceous sputum, singed facial hair, respiratory difficulty, change of voice, inspiratory stridor, and a brassy cough. An arterial blood gas would be able to confirm CO intoxication with elevated carboxyhaemoglobin levels (>10%). Initial management involves administration of 100% oxygen, which reduced the half-life of CO to 45 minutes from 4–5 hours if the patient was breathing room air. Inhalation injury of the lower airways can be confirmed on bronchoscopy. Nebulized bronchodilators and inhaled steroids can be used to relieve bronchospasm and inflammation.

35. E Escharotomy

Full thickness burns across the chest reduces chest expansion and hampers effective ventilation as the chest wall struggles to expand under an unyielding thick eschar. Escharotomy simply means surgically excising through burned skin down to subcutaneous fat. The incision lines are placed longitudinally along the anterior axillary lines from the second to twelfth rib, running into the upper abdomen if necessary. Transverse incisions are made across the upper chest just below the clavicles and upper abdomen, creating a mobile breastplate pattern that improves chest compliance. Circumferential full thickness burns of the extremities cause progressive oedema of the underlying burnt tissue against a rigid overlying eschar, leading to compartment syndrome and eventually an ischaemic limb. Decreased pulses on Doppler ultrasound is the best indicator for escharotomy. Care should be taken when placing escharotomy incisions along the extremities so as not to damage important structures (i.e. ulnar nerve at the medial epicondyle, common peroneal nerve at the neck of the fibula, long saphenous vein and sapheneous nerve at the medial malleolus). It is important to note that escharotomy and fasciotomy are two separate entities. Occasionally, fasciotomies are required to release fascial compartments in patients who have sustained deep thermal injuries or severe electrical burns.

36. G Fluorescein dye

Initial management of any thermal or chemical ocular burn injury involves copious irrigation with water. Fluorescein drops can be used to assess extent of corneal damage and an ophthalmology review is required. In comparison with thermal ocular burns, chemical burns to the eye are far more severe. A strong alkali could cause irreversible blindness within 3 minutes. The corneal epithelium is breached and the alkali causes almost instant opacification of the lens, the pH within the anterior chamber rises and subsequently damages the iris, ciliary body and lens. Extent of ocular injury could be further classified using the Roper–Hall or Dua classifications. As long as there is no conjunctival involvement or limbal ischaemia, the recovery of corneal epithelial defect is generally good. It is important to note that when performing pH testing, the use of eye drops such as fluorescein (alkali) can temporarily alter the pH reading, leading to inadequate first-aid management. Apart from serious complications like cataracts, globe perforation and limbal ischaemia, the inner eyelids can get scarred down to the globe itself, a condition termed as symblepharon.

37. C 10% Calcium gluconate

Hydrofluoric acid is a highly corrosive acid commonly found in industrial sites that manufacture plastics and semiconductors. It is also used in cleaning air-conditioning equipment. Hydrofluoric acid burns produce serious local and systemic effects due to its highly reactive elemental fluoride ion. The fluoride ion combines with calcium or magnesium in the body, depleting intra- and extra-cellular stores. The resultant hypocalcaemia can lead to initial profound bradycardia, tetany, respiratory depression, reduced GCS, seizures and intractable ventricular fibrillation. Due to its severe systemic effects, a TBSA as small as 2% can be fatal. Patients often present with severe pain, oedema and bullae. Initial management include deroofing of the bullae, application of topical 10% calcium gluconate to the burn area to neutralize the fluoride ions and ECG. More severe cases may require intravenous administration of 10% calcium gluconate and early excision of the damaged tissue.

Chapter 56

Hand disorders

Questions

Theme: Differential diagnosis of hand disorders

Options for Questions 1–4:

A	Bouchard's nodes	F	de Quervain's tenosynovitis
B	Boutonnière deformity	G	Rheumatoid nodule
C	Carpal tunnel syndrome	H	Swan neck deformity
D	Ganglion	I	Trigger finger
E	Dupuytren's contracture	J	Wrist osteoarthritis

For each of the following cases, select the single most appropriate diagnosis. Each option may be used once, more than once or not at all.

1. A 50-year-old woman, with a background of diabetes, presents with a history of difficulty in extending her left ring finger at the level of the proximal interphalangeal joint. Full extension of the finger is possible when she uses her other hand to stretch out the finger, with a pop felt. Her symptoms are worse in the morning. On examination, she has a tender nodule with some associated swelling over the flexor aspect of the affected finger.

2. A 43-year-old woman presents with pain and tenderness over the dorsoradial aspect of her right wrist and thumb. On examination, she has tenderness and crepitus in the region of the tendons of the first extensor compartment with a positive Finkelstein's test.

3. A 46-year-old man with a background of epilepsy presents with progressive fixed flexion contractures of the ring and little fingers in both hands. On examination painless nodules and thick cords can be felt on the palmar aspects of both hands and the table top test is positive bilaterally.

4. A 53-year-old woman presents with a known diagnosis of rheumatoid arthritis. On examination the patient is found to have ulnar deviation of the fingers in both hands, tender swellings at the level of the proximal interphalangeal joints, with a flexion deformity of the proximal interphalangeal joint and a hyperextension deformity of the distal interphalangeal joint of the right middle finger.

Theme: Hand trauma

Options for Questions 5–8:

A   Flexor tenosynovitis
B   Mallet finger
C   Mallet thumb
D   Ulnar collateral ligament injury
E   Volar plate injury

F   Zone 1 flexor tendon injury
G   Zone 2 flexor tendon injury
H   Zone 3 flexor tendon injury
I   Zone 4 flexor tendon injury

For each of the following cases, select the single most appropriate diagnosis. Each option may be used once, more than once or not at all.

5.   A 22-year-old man presents with pain, swelling and deformity to the right little finger following an impact with a cricket ball leading to a forced flexion injury. On examination, there is swelling and tenderness at the level of the distal interphalangeal joints in the right little finger, with a correctable flexion deformity at that level. Radiographs are normal.

6.   A 31-year-old woman presents with an injury to her left thumb following a fall whilst skiing. She is found to have tenderness, swelling and ecchymosis over the region of the left thumb thenar eminence and metacarpophalangeal joint, with a decreased range of movement throughout the digit. There is instability of the metacarpophalangeal joint on stress testing, particularly on radial deviation of the thumb. Standard radiographs reveal no fracture.

7.   A 54-year-old woman presents for her 6-week review following a dorsally displaced right distal radius managed conservatively in a Colles' cast. On removal of the cast the fracture site is non-tender and she has a moderate range of movement at the wrist. However, the patient is complaining of an inability to extend her ipsilateral thumb at the level of the inter-phalangeal joint. Radiographs demonstrate no new injury.

8.   A 42-year-old man presents following an accident work with a kitchen knife. On examination he has an incised wound over the palmar aspect of the left index finger at the level of the proximal interphalangeal joint. On examination, the patient is unable to flex the proximal interphalangeal joint of the left index finger when the other fingers are held in extension. The patient also has decreased sensation and sweating over the radial aspect of the digit, but there is no gross vascular deficit found.

Theme: Upper limb nerve lesions

Options for Questions 9–12:

A	Cheiralgia paresthetica		compression
B	Carpal tunnel syndrome	F	Pronator teres syndrome
C	Cubital tunnel syndrome	G	Saturday night palsy
D	Palmar branch of the median nerve	H	Supinator tunnel syndrome
E	Posterior interosseous nerve	I	Ulnar tunnel syndrome

For each of the following cases, select the single most appropriate diagnosis. Each option may be used once, more than once or not at all.

9.   A 30-year-old woman presents with a 2-year history of worsening paraesthesia in the medial one and half digits, with associated weakness, in the left hand. On examination, she has a cubitus valgus deformity secondary to an ipsilateral supracondylar fracture as a child. She has a positive Froment's test but with no evidence of clawing in the hand.

10. A 58-year-old woman presents with an 8-month history of progressive pain and paraesthesia affecting the lateral three and half digits of her right hand, with her symptoms often worse at night. On examination, she has signs of muscle wasting to the thenar eminence and a positive Tinel's test.

11. A 42-year-old alcoholic man presents to the emergency department in police custody wearing handcuffs. He is complaining of a loss of sensation on the dorsoradial aspect of the right hand and wrist. There is no evidence of any motor deficit.

12. A 41-year-old woman presents with an 18-month history of pain and tenderness over the proximal volar aspect of the left forearm, with associated tingling and weakness of the left hand. On examination, there is paraesthesia affecting the lateral fingers and palm of the hand with an associated weakness of the pincer movement.

Answers

1. I Trigger finger

Trigger finger or thumb is characterised by fibrotic thickening of affected tendon sheaths leading to stenosis that ultimately results in the affected flexor tendon being caught within the retinacular pulley system, most commonly at the first annular (A1) pulley. Associated risk factors include middle age, female sex, rheumatoid arthritis, diabetes mellitus and gout. The ring and middle fingers and thumb are most frequently involved.

Diagnosis is made on clinical evaluation with the patient complaining of pain, swelling and difficulty moving the affected digit, with symptoms often worse in the morning. On examination, a tender nodule may be felt on the palmar aspect of the affected digit, and it will remain locked in flexion when passive extension of all digits is attempted. Extension is possible with further effort or with passive force applied, with a pop and triggering of the finger.

Treatment is with conservative (analgesia, physiotherapy, steroid injection) or surgical (release, tenosynovectomy) measures.

2. F de Quervain's tenosynovitis

De Quervain's tenosynovitis was initially described in 1895 by Swiss surgeon Fritz de Quervain. It is characterised by sheath inflammation and stenosis of the tendons of the first extensor compartment (extensor pollicis brevis, abductor pollicis longus). Peak incidence is between 30–50 years of age with a female predominance. The cause is not known, though associations with repetitive overuse and inflammatory arthritis are proposed.

Patients often present with pain, tenderness and swelling of the affected thumb and wrist (dorsoradial). Finkelstein's test is diagnostic as it reproduces the pain in the region of the first extensor compartment. The patient flexes the thumb across the palm, makes a fist and then performs passive ulnar deviation of the wrist. Differential diagnosis includes osteoarthritis of the wrist and/or thumb carpometacarpal joint, which would be found on plane radiographs.

Treatment is either non-operative (rest and avoidance, nonsteroidal anti-inflammatory drugs, splints, steroid injection) or operative (division and release of affected tendon sheaths). Potential complications of surgical treatment are recurrence and neurapraxia of the superficial branch of the radial nerve.

3. E Dupuytren's contracture

Dupuytren's disease was initially documented in 1831 by Parisian surgeon Baron Guillaume Dupuytren, who described the treatment for the disorder. It is characterised by nodules in the palm of the hand, development of cords, progressive fibrotic thickening of the palmar and digital fascia with hyperplasia and contracture (change of collagen from type I to type III), ultimately resulting in fixed flexion deformities of the affected fingers. The incidence rises sharply after 40 years of age and males (10:1) are more commonly affected. Risk factors include:

- Genetics (autosomal dominant)
- Trauma
- Epilepsy, e.g. phenytoin therapy
- Diabetes mellitus
- AIDS/HIV
- Alcohol excess and liver disease/cirrhosis
- Associated disorders:
- Ledderhose disease (plantar fibromatosis)
- Peyronie's disease (penile fibromatosis)
- Garrod's knuckles

The disease often presents in both hands with a symmetrical pattern. The ring and little fingers are most frequently affected (**Figure 56.1**) and pain is rare. The Hueston tabletop test is considered positive when a dorsal aspect of an open hand cannot be placed flat on the table, and is used as an indication for surgery. Treatment includes conservative, collagenase therapy (non-invasive enzyme fasciotomy), fasciotomy, fasciectomy or dermofasciectomy. Complications include recurrence (~30%), infection, neurovascular injury, haematoma, stiffness and complex regional pain syndrome.

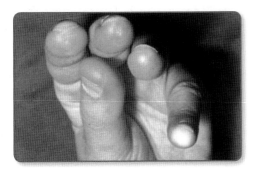

Figure 56.1 Dupuytren's contracture of the little finger.

4. B Boutonnière deformity

Rheumatoid arthritis frequently leads to symptoms involves the joints and soft tissue of both hands. Inflammation and repeated trauma leads to flexor and extensor tendon damage, with potential deformities including:

- Boutonnière deformity is characterised by distal interphalangeal joint hyperextension and proximal interphalangeal joint flexion. Initial disruption of the central slip of the extensor tendon leads to separation and volar subluxation of the lateral bands, followed by dorsal subluxation of the proximal phalanx head. The deformity persists due to contracture of the volar plate, collateral ligaments and oblique retinacular ligament. Stages of the deformity include extension lag followed by flexion contracture

- Swan neck deformity is characterised by proximal interphalangeal joint hyperextension with metacarpophalangeal joint and distal interphalangeal joint flexion and can originate from flexor digitorum superficialis rupture or extensor digitorum communis shortening
- Ulnar and volar deviation of the fingers is secondary to synovial inflammation of the wrist joint and metacarpophalangeal joints
- Z-thumb deformity is often seen due to rupture of the flexor pollicis longus tendon, which in turn is associated with abnormalities within the carpus

5. B Mallet finger

A mallet finger usually occurs following a direct blow to an actively extended finger causing a hyper flexion injury, e.g. attempting to catch a cricket ball. This results in rupture of the distal extensor digitorum tendon slip from its insertion on the distal phalanx, with associated avulsion fractures from the dorsal base possible. Examination demonstrates tenderness and swelling in the region of the distal phalanx, with an inability to actively extend flexed at the distal interphalangeal joint (passive extension possible). Anteroposterior, lateral and oblique radiographs of the affected digit reveal any bony abnormality. Management is with Mallet splint immobilisation (distal interphalangeal joint held in hyperextension) for 6–8 weeks. If there is subluxation of the distal interphalangeal joint or a large amount of the articular surface involved (>50%), fixation with an extension blocking K-wire may be required.

6. D Ulnar collateral ligament injury

The ulnar collateral ligament originates from the head of the thumb metacarpal and inserts on the proximal phalanx of the thumb. Rupture of the ulnar collateral ligament is also known as gamekeeper's thumb (chronic) or skier's thumb (acute). Following a complete rupture, ~80% cases will have a Stener lesion (interposition of the aponeurosis of adductor pollicis muscle between the insertion and the ruptured free edge of the ligament).

Injury commonly occurs following a fall onto an outstretched hand leading to forced abduction of an extended thumb. On examination, there will be tenderness (ulnar aspect), swelling and possible ecchymosis at the thumb metacarpophalangeal joint and thenar eminence, with a restricted range of movement and evidence of instability. Radiographs of the thumb are to exclude an avulsion fracture from the base of the proximal phalanx, with radial stress views (following infiltration of local anaesthetic) demonstrating instability of the metacarpophalangeal joint.

Treatment is with:

- Immobilisation with a thumb spica (partial rupture)
- Operative repair (complete rupture, Stener lesion, avulsion fracture)

7. C Mallet thumb

A mallet thumb is characterised by rupture of the insertion of the extensor pollicis longus tendon at the distal phalanx of the thumb (originates from the middle third of the dorsal ulna surface). Associated avulsion fractures can occur. Causes of a mallet thumb are:

- Acute trauma
- Distal radius fracture
- Late complication (3–12 weeks post injury) due to radial tubercle disruption or fracture fragment
- Rheumatoid arthritis, SLE
- Degeneration as the tendon passes over Lister's tubercle

Examination will reveal tenderness and swelling in the region of the distal phalanx following an acute injury. Patients will have an inability to actively extend the thumb when flexed at the interphalangeal joint, but with passive extension this is often possible. Thumb radiographs are necessary to exclude an associated fracture. Management is with:

- Immobilisation
- Direct operative repair
- Free tendon transfer (e.g. extensor indicis)

8. G Zone 2 flexor tendon injury

Flexor tendon injuries are divided into zones (Verden zones) that guides treatment and prognosis (**Tables 56.1** and **56.2**, **Figure 56.2**). Zone 2, also known as 'no man's land'.

Treatment is with repair, with concomitant repair of the neurovascular structures that are frequently involved.

Table 56.1 Flexor tendon injury zones in the fingers			
Zone	From	To	Contents
1	Mid-point middle phalanx	Finger tip	Flexor digitorum profundus
2	Distal palmar crease (A1 pulley)	Mid-point middle phalanx	Flexor digitorum profundus, flexor digitorum superficialis (sheath)
3	Distal edge carpal tunnel	Distal palmar crease (A1 pulley)	Flexor digitorum profundus, flexor digitorum superficialis
4	Proximal edge carpal tunnel	Distal edge carpal tunnel	Carpal tunnel
5	Forearm and wrist	Proximal edge carpal tunnel	Volar compartment

Table 56.2 Flexor tendon injury zones in the thumb		
Zone	From	To
1	Interphalangeal joint	Finger tip
2	A1 pulley (proximal phalanx)	Interphalangeal joint
3	Thenar muscles	Distal palmar crease
4	Proximal edge carpal tunnel	Distal edge carpal tunnel
5	Musculotendinous junction	Proximal edge carpal tunnel

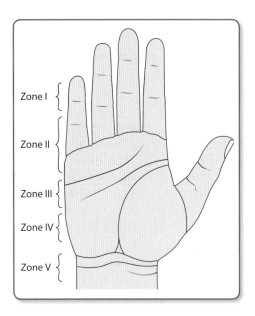

Figure 56.2 Flexor tendon injury zones.

9. C Cubital tunnel syndrome

Cubital tunnel syndrome is the second most frequent neuropathy of the upper limb and is due to a lesion of the ulnar nerve at the level of the elbow. Potential causes/sites include:

- Arcade of Struthers
- Medial epicondyle
- Medial epicondylitis
- Osborne's ligament
- Anconeus epitrochlearis
- Flexor carpi ulnaris aponeurosis
- Tumours or ganglions
- Trauma and deformity
- Cubitus varus or valgus post supracondylar fracture
- Burns

Clinical signs and symptoms are due to proximal ulnar nerve compression with pain and paraesthesia of the medial one and a half digits. Intrinsic muscle weakness and/or atrophy can be found with a positive Froment's sign (adductor pollicis weakness leads to compensatory thumb IPJ flexion). Hand clawing may occur, however, the more proximal the lesion, the less pronounced is the clawing due to the loss of innervation to flexor digitorum profundus medial two digits (ulnar paradox). Therefore, with ulnar tunnel syndrome there is compression of the ulnar at the wrist (Guyon's canal) and thus more pronounced clawing of the hand as innervation to flexor digitorum profundus is preserved. Provocation tests include Tinel's test (tapping over nerve as runs posterior to medial epicondyle) and prolonged elbow flexion test. Nerve conduction studies can confirm the diagnosis. Management options include:

- Non-operative
- Activity modification, splints, anti-inflammatories, steroid injection
- Operative:
    - Decompression (open or endoscopic)
    - Medial epicondylectomy
    - Anterior transposition

10. B Carpal tunnel syndrome

Carpal tunnel syndrome is the most common compressive neuropathy of the upper limb and is due to microvascular compression and neural ischaemia to the median nerve as it passes posterior to the flexor retinaculum of the carpal tunnel. Risk factors include:

- Increasing age (peak incidence middle age)
- Gender (females)
- Obesity, smoking, alcoholism
- Co-morbidities, e.g. diabetes mellitus, hypothyroidism, acromegaly
- Fluid retention, e.g. pregnancy, combined oral contraceptive, congestive cardiac failure
- Inflammatory arthritis, e.g. rheumatoid arthritis
- Trauma, e.g. distal radius fracture, lunate fracture/dislocation
- Occupation (possible links with repetitive movements)

Clinical signs and symptoms are due to median nerve compression within the carpal tunnel; common findings include pain (worse at night, shake hand to relieve) and paraesthesia of thumb, index, middle and the radial half of the ring fingers. Sensation over the radial palm of the hand is preserved as this is innervated by the palmar cutaneous branch of the median nerve. Thenar muscle atrophy and weakness are late signs. Provocation tests include Phalen's test (flex ipsilateral wrist for 1–2 minutes) and Tinel's test (tapping over the nerve at the volar wrist crease). Nerve conduction studies are often used when the diagnosis is unclear. Management options include:

- Non-operative
    - Activity modification, splints, anti-inflammatories, steroid injection
- Operative
    - Carpal tunnel release and decompression (open or endoscopic)

11. A Cheiralgia paresthetica

Cheiralgia paresthetica, also known as Wartenberg's syndrome, is a neuropathy of the superficial sensory branch of the radial nerve. Causes can either be compression (on forearm pronation between extensor carpi radialis longus and brachioradialis) or trauma (external compression from watch or handcuffs). Patients present with pain, burning sensation and paraesthesia over the radio-dorsal aspect of the wrist and hand, but with no motor abnormality present. Provocation tests include Tinel's sign (tapping over the nerve) or resisted forearm pronation for approximately one minute. Treatment options are:

- Non-operative
  - Activity modification, splints, anti-inflammatories
- Operative
  - Decompression

12. F Pronator teres syndrome

Pronator teres syndrome is caused by compression of the median nerve as it passes between the heads of pronator teres on entering the forearm. This disorder is part of the group of disorders known as pronator syndrome. Other potential sites of compression include the:

- Ligament of Struthers
- Bicipital aponeurosis
- Flexor digitorum superficialis aponeurotic arch

The key clinical signs for differentiating pronator syndrome from carpal tunnel syndrome are:

- The loss of sensation over the radial palm of the hand due to the involvement of the palmar cutaneous branch of the median nerve
- Pain at the level of the elbow and/or at the proximal volar forearm
- Phalen's and Tinel's signs at the wrist should be negative
- Weakness of the muscles of the forearm flexor compartment would indicate anterior interosseous nerve involvement
- Provocation test positive on resisted forearm pronation

Management options include:

- Non-operative
  - Activity modification, splints, anti-inflammatories
- Operative
  - Decompression of affected site

Chapter 57

Surgical disorders of the brain

Questions

Theme: Intracranial non-neoplastic lesions

Options for Questions 1–3:

A	Cerebral abscess	**D**	Hydrocephalus
B	Chronic subdural haematoma	**E**	Subarachnoid haemorrhage
C	Extradural haematoma		

For each of the following situations, select the single most likely diagnosis. Each option may be used once, more than once or not at all.

1. A 60-year-old man complains of increasing generalised headache associated with nausea and vomiting for 3 days. He feels feverish and has double vision. In the past he has suffered from and been treated for recurrent sinusitis. He has had type 1 diabetes for 30 years and recently has been on steroids for asthma. On examination, he is pyrexial with a temperature of 39°C and on funduscopy shows early papilloedema.

2. A 25-year-old man is brought into the accident and emergency department while playing in a football match having sustained an injury resulting in gradual drowsiness. During the course of play he collided with another player at the goal-mouth while heading the ball. He was momentarily unconscious but continued playing for some time after the incident. His Glasgow Coma Score is 14, the pupils are equal and reacting to light and he has no papilloedema.

3. A 45-year-old man is admitted with sudden onset of very severe occipital headache which he describes as though somebody has given him a hammer blow to the back of the head. He has vomiting and marked photophobia and is very drowsy. On examination, he has some neck stiffness and oculomotor (3rd nerve) palsy. His blood pressure is 180/100 mmHg and pulse rate is 60 beats per minute.

Theme: Intracranial neoplasms

Options for Questions 4–6:

    A   Acoustic neuroma   D   Meningioma

    B   Cerebral metastases   E   Pituitary tumour

    C   Glioma

For each of the following situations, select the single most likely diagnosis. Each option may be used once, more than once or not at all.

4.   A 70-year-old man is admitted following a seizure that lasted for 10–15 minutes. On admission he complains of severe headache. His Glasgow Coma Score is 15. He complains of having recently suffered from headaches with vomiting. Six years ago, he underwent a right nephrectomy for hypernephroma.

5.   A 45-year-old woman complains of gradual hearing loss and tinnitus of 4–6 months' duration. She has noticed dizziness and feels an illusory sense of her body revolving. She also has right-sided temporal headache which is often associated with vomiting. On examination, she has some facial weakness and numbness in the distribution of the right 7th cranial nerve.

6.   A 42-year-old woman complains of attacks of headache early in the morning as a result of which she is woken up earlier than usual. Recently she noticed that inadvertently she has been bumping into the sides of doorways and into people. Her periods, until recently regular, have been scant and irregular; she has been surprised and embarrassed by secreting milk from her breasts.

Answers

1. A Cerebral abscess

This patient who has long-term type 1 diabetes (and hence is immunocompromised) has features of raised intracranial pressure – headache, nausea and vomiting, and visual disturbances – with signs of infection. Past history of sinusitis gives a clue as to the source of cerebral infection. A localised intraparenchymal abscess begins when bacteria incite an acute inflammatory reaction with oedema, a condition called cerebritis. At this stage death may result from the expanding mass causing transtentorial herniation; secondary abscesses may also form causing death.

In due course as the abscess matures, three layers surround the central core of purulent debris – a layer of granulation tissue, a layer of fibrosis and finally surrounded by gliosis. The bacteria that cause brain abscesses are often anaerobic or microaerophilic. Abscesses are multiple in 15–20%. The condition can also result from haematogenous spread particularly from respiratory and dental infections; in a quarter of the patients no underlying primary infection is found.

On CT scan a ring-enhancing mass lesion is typical of an abscess is seen. Image-guided surgical aspiration under intravenous antibiotic cover is the mainstay of treatment. Aspiration may have to be repeated and the antibiotics continued for 6 weeks. Rarely excision of the abscess wall may be necessary. Steroids may be used in severe oedema but with caution as their use may conflict with the efficacy of antibiotics. Because of the high chance of epilepsy in the long-term, prophylactic anticonvulsant treatment is instituted.

Subdural empyema is less common but more serious and carries a higher mortality. It occurs as a result of acute mastoiditis and rhinosinusitis.

2. C Extradural haematoma

This young man has the typical features of a rapidly forming extradural haematoma (EDH). Presence of a lucid interval is pathognomonic of the diagnosis although this symptom may not always be present. Being the thinnest part of the cranium, the squamous part of the temporal bone is most commonly fractured with tear of the underlying middle meningeal artery as it enters the middle cranial fossa through the foramen spinosum to lie in its groove. As it traverses the groove, fracture of the squamous part of the temporal bone causes the middle meningeal vessels to tear resulting in the haematoma. It can occur in the presence of minor trauma. The classical presentation of EDH of head injury followed by lucid interval with later rapid deterioration in the Glasgow Coma Score is seen only in a minority of patients. If missed, the condition will progress to contralateral hemiparesis, unconsciousness and ipsilateral pupillary dilatation due to uncal herniation. Pupillary dilatation is due to the EDH exerting a space-occupying effect causing the hemisphere to shift to the opposite side resulting in the uncus and the sharp edge of the tentorium to press on the oculomotor nerve.

On CT scan a biconvex hyperdense lesion is seen between the calvaria and the brain. The treatment is prompt evacuation of the EDH by a craniotomy carried out by a neurosurgeon. Evacuation of EDH by making a burr hole at the pterion is often mentioned. This, however, is not a good method for efficient evacuation of an EDH. Ideal treatment is evacuation by a neurosurgeon through a craniotomy by raising an osteoplastic flap.

3. E Subarachnoid haemorrhage

The history of a sudden onset of a severe headache typically described as a hammer blow at the back of the head is characteristic of subarachnoid haemorrhage (SAH) from rupture of a cerebral berry aneurysm. The patient has other typical features: meningism, photophobia and 3rd nerve palsy – the latter is due to rupture of an aneurysm in the posterior communicating artery, which is in close proximity to the oculomotor nerve that is compressed by the haematoma. The immediate past history from his wife of occipital and cervical headache is even more suggestive of the diagnosis. Some patients refer to the initial headache as a 'thunderclap' headache.

These aneurysms typically arise at the bifurcation of the main arteries at the circle of Willis. This is because at the junction (bifurcation) of the arteries, the tunica media is congenitally lacking thus making the particular site weak. Therefore, that particular anatomical site is liable to ballooning by the blood flow creating turbulence and formation of a saccular aneurysm. More than 90% of these saccular aneurysms occur at the circle of Willis being equally distributed at the sites of the junctions of the arteries.

A CT scan confirms the diagnosis in the vast majority if carried out early. If the CT scan is negative a lumbar puncture is carried out. In elective patients with a convincing history and negative lumbar puncture and CT scan, a CT angiogram or cerebral digital subtraction angiogram is done. The treatment is endovascular coiling carried out by an interventional radiologist or craniotomy and clipping by a neurosurgeon.

The commonest cause of non-traumatic SAH is cerebral aneurysm. Clinically SAH is graded according to the World Federation of Neurological Surgeons system. The complications of rupture of cerebral aneurysms are: rebleeding, delayed ischaemic neurological deficit, hydrocephalus and hyponatraemia from cerebral salt wasting.

4. B Cerebral metastases

This 70-year-old man has been admitted as an emergency with an epileptic fit from which he has recovered. There is a history of early morning headache with vomiting, which are symptoms of raised intracranial pressure. A previous history of nephrectomy for renal cell carcinoma is very significant and cerebral metastasis should be considered as the cause of his fit. A thorough neurological examination should be carried out, followed by a contrast CT scan.

Metastatic tumours of the brain far outnumber primary tumours. Routine autopsy shows that 1 in 4 patients with cancers have a brain metastases. The most common site in the brain is the junction of the grey and white matter of the cerebral cortex. The most common primary tumours to metastasise to the brain are lung (in both sexes) followed by breast, melanoma, kidney and the gastrointestinal tract. Brain metastases occurs by haematogenous spread. Over 50% of all cases of metastatic disease of the brain produce multiple metastases.

Adenocarcinoma of the kidney metastasises by the blood stream to the lungs, bones and brain. It is well-known that blood borne metastasis may manifest many years after successful removal of a primary renal cell carcinoma as has happened in this patient whose kidney carcinoma was removed almost 6 years ago. The brain metastasis can have several types of mass effects: raised intra-cranial pressure effects, oedema in surrounding brain tissue (suitable for palliation by steroids), haemorrhage within the tumour (particularly prone in renal cell cancer and melanoma) and obstructive hydrocephalus causing early mass effect.

Multiple lesions are treated by steroids and irradiation. When there is a significant period of recurrence-free interval between removal of the primary and appearance of the secondary, surgical removal of a solitary cerebral metastasis has much to recommend it provided there is no other evidence of the disease.

5. A Acoustic neuroma

This woman has clinical features of raised intracranial pressure with focal neurological deficits suggestive of a tumour in the vicinity of the 8th cranial (vestibulocochlear) nerve. She has tinnitus, deafness and vertigo, symptoms that confirm the suspicion. Facial numbness and weakness point to compression of the 5th (trigeminal) and 7th (facial) cranial nerves. The diagnosis is an acoustic neuroma that arises at the cerebellopontine angle. As it enlarges laterally it may cause erosion of the internal auditory meatus while medially it may extend into the subarachnoid space causing hydrocephalus. In late cases there may be compression of the brainstem and tonsillar herniation which is fatal.

The tumour is a Schwannoma, a benign tumour, arising from the Schwann cells of the nerve sheath of the vestibular component of the 8th cranial nerve. It is slow growing and accounts for 8% of primary intracranial tumours. Most arise within the internal auditory canal or at the meatus causing unilateral sensorial hearing loss, tinnitus and vestibular dysfunction. This is a slow growing tumour and as it enlarges it erodes the internal auditory meatus, extends into the subarachnoid space of the cerebellopontine angle (hence called cerebellopontine angle tumour) compressing the 5th and 7th cranial nerves, brain stem and cerebellum giving rise to symptoms of a posterior fossa mass.

The imaging of choice is gadolinium-enhanced MRI. Excision by open surgery is the treatment of choice. Preservation of facial and auditory nerve function will depend upon the size of the tumour and the preoperative disability. Usually when unilateral, the condition is sporadic. If bilateral, it is a component of neurofibromatosis Type II which may include meningioma, glioma or neurofibroma.

6. E Pituitary tumour

This woman has the clinical features of a pituitary tumour. Her clinical presentation stems from features of raised intracranial pressure, pressure effects on the optic chiasma and hormonal disturbances of hypopituitarism (oligomenorrhoea) and excess prolactin production causing galactorrhoea. Her visual disturbances are due to pressure effects of the adenoma on the optic chiasma causing bitemporal hemianopia, resulting in her bumping into doorways and oncoming people. The bitemporal hemianopia (blindness in the temporal half of both visual fields) occurs because the nasal fibres from both retinas are interrupted; this narrows the outer (temporal) part of both visual fields giving rise to this particular symptom of visual field defect.

The patient needs to be investigated at the outset by baseline investigations of pituitary function such as serum prolactin, FSH, LH, serum oestradiol, TFTs, serum growth hormone and cortisol. Imaging is carried out. Lateral view X-ray of the skull will show widening of the sella turcica and erosion of the posterior clinoid processes from pressure effects of the adenoma. CT scan and MRI are mandatory to identify a macroadenoma or a microadenoma. Visual field defects denote a macroadenoma (>10 mm tumour) in this patient.

Microadenomas are less than 10 mm and more often incidental findings (sometimes endocrine effects may be seen). Prolactinomas constitute 30%, non-functioning tumours constitute 20%, 15% secrete growth hormone and 10% secrete ACTH. Five per cent of pituitary tumours are familial, occurring in association with MEN 1 syndrome. In general, macroadenomas produce visual disturbances whilst prolactinomas are microadenomas. Prolactinomas (the most common endocrinological abnormality) are treated medically with bromocriptine which is a dopamine agonist. Macroadenomas are treated surgically by the trans-sphenoidal route. This patient has a macroadenoma that is also a prolactinoma.

A syndrome may present as an emergency called pituitary apoplexy due to haemorrhagic infarction of a pituitary tumour. The patient presents with sudden headache, visual loss and ophthalmoplegia with impaired consciousness. This requires steroids and urgent decompression.

Chapter 58

The paediatric surgical patient

Questions

Theme: Anatomy

Options for Questions 1–4:

A Greater body surface area to body mass ratio than the adult

B Head is proportionally smaller than in an adult

C Larynx is higher and more anterior in the neck than the adult

D Muscle mass is less than the adult

E Narrowest part of the paediatric airway is at the level of the cricoid cartilage

F Tongue is small relative to the oropharynx

For each of the following situations, select the single most likely answer. Each option may be used once, more than once or not at all.

1. A 3-year-old boy develops respiratory difficulties during the administration of inhalational anaesthesia prior to a minor surgical procedure. The boy is otherwise healthy, with no history of previous respiratory difficulties.

2. A 6-year-old girl is found to be hypothermic during intraoperative monitoring. The surgeon is undertaking adenoidectomy, but there have been numerous delays in theatre and the procedure is taking much longer than planned.

3. An 8-year-old girl is involved in a road traffic accident resulting in intra-abdominal injury. She was a rear seat passenger wearing a seat belt. Her mother was sitting next to her and was also wearing a seat belt but is uninjured.

4. A 7-year-old boy requires a lengthy surgical procedure under general anaesthetic. The patient has no significant past medical history. A cuffed endotracheal tube was used and the anaesthetist is concerned about the risk of pressure necrosis developing due to prolonged intubation.

Theme: Common surgical disorders of the paediatric patient

Options for Questions 5–8:

A	Appendicitis	E	Pyloric stenosis
B	Inguinal hernia	F	Torsion of the testis
C	Intussusception	G	Undescended testes
D	Oesophageal atresia		

For each of the following situations, select the single most likely diagnosis. Each option may be used once, more than once or not at all.

5. A 12-year-old boy presents with acute right iliac fossa pain. On further questioning it is found that the pain initially began in the scrotum but now radiates into the scrotum. On examination, the abdomen is soft and apparently non tender.

6. A 6-week-old boy presents dehydrated and withdrawn. His parents describe forceful vomiting which has increased in severity over the past 7 days. Intermittent vomiting has been present since 2 weeks old. Vomiting occurs immediately after or during feeds.

7. A 7-month-old girl presents with 10 days of increasingly severe episodes of colic, during which she draws up her legs and screams. Over the past 24 hours, she has been vomiting bile-stained fluid.

8. A 10-month-old boy presents with an intermittent lump in his left groin which was noticed by his parents when he was crying. The lump always disappears when relaxed, but appears to be increasing in size when crying. The infant is otherwise well with no suggestion of gastrointestinal upset.

Theme: Neonatal surgical abnormalities

Options for Questions 9–11:

A	Biliary atresia	F	Haemolytic disease of the newborn
B	Diaphragmatic hernia		
C	Exomphalos	G	Meckel's diverticulum
D	Gastric outlet obstruction	H	Oesophageal atresia
E	Gastroschisis	I	Tracheal atresia

For each of the following situations, select the single most likely diagnosis. Each option may be used once, more than once or not at all.

9. A newborn girl is noted to be drooling and coughing. The midwife is concerned. Spontaneous vaginal delivery was uncomplicated. No abnormalities had been detected at the 20 weeks' ultrasound scan. The pregnancy was unremarkable.

10. A newborn boy is noted to have respiratory difficulty and an obvious sunken appearance to the anterior abdominal wall is seen. Prenatal ultrasound scan had demonstrated polyhydramnios but no cause for this had been identified.

Theme: Paediatric oncology

Options for Questions 11–13:

A	Germ cell tumour	D	Rhabdomyosarcoma
B	Hepatoblastoma	E	Wilms' tumour
C	Hepatocellular carcinoma		

For each of the following situations, select the single most likely diagnosis. Each option may be used once, more than once or not at all.

11. A 4-year-old previously healthy boy presents with fever, abdominal swelling and blood stained urine.

12. A 16-year-old girl presents with lump arising from her right thigh. The mass has gradually increased in size over the previous 4 weeks and is non-tender. She is otherwise well and there is no significant past medical history.

13. A 2-year-old boy presents with an obvious swelling at the base of his spine. His parents report that this has gradually increased in size over the past month, but does not appear to cause any discomfort. Past medical history is unremarkable. On examination there is a firm, immobile mass in the sacral region which appears non-tender.

Theme: Paediatric orthopaedics

Options for Questions 14–16:

A	Developmental dysplasia of the hip	D	Osteomyelitis
		E	Perthes' disease
B	Ewing's sarcoma	F	Septic arthritis
C	Juvenile idiopathic arthritis	G	Slipped capital femoral epiphyses

For each of the following situations, select the single most likely diagnosis. Each option may be used once, more than once or not at all.

14. A 7-year-old boy presents with pain in the knee and a limp. His white cell count and C-reactive protein count are normal.

15. A 13-year-old boy with an elevated body mass index presents with hip and knee pain.

16. A 6-month-old girl presents with unequal skin folds between her legs and body.

Theme: Paediatric ear nose throat

Options for Questions 17–19:

A	Acute otitis media	E	Eustachian tube dysfunction
B	Barotrauma	F	Otitis media externa
C	Cholesteatoma	G	Quinsy
D	Chronic otitis media	H	Tonsillitis

For each of the following situations, select the single most likely diagnosis. Each option may be used once, more than once or not at all.

17. A 9-year old boy who has recently come back from Australia presents with right sided ear pain, fluid in the middle ear and conductive hearing loss.

18. A 11-year-old boy presents with pain on swallowing. On examination, he is unable to open his mouth fully due to pain.

19. A 15-year old boy presents with discharge from his right ear, conductive hearing loss and right facial weakness.

Theme: Paediatric urology

Options for Questions 20–22:

A	Anterior ureteral valves	F	Posterior ureteral valves
B	Congenital adrenal hyperplasia	G	Urinary tract infection
C	Enuresis	H	Urolithiasis
D	Hypospadias	I	Vesicoureteral reflux
E	Neurogenic bladder		

For each of the following situations, select the single most likely diagnosis. Each option may be used once, more than once or not at all.

20. A 11-year old boy has urodynamic studies for investigation of his incontinence. Results reveal a large volume, lower pressure bladder with absent contractions. His mother suffers from epilepsy.

21. A 5-year old boy with Lesch–Nyhan syndrome presents and severe back pain.

22. A baby is born at term, however on the initial baby checks the gender is unclear.

Answers

1. C Larynx is higher and more anterior in the neck than the adult

One of the consequences of the larynx being positioned at the level of C3/C4, compared to C4/C5 in the adult, is that the tongue is in closer proximity to the palate. This risks airway obstruction, particularly in the setting of inhalational anaesthesia. Other anatomical predispositions to airway difficulties include a large tongue relative to the oropharynx, vocal cords are at a more antero-caudal angle and the epiglottis is inclined more posteriorly.

2. A Greater body surface area to body mass ratio than the adult

Due to increased body surface area, children are more susceptible to heat loss, especially when they are exposed during surgical procedures or resuscitation. In addition, due to higher basal metabolic rate children have a higher respiratory rate and can become hypoxic more quickly. Children also have a proportionally larger head compared to adults which contributes to greater potential for heat loss.

3. D Muscle mass is less than the adult

In addition to less muscle mass, children generally have less fat, with closer proximity of chest and abdominal organs to the site of impact. In particular, the liver and spleen are proportionally larger than in adults. Injury to these organs can go unrecognised leading to significant blood loss. Combined with the enhanced ability to compensate for intravascular depletion this can result in late recognition of haemodynamic compromise.

4. E Narrowest part of the paediatric airway is at the level of the cricoid cartilage

This can risk pressure necrosis at the level of the cricoid if a cuffed endotracheal tube is used. It should be noted that in the adult the narrowest part of the airway is at the level of vocal cords.

5. F Torsion of the testis

On first impression, the patient may have been triaged as a 'right iliac fossa pain' for repeat abdominal examination considering appendicitis. However, with a full history of the presenting complaint it is clear the diagnosis lies elsewhere. It is important that examination of the scrotum is included in the abdominal examination. Testicular torsion pain is usually present for less than 6 hours. Risk factors may include a malformation of the processus vaginalis where the mesorchium terminates early resulting in mobile testes within the tunica vaginalis, bell clapper deformity and pubertal changes. Cold weather where the cremasteric contraction may induce torsion and anatomical abnormalities such as cryptorchidism (undescended testes are at higher risk of torsion). On examination of the scrotum the affected testes may have a horizontal lie, and the cremasteric reflex may be absent.

This is a surgical emergency, if treated within 6 hours there is a high chance of saving the testes, but this falls to 50% between 6 and 12 hours. In younger boys (< 10 years) the hydatid of Morgagni (present in around 90%) can become contorted and present with similar pain. This may be difficult to differentiate clinically and surgical exploration is likely to be indicated.

6. E Pyloric stenosis

Infants with pyloric stenosis usually present within the first 8 weeks of life. The pylorus is thickened causing gastric outlet obstruction with non-bilious, projectile vomiting. Patients usually present dehydrated with a hypochloraemic metabolic alkalosis. The underlying aetiology is unknown although there may be a genetic background as children with parents of the condition are more likely to be sufferers. It is more common in boys than girls and is rare past 6 months of age. On examination a 'pyloric olive' may be palpable in the epigastrium. Diagnosis is made by ultrasound scan which demonstrates the thickened pylorus.

7. C Intussusception

This is the invagination of one part of the intestine into another. Infants present with intermittent severe cramping abdominal pains or colic. During an episode the child may scream, draw up their legs, or fall asleep between episodes. Later in the course the infant may develop bilious vomiting and 'redcurrant jelly stools' or rectal bleeding. In approximately one-third of patients the intussuscepted segment is palpable as a sausage shaped mass. Late complications include perforation and peritonitis. In infants the majority occur in relation to a viral infection where the lead point is an enlarged Peyer's patch. In older patients the underlying aetiology is likely to be pathological, including a tumour, polyp or Meckel's diverticulum. Ultrasound scan may show a typical 'target sign'. Small bowel obstruction may be seen on abdominal X-ray. If the patient is unstable laparotomy is indicated given the potential for bowel ischemia or perforation. In the stable patient, a barium enema which shows a 'crab-claw' deformity confirms the diagnosis (**Figure 58.1**); the procedure could also be used to relieve the intussusception. A successful outcome is indicated by reflux of barium into the terminal ileum.

8. B Inguinal hernia

In children, inguinal herniae are invariably indirect and more often occur on the right side due to the later descent of the right testes. There is a male preponderance. In females the lump is present in the upper part of the labia majora. Risk of

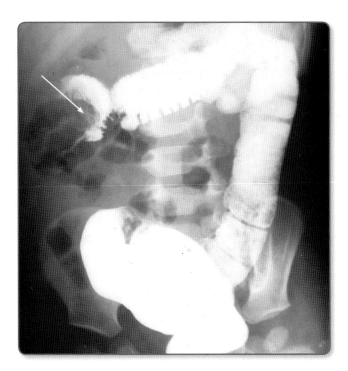

Figure 58.1 Barium enema showing typical crab claw appearance (arrow) in ileocaecocolic intussusception in a baby.

incarceration is high in infants (less than 1-year-old) and so surgery should be undertaken within around 2 weeks, as an 'urgent elective' case. After one year of age the risk of incarceration is reduced and surgery may be less urgent.

Inguinal hernia repair is a common operation in young children, especially ex-premature infants and low birth weight babies. In the latter patients the abdominal wall is weak and the normal obliteration of the sac has not occurred.

In terms of management, in the case of the irreducible hernia gentle pressure may be applied in an attempt to reduce the hernia. Attempting reduction with firm pressure under anaesthesia is contraindicated. However, evidence of intestinal obstruction or suggestion of ischemia necessitates emergency surgery.

9. H Oesophageal atresia

This is a congenital defect whereby the oesophagus terminates before reaching the stomach, leading to two blind ending pouches. The condition may be associated with a fistula to the trachea (tracheoesophageal fistula). The condition is noticed and treated soon after birth. Rarely an emergency procedure is required as nutritional supplements and fluids can be provided parenterally allowing for further investigations to exclude other abnormalities. Associated defects may include cardiac, spinal and/or renal abnormalities. The presence of multiple abnormalities in this context is known as VACTERL syndrome (vertebral column, anorectal, cardiac, tracheal, oesophageal, renal and limbs). Oesophageal atresia can be diagnosed from around 26 weeks' gestation by ultrasound scan. Treatment is surgical, usually requiring primary anastomosis or occasionally colonic transposition if the two sections of oesophagus cannot be approximated. Infants with tracheal atresia present with stridor. Although present from birth tracheal atresia may not cause significant symptoms until later in life.

10. B Diaphragmatic hernia

This sunken appearance to the anterior abdominal wall is also known as a 'scaphoid abdomen'. It takes its appearance due to the position of upper abdominal viscera which have moved into the thorax secondary to a large diaphragmatic hernia. Around 50% of diaphragmatic hernias are detected on prenatal ultrasound scan and polyhydramnios may be detected. The condition is associated with a variable degree of pulmonary hypoplasia and in severe cases left ventricular hypoplasia may also be seen. **Figures 58.2** demonstrates an X-ray finding of a diaphragmatic hernia.

The most common type of congenital diaphragmatic hernia is Bochdalek's hernia which is a posterolateral defect. Other types include Morgagni's, a rare anterior diaphragmatic defect, and diaphragm eventration where an otherwise intact diaphragm is displaced within the chest.

Initial management includes the placement of an orogastric tube and intubation to protect the airway followed by surgical intervention as appropriate.

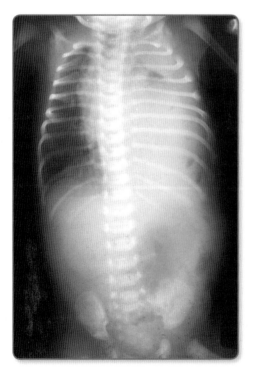

Figure 58.2 Plain X-ray in a neonate showing no left lung shadow and no left dome of diaphragm as a result of a congenital diaphragmatic hernia.

11. E Wilms' tumour

This renal tumour represents the most common primary malignant renal tumour of childhood (approximately 8% of solid tumours). Up to 10% of tumours are bilateral. Potential for lung metastases and involvement of the renal vein and vena cava should be investigated with CT and ultrasound scanning respectively. First presentation usually relates to a large abdominal mass which is easily palpable. Patients may also experience abdominal pain, fever, nausea/vomiting, haematuria in approximately 20% and occasionally hypertension. Most are chemosensitive, with patients undergoing preoperative chemotherapy followed by delayed resection. Often the kidney can be preserved where there is a pseudocapsule around the tumour. If the tumour is not completely microscopically excised radiotherapy may be applied. For early stages survival is greater than 90%. Neuroblastoma is a differential diagnosis for malignant cause of abdominal swelling. It usually effects a younger age group (<2 years). Neuroblastoma tends to encase vascular structures, rather than invade.

12. D Rhabdomyosarcoma

This is a rare tumour which generally arises from skeletal muscle. Incidence is highest in children aged 1–5 and 15–19 years old. A combination of surgery and either pre- or postoperative chemotherapy and/or radiotherapy is used depending on tumour subtype and extent. Cure is dependent on the type, location and extent of tumour, although survival is usually long-term.

13. A Germ cell tumour

Germ cell tumours originate from primordial or pluripotential germ cells. The commonest type of germ cell tumour is a sacrococcygeal teratoma. Presentation is usually with an obvious mass in the sacral region, although some can be entirely presacral with no obvious external mass. Presacral tumours may present with lower gastrointestinal or urinary symptoms.

The preferred treatment is surgical resection, which should include the sacrum and coccyx. While the majority of germ cell tumours are benign the malignant potential requires long-term oncological follow-up.

14. E Perthes' disease

Also known as Legg–Calvé–Perthes' disease. This condition is an avascular necrosis of the proximal femoral head. The most common age group is 5–10 years of age. It is more common in boys. Patients present with an intermittent limp. Pain may also be present down the anterior thigh but the limp can also be painless. Diagnosis is by X-ray of the pelvis with anterior posterior views and lateral leg view which typically presents with a flattened femoral head. MRI can be used when the X-ray images are inconclusive.

15. G Slipped capital femoral epiphysis

Slipped capital femoral epiphysis results from a Slater-Harris fracture through the proximal femoral physis. It is thought to be caused by increased pressure from the hip on the growth plate. It most commonly presents in obese adolescent boys. Diagnosis is by X-ray of the pelvis with anterior posterior views and lateral leg views. The femoral head looks similar to a melting ice cream cone. Patients are at risk of avascular necrosis. Management usually involves bed rest and internal fixation of a cannulated screw.

16. A Developmental dysplasia of the hip

DDH is present in around 2 in every 1000 babies. It normally presents at birth but can also be seen in the first year of life. It can affect one hip or both sides.

Risk factors for developing DDH include being female, a firstborn child, family history, oligohydramnios and breach delivery. If you have the risk factors for DDH or the hip feels unstable then an ultrasound scan is normally recommended. The condition can initially be picked up at the newborn checks when the hips are tested using Ortolani and Barlow's test. Ortolani's test tests for a dislocated hip by putting gentle forward pressure to each femoral head to see whether it is possible to see whether there is any movement suggesting a dislocated or sublimed hip joint. In Barlow's test backward pressure is applied and to the head of each femur and if there is movement of the head to suggested subluxation of the hip.

If diagnosed early a Pavlik harness is recommended, which stabilises the baby's hips and holds them in position. The harness is worn for several weeks and eventually can start to be taken off. Surgical reduction can also be done if DDH is diagnosed after six months or the harness has not corrected the hip joint. Patients, especially those that are not treated early can develop osteoarthritis and a limp.

17. B Barotrauma

This patient has just returned from a flight from Australia making barotrauma of the ear the most likely diagnosis. This can occur when the plane descends for landing. The pressure change creates a vacuum pushing the eardrums inwards. Increased water pressure from scuba diving is also another presentation for barotrauma. Prognosis is generally very good.

18. G Quinsy

This patient is suffering from odynophagia and trismus making quinsy the most likely diagnosis. Quinsy is a peri-tonsillar abscess. It is commonly a complication of tonsillitis. Treatment is by intravenous antibiotics and drainage of the pus.

19. C Cholesteatoma

Cholesteatoma is an expanding, destructive squamous epithelial growth which typically presents with conductive hearing loss, recurrent middle ear infections and symptoms relating to invasion into nearby structures. Management is usually surgical excision of the cholesteatoma.

20. E Neurogenic bladder

This patient has a flaccid neurogenic bladder with no evidence of detrusor activity. In children it is commonly caused by neurological birth defects, such as spina bifida. This patient's mother suffers from epilepsy and many anticonvulsants are associated with neural tube defects. Any disease of the central or peripheral nervous system can lead to a neurogenic bladder.

21. H Urolithiasis

This patient is suffering from a metabolic disease which pre-disposes children to urolithiasis. Urolithiasis is relatively rare in children. It can present with metabolic, endocrine, and renal disorders. Some chemotherapy drugs also predispose patients to urolithiasis.

Lesch–Nyhan syndrome is an X-linked inherited disorder which results in a build-up of uric acid in the body. The excess uric acid results in neurologic, cognitive dysfunction as well as self-injuring behaviour. This also results in gout, arthritis and urolithiasis.

22. B Congenital adrenal hyperplasia

Congenital adrenal hyperplasia is an autosomal recessive disorder involving a deficiency in adrenal enzymes that are responsible for the production of adrenal hormones. Most commonly, congenital adrenal hyperplasia is due to a deficiency in 21-hydroxylase. 21-hydroxylase deficiency leads to virilisation and ambiguous genitalia in genetically female neonates. Salt wasting is another complication due to a deficiency in mineralocorticoid steroids.

Chapter 59

Upper limb trauma

Questions

Theme: Upper limb trauma

A Anterior dislocation of shoulder
B Barton's fracture
C Colles' fracture
D Compartment syndrome
E Galeazzi's fracture
F Humerus shaft fracture
G Monteggia's fracture–dislocation
H Posterior dislocation of shoulder
I Scaphoid fracture
J Supracondylar fracture of the humerus

For each of the following cases, select the single most appropriate diagnosis from the options listed above. Each option may be used once, more than once or not at all.

1. A 7-year-old boy presents to the emergency department following a fall from a swing while playing in the park. There is obvious swelling around his left elbow with loss of distal pulses.

2. A 72-year-old woman slipped in the kitchen and presented with pain around her right wrist. On examination she had a 'dinner-fork' deformity and the type of injury confirmed on X-ray. The fracture was reduced and a plaster cast applied which was removed after 6 weeks.

3. A 24-year-old man who sustained a fall from his motorbike was found to have a closed fracture in his forearm which was treated with a long arm splint. Two hours later, the man complains of worsening pain, which is not relieved even after an injection of morphine.

4. A 21-year-old man who was injured while playing rugby is brought to the emergency department. He supports his right arm at the elbow using his opposite hand. He remembers having suffered a similar injury 2 years ago during a game. He is in severe pain, and refuses to move his arm.

5. A 34-year-old electrician sustained a high voltage electric shock while at work and was admitted to the burns unit for management. A day after admission, the orthopaedic team is consulted for pain and difficulty in movement of his right shoulder.

6. A 30-year-old man sustains a fracture of his left upper limb. After reduction and application of a U-slab, he develops a wrist drop.

7. An 18-year-old basketball player fell on his hand while playing and injured his right wrist 8 months ago. His initial X-rays appeared normal, and he did not seek any further medical advice. He presents now with persisting pain in his wrist. X rays reveal a fracture that has not united.

8. A 27-year-old man sustained a fracture in his forearm after a car accident. A fracture of the distal radius shaft is fixed with plates and screws, and the distal-radio ulnar joint is pinned with a K-wire. Postoperatively the forearm is immobilised in supination.

Answers

1. J Supracondylar fracture of humerus

Supracondylar fracture of the humerus is common in the 5–9-year age group, and occurs from a fall onto the outstretched hand. Two types are recognised – the extension type, which is far more common (98%), and the flexion type (2%). In the extension type of supracondylar fracture, the distal fragment is displaced posteriorly. The spike of the proximal fragment can impinge on the brachial artery anteriorly and cause vascular insufficiency (**Figure 59.1**).

The other structures liable to be injured in a supracondylar fracture are the median, radial and ulnar nerves. Clinically, the child presents with a painful and swollen elbow after a fall. The S-shaped deformity at the elbow is typical in a displaced extension type fracture (**Figure 59.2**).

It is critical to ascertain the distal neurovascular status of the limb because of the risk of injury to the structures mentioned above. The limb is initially splinted in a position of 30° flexion at the elbow. Treatment is usually by closed reduction, which is achieved by traction, and hyperflexion of the pronated forearm. The fracture (unless undisplaced) is usually held with two or three K-wires, and a cast applied.

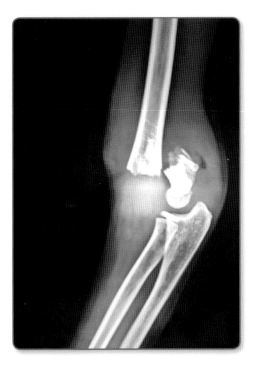

Figure 59.1 An extension type supracondylar fracture of humerus. The brachial artery is at risk of impingement by the proximal fragment.

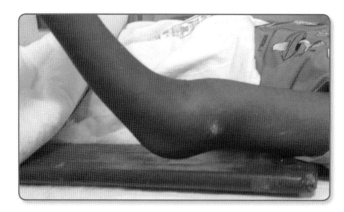

Figure 59.2 The typical deformity of a displaced supracondylar fracture.

2. C Colles' fracture

A Colles' fracture is a fracture of the distal radius at the cortico-cancellous junction, which usually occurs in osteoporotic bone. It is more common in elderly women, owing to post-menopausal osteoporosis. The mechanism of injury is a fall on an extended wrist. The displacement of the fracture (described by the relative position of the distal fragment in relation to the proximal) is typical as shown in **Figure 59.3** and consists of:

- Radial deviation
- Radial tilt
- Dorsal displacement
- Dorsal tilt
- Supination
- Impaction of the fragments

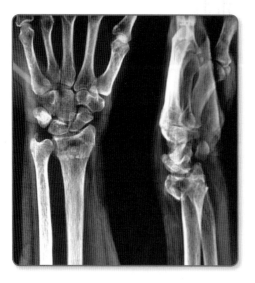

Figure 59.3 X-rays showing the typical displacement in a Colles' fracture.

The displacement results in the typical 'dinner-fork' deformity of the wrist. The fracture is reduced by traction, pronation and ulnar deviation of the wrist, and is then immobilised in a below-elbow plaster cast (**Figure 59.4**) for a period of 6 weeks.

Complications of a Colles' fracture are:

- Malunion
- Stiffness of the wrist
- Reflex sympathetic dystrophy (Sudeck's dystrophy)
- Rupture of the extensor pollicis longus tendon
- Median nerve palsy due to carpal tunnel compression (rarely)

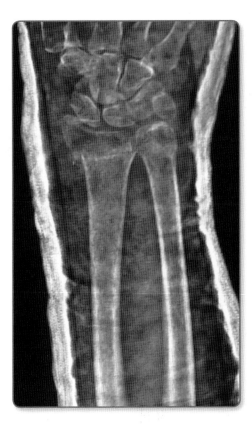

Figure 59.4 A Colles' fracture reduced and immobilised in a plaster cast.

3. D Compartment syndrome

This man is developing compartment syndrome, which is obvious from the unrelenting pain, not settling with analgesics, and out of proportion to the magnitude of injury. Compartment syndrome develops from increased pressure in a closed osteo-fascial compartment, which compromises tissue perfusion. This happens because of muscle oedema, bleeding into the closed compartment, burns, tight casts or bandages. A vicious cycle of increasing pressure and decreasing capillary perfusion develops. Unless treated promptly, the muscles undergo necrosis leading to Volkmann's ischaemic contracture.

The limb appears swollen, tense and blistered. There is extreme pain on passive stretch of the affected muscles.

Timely intervention is crucial to prevent muscle necrosis. Any splints or tight dressings should be removed immediately. Compartment pressure can be monitored, and if it rises to within 30 mmHg of the diastolic pressure, it is an indication for urgent surgical intervention. A fasciotomy is performed to relieve the compartment pressure.

4. A Anterior dislocation of the shoulder

Anterior dislocation is the most common type of shoulder dislocation. The mechanism of injury is forceful abduction and external rotation of the shoulder. The patient presents in severe pain, often with the affected arm supported at the elbow by the opposite hand. There is loss of the rounded contour of the shoulder on the affected side (**Figure 59.5**), and attempted movements are extremely painful. X-rays reveal the humeral head has been forced out of the glenoid cavity (**Figure 59.6**).

Treatment of an acute dislocation entails immediate reduction, which can be carried out by a number of methods – the Kocher, Hippocratic and Stimson's techniques being the important ones.

The most common complication of an anterior dislocation of the shoulder is recurrent anterior instability. Recurrent instability is more common when the first dislocation occurs at a younger age. Recurrent anterior instability can be addressed by an arthroscopic repair of the glenoid labrum – the Bankart's repair.

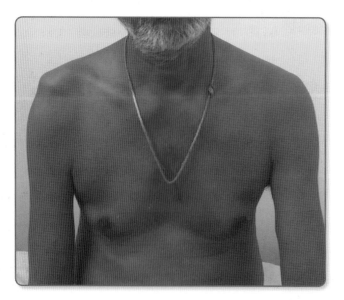

Figure 59.5 Loss of the normal contour of the shoulder can be appreciated on the right side compared to the left. The head of the humerus can be seen to bulge anteriorly on careful inspection.

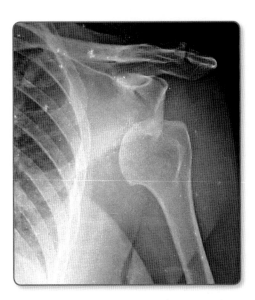

Figure 59.6 X-ray showing an anterior dislocation of the shoulder.

5. H Posterior dislocation of the shoulder

Posterior dislocation of the shoulder is much less common than anterior dislocation, and comprises about 2% of all shoulder dislocations. The mechanism of injury is exactly the opposite of an anterior dislocation. A very strong force is required to dislocate the shoulder posteriorly, and this happens with forceful adduction and internal rotation. The magnitude of force required to produce this usually occurs in a patient who has suffered a seizure, or has convulsed from an electric shock.

Clinically, there is pain and a restriction of lateral rotation of the arm. The X-rays are frequently passed off as normal, resulting in the diagnosis being commonly missed. A true lateral view of the shoulder reveals the dislocation. Treatment is by closed reduction, which is achieved by applying traction to the adducted arm and then laterally rotating it.

6. F Humerus shaft fracture

The patient has sustained a fracture of the shaft of the humerus. The radial nerve is intimately related to the bone as it winds around it in the spiral groove. The nerve is particularly at risk in a fracture occurring at the junction of the middle and distal third of the humerus. This is because, at this level, the nerve pierces the lateral inter-muscular septum to pass anteriorly, and is relatively tethered and immobile. In all cases of humerus shaft fractures, the radial nerve function should be specifically examined by asking the patient to extend the metacarpophalangeal and wrist joints. In this case, radial nerve palsy has developed after manipulation of the fracture, and this is an indication for open reduction and exploration of the nerve.

Fractures of the humeral shaft do well with non-operative treatment, while being immobilised in a U-slab or a hanging cast initially for 2 weeks (**Figure 59.7**) and thereafter in a functional brace.

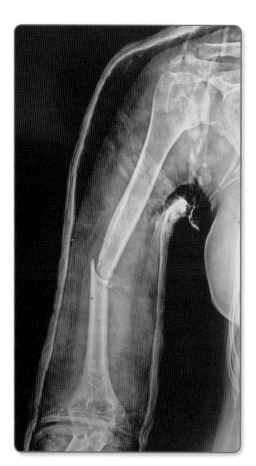

Figure 59.7 A fracture of the humerus shaft, immobilised in a U-slab.

7. I Scaphoid fracture

Fractures of the waist of the scaphoid are at a high risk of non-union and avascular necrosis of the proximal fragment. This is because of the nature of vascular supply to the scaphoid. 80% of the proximal scaphoid is supplied via retrograde blood flow and hence is predisposed to non-union and avascular necrosis.

Clinically, a scaphoid fracture should be suspected when tenderness is elicited in the anatomical snuff box and at the base of the thumb. Frequently, the fracture cannot be picked up on X-rays in the acute setting, and the fracture is missed (**Figure 59.8**). An ulnar deviated PA view of the wrist provides a much better assessment of the scaphoid. When a fracture is strongly suspected clinically but not visible on radiographs, the wrist should be immobilised in a thumb spica cast and radiographs repeated at 2 weeks. When X-rays are ambiguous, MRI is the best imaging modality.

8. E Galeazzi's fracture

Single bone fractures of the forearm are rare. Therefore, an associated injury to the proximal or distal radio-ulnar joints should be strongly suspected where a single bone fracture has occurred. Patterns of injury with a single bone fracture and proximal/distal radio-ulnar joint injury are well known by their eponyms. A Galeazzi's fracture is a fracture of the radius (usually occurring in the distal third of the shaft) with a disruption of the distal radio-ulnar joint (**Figure 59.9**). Similarly, a fracture

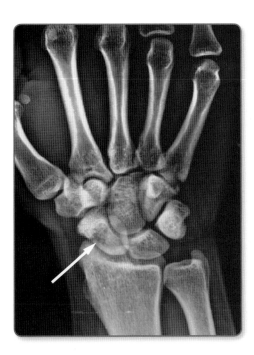

Figure 59.8 A neglected fracture of the scaphoid. Before treatment is planned, an MRI should be performed to rule out avascular necrosis of the proximal fragment

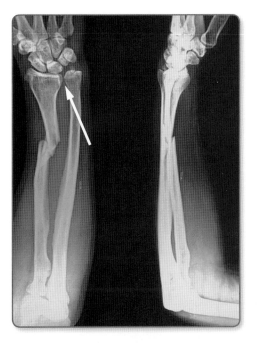

Figure 59.9 A Galeazzi's fracture. The distal third of the radius is fractured, and the disruption of the distal radio-ulnar joint (DRUJ) is evidenced by the opening up of the space as pointed out by the arrow.

of the proximal ulnar shaft along with dislocation of the radial head is known as a Monteggia's fracture–dislocation.

In a Galeazzi's fracture, after the distal radius is fixed, the DRUJ is assessed for the presence of persistent dorsal subluxation of the ulna (the piano-key sign). If found unstable, the DRUJ is reduced and held with a K-wire, and the forearm immobilised in supination.

Chapter 60

Lower limb and spine trauma

Questions

Theme: Lower limb and spinal trauma

A   Anterior cruciate ligament tear
B   Common peroneal nerve injury
C   Deep peroneal nerve injury
D   Fat embolism syndrome
E   Fracture of the C6 vertebra
F   Fracture of the L1 vertebra
G   Neck of femur fracture

H   Intertrochanteric fracture
I   Jones' fracture
J   March fracture
K   Medial meniscus tear
L   Posterior dislocation of the hip
M   Prolapsed intervertebral disc

For each of the following cases, select the single most appropriate diagnosis from the options listed above. Each option may be used once, more than once or not at all.

1. A 52-year-old man presents with acute onset pain in the lower back which started after he stooped down to lift a bucket of water. The pain radiates down the posterior aspect of his right thigh, and a straight leg raising test elicits pain at 30º.

2. A 25-year-old professional footballer sustained an injury during a match and presents to the emergency department with a painful effusion of his left knee. He complains of having landed awkwardly on his knee, and 'feeling a pop' at the time of the injury. A Lachman's test reveals laxity of the knee.

3. A 32-year-old man who was involved in a motorbike collision was admitted to the orthopaedic ward with a fracture in his right lower limb. 72 hours after the injury, he was found to be drowsy, tachypnoeic, with a pulse rate of 124 bpm and a fine rash over his chest. Arterial blood gas analysis shows his PaO_2 levels to be 58.3 mmHg.

4. An 85-year-old woman slipped in the bathroom 4 days ago and developed pain around her right hip. She managed to walk with the pain until a day prior to presentation when the pain worsened, and she was unable to bear any weight on the affected limb. The orthopaedic consultant reads her X-rays and advises a partial hip replacement.

5. A 28-year-old woman who was a front seat passenger in a high velocity car collision, presents with pain and inability to move her left hip. In the emergency department, the affected limb is adducted and internally rotated, with any attempt at movement being extremely painful.

6. A 22-year-old hockey player was involved in an altercation with an opponent who struck him with his hockey stick around the knee. Subsequently, he is unable to actively dorsiflex his foot, and knee radiographs reveal a fracture of the neck of the fibula.

7. A 72-year-old woman slipped in the bath and has been unable to stand since the fall. She complains of severe pain around the right hip. The affected limb is shortened and externally rotated, with ecchymosis around the hip region. A day later, she undergoes internal fixation using a dynamic hip screw.

8. A 27-year-old man presents to the emergency department with pain and swelling over his left foot, which he accidentally twisted while running on an uneven path. Examination reveals swelling over the lateral border of the foot, with marked tenderness at the base of the 5th metatarsal.

9. A 24-year-old man was brought to the emergency department after a motorbike collision. On presentation his Glasgow Coma Score is 9/15. His pulse rate is 58 beats per minute with a blood pressure of 90/60 mmHg, but warm extremities. He is not moving his lower limbs. A rigid cervical collar is applied and the patient placed on a rigid spinal board.

Answers

1. M Prolapsed intervertebral disc

This patient has an acute intervertebral disc prolapse. The prolapsed disc causes nerve root irritation resulting in pain, which radiates from the lower back, down the posterior aspect of the thigh and leg. There may be weakness of the muscles supplied by the affected nerve root. These are the great toe extensors in an L5 affliction, and ankle and toe plantar flexors in a S1 affliction.

On examination, the patient stands with a 'list' to one side to avoid pressure on the affected nerve root (**Figure 60.1**). A straight leg raise produces tension in the sciatic nerve and causes severe pain.

An MRI is the best investigation to diagnose a herniated disc (**Figure 60.2**). Unless there is cauda equina compression, treatment involves bed rest with analgesics. Patients with cauda equina syndrome, and those with neurological deficits or persistent radicular symptoms, require decompression by laminotomy or a microdiscectomy.

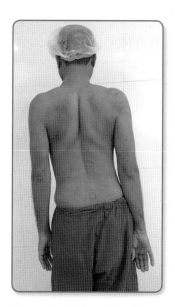

Figure 60.1 Note that this patient with a herniated disc stands with a 'list', in order to prevent impingement on the involved nerve root.

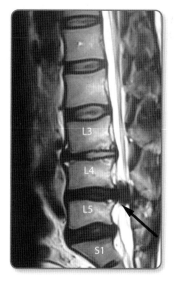

Figure 60.2 MRI showing L4/L5 herniated intervertebral disc.

2. A Anterior cruciate ligament tear

The anterior cruciate ligament (ACL) runs upwards, backward and laterally from its attachment anteriorly on the tibial plateau, to the medial surface of the lateral femoral condyle. The major function of the ACL is to prevent excessive anterior translation of the tibia relative to the femur, providing antero-posterior stability to the knee joint.

The mechanism of an ACL tear involves landing on one leg, with the femur rotating forcefully over the fixed tibia. The most sensitive test to perform in the acute setting is the Lachman's test. With the knee flexed to 20°, the proximal tibia is grasped and pulled anteriorly relative to the femur (**Figure 60.3**). The ruptured ACL provides no resistance to the examiner's force, and anterior laxity is evident.

The investigation of choice is an MRI. In high-demand athletes, the treatment is ACL reconstruction performed arthroscopically (**Figure 60.4**).

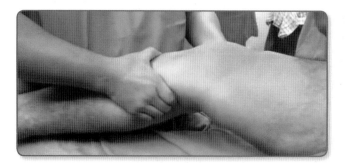

Figure 60.3 The Lachman's test. The knee is flexed to about 20°, and the proximal tibia pulled anteriorly by the examiner, while stabilising the femur with the opposite hand.

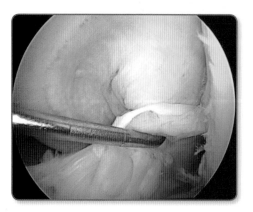

Figure 60.4 The native anterior cruciate ligament as seen during an arthroscopic procedure.

3. D Fat embolism syndrome

This clinical scenario is classical of fat embolism syndrome, a well-known complication after a fracture of the femoral shaft. Fat embolism syndrome develops 48–72 hours after the injury and is heralded by typical signs. A patient who undergoes reamed intramedullary nailing of the femur (**Figure 60.5**) in this critical period is at a very high risk of developing fat embolism and hence this procedure should be delayed until 4–5 days after injury, if it has not been performed in the acute setting.

The patient becomes drowsy, and there may be altered sensorium. In severe cases, there may be seizures. There is hypoxia on arterial blood gas analysis, and a petechial rash develops over the chest wall, mainly in the region above the nipples. Rarely, there may be fat globules in the urine, on fundus examination and in the sputum. A chest X-ray reveals a 'snow-storm' appearance (**Figure 60.6**).

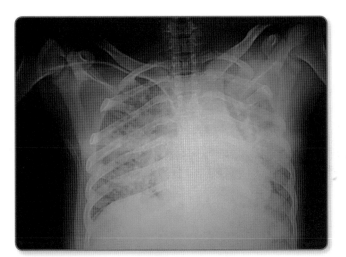

Figure 60.5 The typical 'snow-storm' appearance on a chest X-ray seen in fat embolism syndrome.

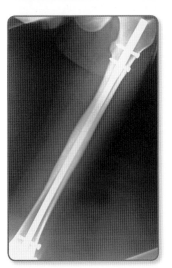

Figure 60.6 A femoral shaft fracture (here already united) treated with an intramedullary-interlocked nail, which is the current gold standard in the management of these fractures.

4. G Neck of femur fracture

This elderly woman has sustained a neck of femur fracture which was an incomplete fracture to begin with and later developed into a complete fracture.

Femoral neck fractures are low energy injuries in elderly osteoporotic individuals, which can develop even after trivial twisting forces to the hip. They are classified according to the Garden's classification:

- Type 1 – incomplete fracture, undisplaced
- Type 2 – complete fracture, undisplaced
- Type 3 – complete fracture, partially displaced
- Type 4 – complete fracture, completely displaced (**Figure 60.7**)

Non-union and avascular necrosis of the femoral head are the two most significant complications associated with a femoral neck fracture.

Treatment depends on the 'physiological age' of the patient. Broadly, patients younger than 65 years of age are treated as an emergency with internal fixation using multiple cannulated screws, whereas elderly patients are treated with either a total or partial hip replacement (**Figure 60.8**).

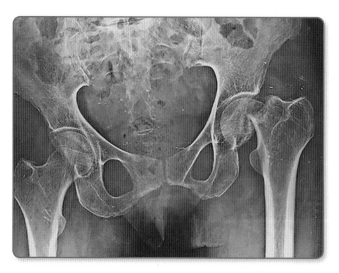

Figure 60.7 A Garden's type 4 fracture of the neck of the femur.

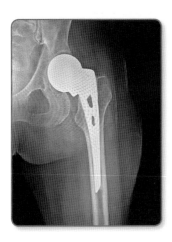

Figure 60.8 A fracture neck of femur in an elderly patient treated with hemiarthroplasty.

5. L Posterior dislocation of the hip

The diagnosis is posterior dislocation of the hip because of the typical mechanism of injury (patient being a front seat passenger of a car) and the classical type of deformity of the hip (adduction and internal rotation). The mechanism involves striking the flexed knee against the dashboard of a car during a collision, or against the road in motorcycle accidents.

An X-ray of the pelvis confirms the diagnosis (**Figure 60.9**). Fractures of the acetabular wall and femoral head should be carefully looked for in such injuries.

Traction applied to the femur with the hip flexed 90° along with gentle rotatory movements while an assistant stabilises the pelvis, reduces the hip. A post-reduction CT image should be obtained to exclude intra-articular fragments, which, if present, should be removed.

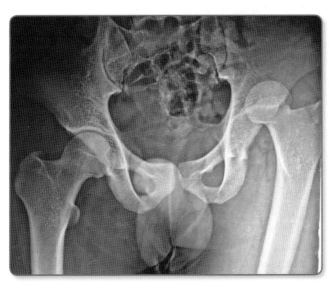

Figure 60.9 A posterior dislocation of the hip. Although the femoral head and acetabulum appears intact, it is important to obtain a post-reduction CT film to rule out intra-articular fractured fragments.

Immediate complications include injury to the sciatic nerve and superior gluteal artery; avascular necrosis of the femoral head may be a late complication.

6. B Common peroneal nerve injury

The common peroneal nerve is a branch of the sciatic nerve. It lies on the medial side of the biceps femoris tendon, and descends obliquely between the biceps femoris and lateral head of the gastrocnemius. It then winds around the neck of the fibula, lying under the peroneus longus, and then divides into the superficial and deep peroneal nerves. The superficial peroneal nerve supplies the muscles of the lateral compartment of the leg – peroneus longus and peroneus brevis, which are evertors of the ankle. The deep peroneal nerve supplies the muscles of the anterior (extensor) compartment of the leg. Hence, injury to the common peroneal nerve by a direct blow at the back of the knee causing fracture of the neck of the fibula (**Figure 60.10**) produces a foot drop due to loss of active dorsiflexion at the ankle.

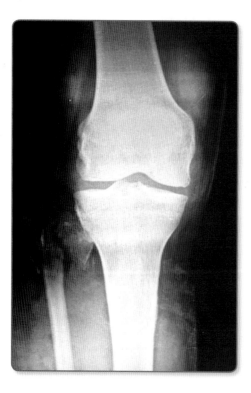

Figure 60.10 The type of fracture of the neck of the fibula that should arouse suspicion of a common peroneal nerve injury.

7. H Intertrochanteric fracture

This woman has sustained an intertrochanteric fracture (**Figures 60.11** and **60.12**) as shown by the limb being shortened, externally rotated with ecchymosis around the hip region and treated with a dynamic hip screw. An intertrochanteric fracture should be differentiated from fracture of the neck of the femur by the following features:

- A femoral neck fracture is intracapsular, an intertrochanteric fracture is extracapsular
- Because of the restraining effect of the capsule, the shortening and external rotation are less evident in femoral neck fractures than in intertrochanteric fractures
- A femoral neck fracture is at a high risk of complications of non-union, and avascular necrosis of the femoral head. Union is seldom an issue in intertrochanteric fractures. These usually mal-unite in varus and external rotation
- In elderly individuals, the treatment of choice in a femoral neck fracture is partial or total hip replacement, whereas intertrochanteric fractures are fixed using a dynamic hip screw or proximal femoral nail

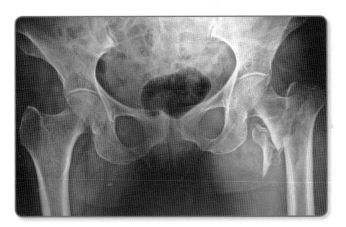

Figure 60.11 An intertrochanteric fracture of the left hip.

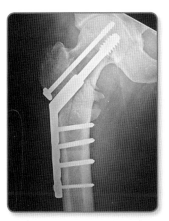

Figure 60.12 An intertrochanteric fracture fixed using a dynamic hip screw.

8. I Jones' fracture

This patient has a fracture of the base of the 5th metatarsal – Jones' fracture (**Figure 60.13**). It was originally described by Sir Robert Jones as a fracture of the 5th metatarsal occurring three-quarters of an inch above its base. The 5th metatarsal base provides insertion to the tendon of the peroneus brevis and the lateral band of the plantar fascia. These, therefore, are the important deforming forces for this fracture. The mechanism of injury is usually forced inversion of the foot, which can occur during dancing, stepping over a pothole, or running over uneven ground.

The proximal metaphysio-diaphyseal junction of the 5th metatarsal has a precarious blood supply, which predisposes fractures in this region to non-union. Most cases of Jones' fractures can be managed conservatively in a plaster cast.

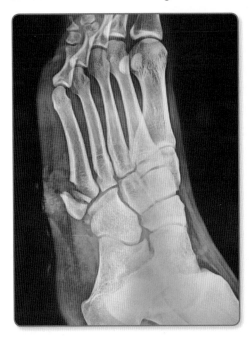

Figure 60.13 A Jones' fracture.

9. E Fracture of the C6 vertebra

In this patient, a cervical spinal injury is the diagnosis because:

- High velocity trauma with head injury and a low GCS (Glasgow Coma Score)
- Suspicion of a neurological deficit – the patient is not moving his lower limbs
- Bradycardia in the presence of hypotension. In hypovolemic shock, the heart rate increases, hypotension ensues, and the extremities are cold. In this scenario, however, the extremities are warm and there is hypotension with bradycardia. This is indicative of spinal shock rather than hypovolemic shock. The cause is the loss of thoraco-lumbar sympathetic outflow due to a cord injury from the cervical vertebral fracture.

It is extremely important to immobilise the cervical spine in a multiply-injured patient, until a cervical spinal injury has been excluded after radiological examination. An AP and lateral view showing all seven cervical vertebrae clearly must be seen before excluding injury to the cervical spine.

Chapter 61

Elective orthopaedics

Questions

Theme: Elective orthopaedics

A   Avascular necrosis of the femoral head
B   Calcific tendinitis of the supraspinatus
C   Congenital talipes equinovarus
D   Congenital vertical talus
E   Frozen shoulder
F   Flat foot
G   Golfer's elbow
H   Osteoarthrosis of the hip
I   Osteoarthrosis of the knee
J   Perthes' disease
K   Slipped capital femoral epiphysis
L   Spinal canal stenosis
M   Spondylolisthesis
N   Tarsal tunnel syndrome
O   Tennis elbow

For each of the following cases, select the single most appropriate diagnosis from the options listed above. Each option may be used once, more than once or not at all.

1. The orthopaedic team is consulted to assess a newborn baby boy with a deformity in both his feet. The forefoot is found to be adducted, with the hindfoot in varus. The team plans to start manipulation of the foot with weekly serial casts for correction of the deformity.

2. A 63-year-old man complains of pain in his right gluteal region, which comes on when he starts walking. It is associated with heaviness and paraesthesias in his right thigh and calf. He can however, ride a bicycle and climb stairs fairly comfortably.

3. A 14-year-old obese boy is brought to the orthopaedic clinic with complaints of persisting pain in his right thigh and knee, which is worse while walking and running at school. His parents have noted that he has been walking with his foot rotated outwards for the past few months. After obtaining X-rays, he is admitted for emergent surgery the following day.

4. A 30-year-old woman presents with pain in her right foot of gradual onset, which is now disturbing her sleep. She complains of waking up with the sole of her foot feeling heavy and numb, which resolves only after she walks around the room for a few minutes.

5. A 32-year-old man complains of pain in his left elbow. On examination there is tenderness at the lateral humeral epicondyle. Resisted dorsiflexion of the wrist is painful.

6. A 47-year-old man who has been on low dose prednisolone for several years for treatment of myasthenia, complains of pain in his left hip which has gradually worsened to the point of causing a marked limp while walking. After staging the disease with an MRI, he is planned for a core decompression of his left hip.

7. A 58-year-old woman who has diabetes and is known to have poor glycaemic control presents with complaints of pain in her right shoulder. This pain was mild initially (a few months ago), but has worsened over time. She now finds it very difficult to lift her arm to dress herself and do her hair. Examination reveals a global loss of movements at the glenohumeral joint.

8. A 65-year-old obese woman presents with long standing pain in both her knees, which is worse with weight bearing. Examination reveals fixed flexion and varus deformities at both knees. X-rays show a decreased medial joint space bilaterally.

Answers

1. C Congenital talipes equinovarus

The attitude of the feet described in the scenario is typical of CTEV (congenital talipes equinovarus).

The major deformities are: equinus at the ankle joint, inversion (or varus) at the sub-talar joint, and adduction and supination of the forefoot. The soft tissue structures on the posterior and medial aspect of the foot and ankle are contracted.

The foot can seldom be dorsiflexed beyond the neutral position. The lateral border of the foot is curved, with a prominent talar head (**Figure 61.1**). Deep skin creases are seen on the medial aspect of the sole and the posterior part of the ankle.

CTEV is managed by the Ponseti method of manipulation of the foot with application of weekly plaster casts. The foot is passively stretched and rotated into abduction and eversion using the talar head as a fulcrum.

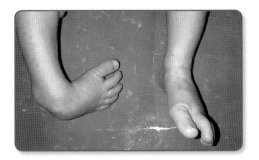

Figure 61.1 The typical attitude of a clubfoot in a newborn (right foot). Note the prominence of the talar head and the convex lateral border of the right foot.

2. L Spinal canal stenosis

This patient has neurogenic or spinal claudication. The cause is narrowing of the lumbar vertebral canal, which results in a compression on the neural structures present within the canal. It occurs quite commonly in the setting of degenerative spinal disease in older individuals.

The capacity of the spinal canal is maximum in flexion of the lumbar spine. It follows that on assuming postures involving flexion of the spine (e.g. sitting, cycling, walking upstairs etc.), the neural compression is relatively less, and is exacerbated with spinal extension (e.g. walking downhill). Neurogenic claudication must be distinguished from vascular claudication where the cause of pain is ischemia of the limb.

Lumbar canal stenosis is best evaluated with an MRI of the lumbar spine, which enables accurate measurements of the canal diameter at various levels. Management involves posture care and physiotherapy. Patients with severe symptoms not controlled by conservative means require spinal decompression.

3. K Slipped capital femoral epiphysis

The boy's symptoms, his age (adolescent at puberty), obesity and external rotation of the affected limb all point towards the diagnosis of a slipped capital femoral epiphysis (SCFE).

Clinically, the pain is frequently referred to the thigh and knee. When the slip is mild, the only clinical sign may be that the hip, when passively flexed, falls into external rotation, and internal rotation is restricted (**Figure 61.2**).

The most sensitive view to diagnose a slip is the frog-leg lateral view taken with both hips in external rotation. A line drawn through the superior aspect of the femoral neck usually intersects a portion of the epiphysis; however, in SCFE this line crosses superior to the epiphysis. This is called the Trethowan's sign and is diagnostic of a slip (**Figure 61.3**).

The usual course of treatment is to perform an emergent in-situ pinning to prevent further slip.

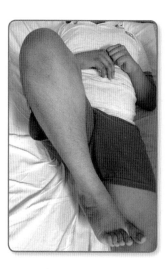

Figure 61.2 Flexion of the hip in SCFE causes it to assume an attitude of external rotation.

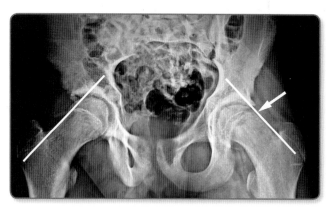

Figure 61.3 Trethowan's sign. A line drawn through the superior aspect of the femoral neck intersects a small portion of the physis on the normal hip (to the left in this figure), but passes superior to it on the affected hip (arrow).

4. N Tarsal tunnel syndrome

The symptoms of heaviness and paraesthesias/numbness in the foot are suggestive of tarsal tunnel syndrome. The posterior tibial nerve may occasionally get compressed at the ankle below the medial malleolus, under the flexor retinaculum. There may sometimes be an identifiable mass responsible for this compression (e.g. a ganglion cyst), but frequently there is no identifiable cause.

In more severe cases, the pain disturbs sleep when venous return from the lower limb is decreased, resulting in congestion in the tunnel. The patient wakes up with the foot feeling heavy and painful and may need to walk for some time before the pain subsides.

Initial management should be conservative with alteration of footwear and the use of orthotic devices, along with analgesics and neurolytics. In cases where an identifiable cause of compression is present, and in those who fail to improve with conservative therapy, the nerve is decompressed in the tarsal tunnel.

5. O Tennis elbow

The examination findings described are typical of lateral epicondylitis or tennis elbow. The condition usually arises from unaccustomed activity that strains the extensors of the wrist, whose common origin is at the lateral humeral epicondyle. Pathologically, the origin of common wrist extensors (mainly the extensor carpi radialis brevis), show degenerative changes like calcification, congestion, and tear of the fibres.

The diagnosis is fairly straightforward. The pain is usually well localised to the lateral side of the elbow and palpating the tendinous origin of the wrist extensors elicits tenderness. Straining these muscles by asking the patient to dorsiflex the wrist against the examiner's resistance causes pain and discomfort.

Management is mainly conservative with non-steroidal anti-inflammatory drugs and restriction of painful wrist activity. If this does not suffice, a local steroid injection around the common extensor origin may be used. Ultrasonic therapy to the elbow is very helpful to relieve the pain.

6. A Avascular necrosis of the femoral head

The history of hip pain following long-term steroid use should arouse suspicion of avascular necrosis (AVN) of the femoral head. Other recognised causes include chronic alcoholism, glycogen storage disorders, sickle cell disease and Caisson's disease (the bends).

As the femoral head loses its blood supply, it becomes sclerotic, weak and prone to deformity and collapse (**Figure 61.4**). The patient complains of pain in the hip on standing and walking, and may note restriction of hip movements. As the disease progresses and the femoral head collapses, there may be fixed deformities at the hip and marked limitation of ambulation.

An MRI is the gold standard investigation to evaluate osteonecrosis of the femoral head in the early stages. Early osteonecrosis is managed by drilling multiple holes

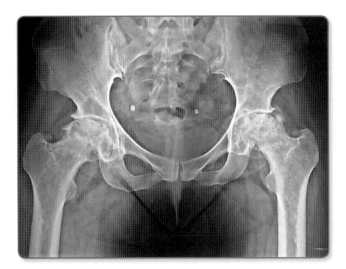

Figure 61.4 X-ray of a 42-year-old woman with bilateral osteonecrosis of the femoral head. Note the irregular shape of the head with areas of varying density.

in the head of the femur, or drilling the head with a large sized reamer – core decompression. Advanced disease is best managed by total hip replacement.

7. E Frozen shoulder

The scenario is suggestive of a progressive painful disorder of the shoulder, with associated stiffness that has developed over time. This is typical of frozen shoulder, which is also known as adhesive capsulitis, or periarthritis of the shoulder. It is seen commonly with thyroid disorders, diabetes and Dupuytren's disease. The basic underlying pathology of the disease is inflammation and eventual fibrous contracture involving mainly the capsule, but also the synovium and other structures around the shoulder.

Management is conservative with anti-inflammatory drugs and analgesics to relieve the pain, and range of motion exercises of the shoulder to reduce the period of stiffness. A steroid injection into the capsule has been shown to be of benefit. Cautious manipulation of the joint under general anaesthesia tears the fibrous adhesions in the capsule, and improves range of motion.

8. I Osteoarthritis of the knee

Osteoarthrosis of the knee is an extremely common degenerative disease. The primary pathology is the loss of articular cartilage lining the joint surfaces, which exposes subchondral bone. On weight bearing, the articular surfaces with frayed, denuded cartilage come into contact, causing marked pain. The arthritic process affects most the medial compartment of the knee through which the weight-bearing axis, of the lower limb passes.

On examination, the knees appear to be in varus (**Figure 61.5**). The medial joint line of the knee is tender to palpation. There is frequently a fixed flexion deformity, and

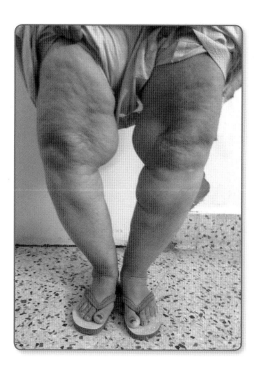

Figure 61.5 The typical varus deformity of the knees is seen in this obese woman with advanced osteoarthrosis of both knees.

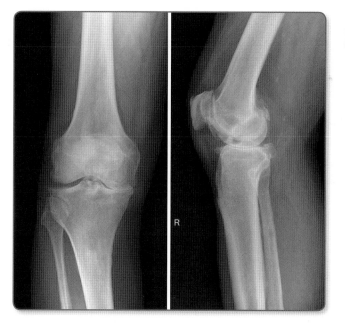

Figure 61.6 X-rays of osteoarthrosis of the knees. The knees are in varus, the medial joint space is obliterated and osteophytes are seen at the medial margin of the tibia. There is sclerosis of the subchondral bone.

crepitus is felt while moving the knee. The range of flexion is reduced and deep flexion causes marked pain.

X-rays (**Figure 61.6**) reveal reduction or obliteration of medial joint space with obvious varus deformity. Management in the early stages consists of weight reduction and physiotherapy. Patients with severe symptoms will require a knee replacement.